Behavioral Pharmacology

Behavioral Pharmacology

Second Edition

Susan D. Iversen
Department of Experimental Psychology
University of Cambridge

Leslie L. Iversen
MRC Neurochemical Pharmacology Unit
Department of Pharmacology
University of Cambridge

New York   Oxford
OXFORD UNIVERSITY PRESS
1981

Library of Congress Cataloging in Publication Data

Iversen, Susan D   1940–
    Behavioral pharmacology.

    Bibliography: p.
    Includes index.
    1. Psychopharmacology. I. Iversen,
Leslie Lars, joint author. II. Title.
[DNLM: 1. Behavior—Drug effects. 2. Psycho-
pharmacology. QV77 I94b]
RC483.I93 1981   615'.78   80–18630
ISBN 0–19–502778–7
ISBN 0–19–502779–5 (pbk.)

9 8 7 6 5 4 3 2

Preface to the Second Edition

Since the publication of the first edition there have been rapid advances in the field, especially in understanding of basic neuropharmacology. Thus, a new family of possible chemical transmitters in brain—the neuropeptides—has been discovered, and rapid advances in neurochemical studies of brain receptors for drugs and transmitters have been made. These topics have been incorporated into the second edition, with special attention being given to the opioid peptides with regard to both their analgesic and their reinforcing properties. The second section of the book, dealing with the actions of particular groups of drugs on behavior, has been completely restructured, so that drug effects on different facets of behavior are now treated in a series of separate chapters. Wherever possible, some discussion of the practical application of this research to the use of psychoactive drugs in man has been included. The second edition proved to be a far larger undertaking than at first envisaged, but we hope it represents a substantial improvement on the coverage and structure of the original text.

Cambridge   S.D.I.
August 1980   L.L.I.

Preface to the First Edition

Neuropharmacology is concerned with the study of the effects of drugs on nervous tissue; psychopharmacology is concerned with the study of the effects of drugs on behavior. The discovery, in recent years, of highly effective drugs for treating various categories of mental illness in man has stimulated research in both areas and encouraged closer ties between them. In several instances, these drugs are now known to have specific neuropharmacological actions, and this has provided an added impetus to efforts to define the effects of such drugs on normal animal behavior precisely and to devise animal model behavior systems for discovering and assessing modifications of these clinically valuable drugs.

In this book we describe the achievements of psychopharmacology in providing behavioral methods for assaying drug action, and we give a brief resumé of the subject matter of neuropharmacology. The major classes of psychoactive drugs are described from both of these points of view. In the final section, examples are described where the marriage of neuro- and psychopharmacology is throwing new light on some old clinical problems.

Cambridge   S.D.I.
January 1975   L.L.I.

Contents

II.   Drugs and Behavior

I. Principles of Behavioral Pharmacology

1. The Analysis of Behavior

There are many ways of studying behavior, and opinions differ as to which are the most useful assays for assessing pharmacological effects. In this chapter we will confess ourselves immediately to be advocates of the descriptive behaviorism originally expounded by B. F. Skinner. This approach is grounded in the belief that by selecting a clearly defined element of behavior and objectively describing its occurrence under a variety of conditions, a predictive explanation of behavior emerges. This approach avoids any subjective and anthropomorphic interpretations of animal behavior. Many have found such an approach to behavior unacceptable. As we shall see later, for example, if one is interested in the effects of drugs on memory processes, performance levels of free-operant responses are not relevant measures of the behavior. Other critics view lever pressing in the rat or key pecking in the pigeon both as unnatural behaviors and as artificially selected elements of a much more complex behavior pattern. The relevance of studies of animal behavior to an understanding of human behavior, whether normal or abnormal, appears to reinforce the conviction that we should be concerned with "whole" behavior patterns rather than their individual elements. As Dews (1958) remarked, "why is it, that when somebody learns how to study a single nerve cell or a single renal tubule or to isolate a single enzyme everyone (rightly) says 'Bravo'; but when attempts are made to isolate functional units of behaviour for study many people say 'Ah, but you are neglecting all other concurrent behaviour and therefore your results are meaningless.'"

We hope to show, however, that the methods devised by Skinner have played a historic role in the development of psychopharmacology and have served it well (Dews, 1978). This is not to say that there is no room for other behavioral methods in the analysis of drug action. In Chapters 1 and 3 the variables that determine patterns of responding are described, and in Section II (Chapters 4–10) we go on to show how the major classes of psychoactive drugs can be identified by the manner in which they modify the control these variables have over behavior. A more detailed discussion of some of the behavioral issues and further definition of terms may be found in Blackman (1974), Rachlin (1970), and Reynolds (1968).

NORMAL BEHAVIOR
Classical and operant conditioning

In this chapter we will review some of the principles and techniques used in the experimental analysis of animal behavior. Under natural conditions, an animal is observed to make two kinds of behavioral responses, ELICITED and EMITTED. Elicited responses are those that can be induced reliably by a specific stimulus and under normal conditions only by that stimulus or one very similar to it. Such responses are reflexive; for example, withdrawal of a limb to a painful stimulus, pricking of the ear to sound, contraction of the pupil to light, and salivation to food. Elicited responses are precisely determined by the properties of the eliciting stimulus (its frequency of presentation, duration, and intensity) and are objectively quantified by their latency of onset, their amplitude, and the intensity of eliciting stimulus required to induce them. Emitted responses, by contrast, are not induced by any identifiable stimulus. Rats, for example, placed in an activity box run about. The amount of running characteristically decreases gradually with time, and many variables, such as time of day, degree of deprivation, estrous state in the female, temperature, and experience with the box, influence the characteristics of this habituation. Yet in such conditions, eliciting stimuli are not readily identified, and the behavior cannot therefore be controlled. If one is interested in using baselines of spontaneously emitted behavior for evaluating drug actions, one must resort to the observational methods of the ethologist, recording all the elements of behavior, as far as they can be defined, and their sequence. The studies of Chance and Silverman (1964) on rat social behavior provide an example of this method.

In certain natural patterns of behavior the relationship between emitted and elicited responses is complex. In many animals, for example, courtship and mating involve predominantly emitted behavior initially. Gradually, however, elicited behaviors under precise stimulus control emerge in sequence, and, finally, copulation, a reflexive action controlled primarily by the autonomic nervous system, occurs.

Elicited and emitted responses may be modified by conditioning. There are two kinds of conditioning—CLASSICAL (respondent or type 1) and OPERANT (instrumental or type 2)—and it is generally accepted that elicited responses are most easily conditioned classically and emitted responses operantly. Classical conditioning was originally described by Pavlov and is a process of stimulus substitution achieved by stimulus contiguity. A given response (the unconditioned response, UR) is elicited by a certain stimulus (unconditioned stimulus, US). A neutral stimulus (conditioned stimulus, CS) that would not normally elicit the response (UR) is presented at the same time as the natural elicitor (US), and, after the response to the paired stimuli has occurred, the previously neutral stimulus (CS) will now elicit that response (CR). If, for example, the sound of a bell (CS) is paired with the presentation of food (US), salivation (UR) can be elicited eventually by the bell alone (CR). It has been suggested that the UR and CR, although superficially similar, actually differ basically; for example, the chemical composition of saliva is different when it is naturally elicited than when it is conditioned to occur.

Classically conditioned responses have clearly defined properties, which distinguish them from operantly conditioned responses (Kimble, 1961). Stimulus parameters of the CS such as its intensity and duration are crucial, and the way in which the US and CS stimuli are paired, the interval between conditioning trials, and the regularity of the pairing also influence the CR. For example, short weak stimuli, which do not reliably occur together, constitute less than ideal conditions for classical conditioning. Even if strongly established, conditioned responses may quickly disappear (EXTINGUISH), once the stimulus contiguity is broken. When stimulus pairing is irregular, and conditioning accordingly weaker, extinction is even more rapid.

Operant conditioning, by contrast, is not concerned with modifying the eliciting conditions for behavior but with the processes by which the consequences of present behavior determine future behavior. If a response is followed by a pleasant or an unpleasant consequence, the probability of that response occurring again is changed. A pleasant consequence is called REINFORCEMENT and an unpleasant one PUNISHMENT. The former increases the probability of responding and the latter decreases it.

The basic concepts of operant conditioning were developed by the American school of behavior theory initiated by Thorndike. The original experiments were largely concerned with the learning of such complex tasks as mazes for rats or puzzle boxes for cats. The properties of operant conditioning, however, were most clearly defined by B. F. Skinner. In contrast to other theorists, who studied complex learned responses, Skinner believed that the principles of operant conditioning could be demonstrated most clearly when a simple response was studied. The lever press of a rat or the key peck of a pigeon served well for this purpose, and an automated apparatus for recording such behavior was developed, the so-called Skinner box. When placed in a small chamber with a lever on one wall, the rat emits a whole variety of responses, none of which is obviously elicited by stimuli in the environment. The lever is electrically connected so that when it is pressed a food reward drops into the cup below. Often the rat manipulates the lever by chance, and the process of reinforcement begins to operate. To speed this up, "free" reinforcements are given in the food well to encourage the rat to emit most of its behavior in the vicinity of the lever. Following "shaping" with reinforcement, further bar presses are likely to occur.

The development of apparatus for automating reinforcement delivery and recording responses has played a large role in advancing experimental analyses of operant conditioning. Electromagnetic or solid-state switching circuits are used to control the stimuli in the testing chamber, the schedule of reinforcement, and the delivery of reinforcement when appropriate responses have been made. The responses to the lever, the key or other device are counted, and, if required, their rate distribution over time can be plotted on cumulative recorders. This is a pen and paper recording method; the paper moves over a drum at a given speed, and each response moves the recording pen one step across the paper. The pen resets after crossing the paper. The rate and pattern of responding can be seen immediately: with high, regular rates of responding, the pen crosses the paper within a short time, whereas, with slow rates, the slope of the response line is proportionately less steep (Fig. 1–1). There are two major approaches to quantifying operantly conditioned responses and both are valuable in behavioral pharmacology. First, there is the FREE OPERANT method derived directly from Skinner's work, in which the main dependent variable is the *rate* of performing a specific act, such as key pecking in the pigeon. Rates of responding are sensitive indices of motivation, emotion, and drug-induced changes. Coupled with the use of schedules of reinforcement which influence rate of responding over time, free-operant methodology has much to

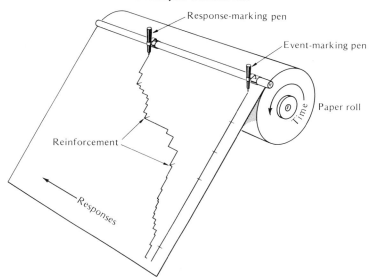

Fig. 1–1 A schematic drawing of the cumulative recorder. The paper unrolls under the two pens with time. Each occurrence of the response moves the response-marking pen up one unit toward the top of the paper. Reinforcement is indicated by a hatch-mark on the cumulative record. Additional events during an experimental session can be indicated along the horizontal line at the bottom (or top) of the record by the event-marking pen. (Reproduced from Reynolds, 1968.)

offer quantitative behavioral pharmacology. However, some drug effects are not readily reflected in changes in the rate or pattern of responding. Within this category fall changes in sensory thresholds, discrimination, and memory processes. Here it is sufficient to present a stimulus and to determine the *probability* and *accuracy* of the response to that stimulus. Failure to detect the stimulus, discriminate it from others, or to retain the information results in loss of performance. The physical characteristics of the stimulus or the period of time for which it has to be retained can be varied to assess the limits of threshold, discriminability, and memory. DISCRETE TRIAL PROCEDURES serve these purposes (Heise, 1975). In these procedures a single response to a stimulus is all that is required for reinforcement. Performance is measured in terms of probability; in other words the proportion of times the subject identifies the stimulus and makes the required response. Such methods are widely used in human experimental psychology, and sophisticated methods of analyzing response probabilities are available. Signal detection theory allows one to differentiate changes in sensitivity from response bias (Appel and Dykstra, 1977) and offers a powerful new analytic tool to behavioral pharmacology. Some of these procedures are mentioned in Section II (Chapters 4–10) in relation to particular drug groups.

Evaluation of classical and operant conditioning procedures

Although much has been made of the distinction between classical and operant conditioning, recent experimental evidence brings this emphasis into question (Mackintosh, 1974; 1978). Classical conditioning involves the relationship between a stimulus and a reinforcer, whereas operant conditioning is defined in terms of the relationship between a response and a reinforcer. There is no doubt that *procedurally* the two are different. The distinction becomes blurred, however, when conditioning situations are examined more closely. It is clear that stimulus–reinforcer (S–Re) relations can be modified during operant conditioning and similarly that response–reinforcer (R–Re) relations can be modified during classical conditioning. If a pigeon learns to press an illuminated key for food, the assumption is that the probability of the key press response increases because it is followed by reinforcement. Equally possible in such a situation, however, is that illumination of one key is reliably associated with the delivery of food. It is possible, therefore, that the emergence of key pecking is controlled by stimulus–reinforcer concurrence rather than by, or in addition to, the response–reinforcer contingency. To cite the opposite case, one may consider classical conditioning of leg withdrawal to shock. The dog reliably withdraws its leg to a conditioned stimulus, having been exposed to the CS paired with shock to the foot. However, it is possible that in addition to control by a stimulus–response contingency, behavior is also modified by the operant conditioning (response–reinforcer) contingency. When the dog withdraws its leg, the shock to the paw becomes less painful, that is, the leg withdrawal response is negatively reinforced and this response–reinforcement contingency may well contribute to the maintenance of behavior.

Another difference between the two procedures concerns the widely held belief that visceral responses controlled by the autonomic nervous system are *always* elicited rather than emitted and that only emitted behavior is controlled by the so-called voluntary motor nervous system. Considering the nature of the two conditioning procedures, it was reasoned that involuntary responses were modified by classical conditioning and voluntary responses by operant conditioning procedures. Thus, it was assumed that involuntary responses could not be modified with operant conditioning contingencies. Presumably the opposite was also true; therefore, voluntary responses were not thought to be sensitive to classical conditioning contingencies. The former position attracted the greater interest as it raised the question of whether or not bodily functions could be brought under voluntary control. Within this framework Miller and his colleagues worked tenaciously to demonstrate operant conditioning of involuntary responses in animals.

First, Miller and Carmona (1967) were able to show in dogs that spontaneous increases or decreases in saliva output could be maintained by appropriate reinforcement. The parotid duct was canulated to allow measurement of saliva, the dogs were made thirsty by water deprivation, and water was used as the reinforcer. Such results, however, are inconclusive evidence of instrumental conditioning of autonomic responses. The skeletal muscles are operative in the animal, and the observed visceral changes could have been mediated via skeletal responses known to be instrumentally conditioned. To counter this criticism, Miller and DiCara (1967) subsequently prepared a curarized rat preparation in which all skeletal responses were eliminated. Spontaneous increases or decreases of heart rate were conditioned with electric stimulation at medial forebrain bundle sites known to show intracranial self stimulation in the rat (Fig. 1–2). In view of these findings, a potential value of operant autonomic conditioning for the treatment of psychosomatic illness has been proposed; patients might be trained to control their own aberrant heart rate or blood pressure, for example.

Unfortunately, these results have proved difficult to replicate. There are, undoubtedly, many factors that must be controlled and it may take a long time to define precisely the conditions under which voluntary autonomic control may occur. Thus, in any conditioning situation it is very likely that S–Re and R–Re contingencies are operating and, at least theoretically, both voluntary and involuntary responses may be modified by either procedure. Looking at a given situation, it is difficult to specify all the responses which have been conditioned and the ways in which this happened. Shapiro (1961) illustrated how the fabric of conditioned behavior consists of interrelated patterns of involuntary or voluntary responses geared to the requirements of the organism. Dogs were surgically prepared with chronic indwelling catheters in the duct of the parotid gland. In these dogs, a continuous record of salivary secretion was obtained while they were being reinforced with food for lever pressing. Reinforcement was given every 2 min, and the dogs

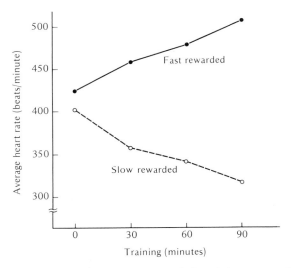

Fig. 1–2 Instrumental learning in groups rewarded with brain stimulations for fast or slow heart rates. (Each point represents average beats per minute during 5 min.) (Reproduced from Miller and DiCara, 1967.)

salivated not only, as expected, after the food reinforcement, but also toward the end of the 2-min fixed-interval period (Fig. 1–3). Furthermore, a high correlation between the magnitude of conditioned salivation and the number of lever presses during the fixed interval was observed. Clearly, this anticipatory salivation is closely tied to the operantly conditioned lever press, and it becomes meaningless to try to distinguish between elicited and emitted responses in a composite behavior of this kind.

Nevertheless, having demonstrated that there appear to be no absolute relationships between stimuli, responses, and reinforcers—only in the manner in which they are presented—one is forced immediately to cite the exceptions. Some responses apparently can be modified reliably only in one manner. Eyeblink in the rabbit cannot be modified with operant contingencies nor can autoshaped key pecking in the pigeon; yet autoshaped lever pressing in the rat is very sensitive to the omission of food. In summary:

Some responses appear to be readily modifiable by their consequences while others do not; stimulus–reinforcer relationships appear sufficient to generate some changes in behaviour but not others. The distinction is surely not an absolute one: although many responses may be affected more by one process than the other, many are affected by both . . . at present the most plausible suggestions seem to be that more reflexive responses are likely to be more subject to classical contingencies, and responses providing substantial intrinsic feedback are likely to be more subject to instrumental contingencies.

(MacIntosh, 1978).

Characteristics of reinforced behavior

Despite the fact that elicited and emitted responses are so closely bound together in the fabric of normal behavior, classical conditioning procedures have hardly been used in the study of the effects of drugs on behavior. Most of the rest of this chapter is, therefore, restricted to a consideration of the characteristics of operant conditioning.

Concepts of reinforcement
An event is identified as a reinforcer when it follows a response and there is

Fig. 1–3 Cumulative salivary responding and lever pressing by a dog, reinforced with food for lever presses on an FI 2 schedule. *Upper:* cumulative salivary responses; *lower:* discrete lever presses. Reinforcements are designated by the diagonal downstrokes of the cumulative pen. The salivary response clearly covaries with the schedule of food reinforcement. (Reproduced from Shapiro, 1961.)

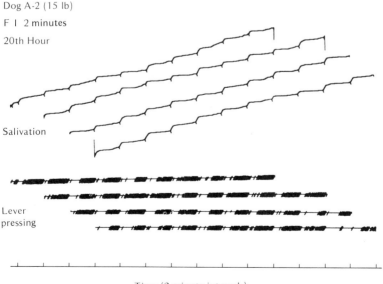

Dog A-2 (15 lb)

F I 2 minutes

20th Hour

Salivation

Lever
pressing

Time (2-minute intervals)

a subsequent increase in the occurrence of that response or closely related ones. Reinforcement increases the probability of the recurrence of the immediately preceding behavior and may act as such either when a pleasant event is presented (e.g. food) or an unpleasant one is terminated (e.g. electric shock).

There are a number of ways in which the termination of unpleasant events may be used to control behavior. Animals will learn to ESCAPE or remove themselves from the unpleasant events or from stimuli predicting the occurrence of unpleasant events. Alternately, they will learn responses which prevent the occurrence of the unpleasant event. This is called AVOIDANCE behavior. However, it should be emphasized that, while procedurally these can be distinguished, the theoretical relationship between escape and avoidance remains unresolved (see Blackman, 1974, Chapter 12).

The terms POSITIVE REINFORCEMENT for the presentation of pleasant events and NEGATIVE REINFORCEMENT for the removal of unpleasant events are commonly used. These terms are opposites, but since under both conditions the probability of responding increases, they can be misleading. It is perhaps better to simply talk of reinforcers and to describe the particular event. The concept of reinforcement is central to all behavior theory. Controversy centers rather on the nature of the responses that are strengthened and on the strengthening processes themselves. One school believes that animals learn relationships between external events and that reinforcement, although it generally increases the probability of learned behavior occurring, is not a prerequisite for the learned associations to be formed. By contrast, others view reinforcement as the means of forming learned associations. It is further contended that animals learn relationships between external events rather than the responses made to those events. The former theories are described as "cognitive" or "map in the head" and the latter "stimulus–response associative." Students are often asked, "do rats learn where to go or what to do." The behavior theories of Tolman and Hull polarize these controversies (Hilgard and Bower, 1966), but they are not our immediate concern. The demands of behavioral pharmacology are more consistent with Skinner's approach to behavior, which is basically a description of the variables influencing behavior in a particular situation, with no recourse to explanation. This is not to say that there are no underlying reasons for behavior, but simply that if behavior can be defined, described, and consistently manipulated, these reasons are irrelevant. Furthermore, as we shall see, explanations in terms of such internal variables as the motivation of fear or hunger can encourage parsimonious interpretations of behavior, which may be misleading. A rat presses a lever, obtains food, and subsequently presses the lever more frequently. To traditional behavior theorists, the animal is MOTIVATED to obtain food and learns the bar-pressing response because its INTERNAL DRIVE STATE is reduced by the food. To the Skinnerian, the probability of a bar-pressing response by a hungry animal increases if that response is followed by reinforcement.

Properties of reinforcers

The terms SATISFIER and ANNOYER from Thorndike's writings crystallize the nature of reinforcement. Certain events, innately or after experience, satisfy basic needs, and other events, by contrast, induce withdrawal. The tendency to withdraw from unpleasant events is innately strong and can be reliably induced in animals under experimental conditions. Species vary in what they find aversive; electric shock is effective in most species, but some species have particular aversions, which are useful experimentally, e.g., puffs of air to the cat. The need for satisfiers, because of the general physiological characteristics of the animal, is variable, and DEPRIVATION is often used to ensure the potency of a satisfier for experimental purposes. The animal is deprived of a satisfier for a period of time, thus ensuring its reinforcing properties under experimental conditions. Food and water are most commonly used, but access to a receptive female for the male rat, salt, heat, electric stimulation of the brain, and infusion of such mood-changing drugs as amphetamine, cocaine, or morphine have all been used as reinforcing stimuli. For practical reasons, food deprivation and the use of food as a satisfier and electric shock as an annoyer dominate the experimental literature, and work is needed to demonstrate that the effects on behavior obtained by the presentation of food or withdrawal of shock are common to all reinforcers.

There are no set parameters for reinforcers and among other variables attention must be given to the magnitude of the reinforcers used. If large food rewards are given the animal performs for fewer trials and performance may be disrupted in the process of eating those rewards. When the termination of shock or other noxious stimuli is used to maintain behavior, the intensity of that stimulus is crucial. If too intense, all behavior may be eliminated and the animal withdraws totally from the situation.

As mentioned earlier, two procedurally different ways of using reinforcement may be identified. It may be programmed on various *schedules* to control different rates and patterns of responding or it may be used to control choice behavior in *discrete trial situations*. For example, in mazes, on each trial the correct response is rewarded and the incorrect unrewarded. In sensory discrimination tasks, two or more stimuli are presented on each trial and only the correct response is reinforced. In studying negative reinforcement, discrete trial escape and avoidance tasks have been very widely used in behavioral pharmacology.

If every response is reinforced, CONTINUOUS REINFORCEMENT (crf) is said to be operating and the probability of responding increases quickly. But reinforcement may be presented intermittently *on schedules* and this reveals clearly its ability to control behavior. Skinner and his collaborators in the 1930's and 1940's laid the groundwork for such studies by describing two basic manipulations or SCHEDULES of reinforcement, one determined by time and the other by frequency of responding.

The fixed-interval schedule (FI). On this schedule, reinforcement becomes available at regular temporal intervals, e.g. every 5 min provided the animal makes an appropriate response. Irrespective of the animal's behavior during the interval, the first response that occurs after the 5 min have elapsed is reinforced. The animal could, therefore, make one response every 5 min and receive maximum reinforcement. After responding for a short period of time on such a schedule, animals do not do this, nor do they respond throughout the period. Their response pattern is said to be scalloped (Fig. 1–4). Immediately after a reinforcement, responding virtually ceases and then accelerates as the time for the next reinforcement approaches.

Fixed-ratio schedule (FR). By contrast, on ratio schedules, a fixed *number* of responses must be made before the reinforcement occurs, and thus, frequency of reinforcement is determined by frequency of response. Hence, FR schedules result in high regular response rates with only a short post-reinforcement pause (Fig. 1–4).

The variable-interval schedule (VI). Under these conditions, time again determines reinforcements, which occur at variable time intervals. A VI schedule has a range of inter-reinforcement delays around a mean value, which is used to designate the schedule (e.g. VI 1 min has a mean inter-reinforcement time of 1 min). This schedule generates a very high and sustained rate of responding due, it is said, to the uncertainty of the reinforcement.

The variable-ratio schedule (VR). This schedule presents each reinforce-

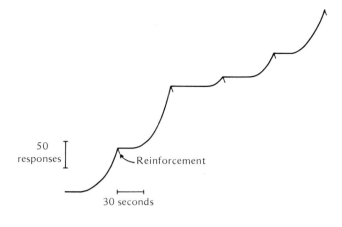

50
responses

Reinforcement

30 seconds

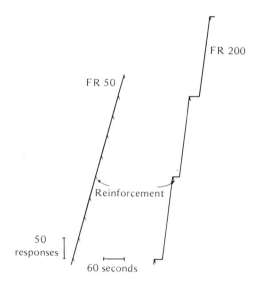

FR 200

FR 50

Reinforcement

50
responses

60 seconds

Fig. 1–4 *Upper:* Performance generated by a 1-min, fixed-interval schedule; *lower:* performance generated by two different fixed-ratio (FR) schedules. (Reproduced from Reynolds, 1968.)

ment after a variable number of responses, and, again, there is a mean ratio-value used to designate the schedule. It generates a high regular rate of responding until the ratio demands become very large; then a waning of response, called straining, begins to appear as the animal has difficulty in meeting the response requirement.

It is important to emphasize that the schedule of reinforcement is more important than the nature of the reinforcement. It is impressive how similar the response patterns are across species, across reinforcers, and across responses when reinforcement is programmed to become available in the same way. This is illustrated in Fig. 1–5 using the fixed-interval schedule. The generality of reinforcement in controlling behavior is further emphasized by the fact that presentation of food or removal of electric shock, when programmed on an FI schedule, yields indistinguishable patterns of responding (Fig. 1–6). Such observations, incidentally, undermine motivational explanations of behavior. It is difficult to explain, using the intervening variable of motivation, how food and fear can produce the same behavior. The explanation of the similarity of behavior lies not in the nature of the reinforcer but in the way it is programmed to occur.

The multiple schedule illustrated in Fig. 1–6 also includes a useful manipulation termed TIME OUT. Under this condition there are no programmed contingencies in operation or, in other words, the apparatus is dead. With removal of the schedule of reinforcement and the associated test chamber stimuli, all behavior ceases. This is to be contrasted with EXTINCTION where the reinforcer no longer follows the operant response, but the general test stimuli are otherwise the same as during training.

Other reinforcement schedules. In addition to these commonly used schedules, a variety of modifications are used, constituting the subject matter of much operant conditioning research. The DRL (differential reinforcement of low rate of responding), for example, is now being used to greater extent in such applied research as behavioral pharmacology. The DRL is a *free-operant* schedule insofar as behavior is not parceled into discrete units by regular reinforcement. Reinforcement is programmed to occur after a certain period of time has elapsed since the previous response, but is actually given only when fewer than a specified number of responses has occurred during that period. If more than this number of responses has occurred, reinforcement is delayed until this low rate of responding has been achieved. The response requirement is stringent. A precise and steady rate

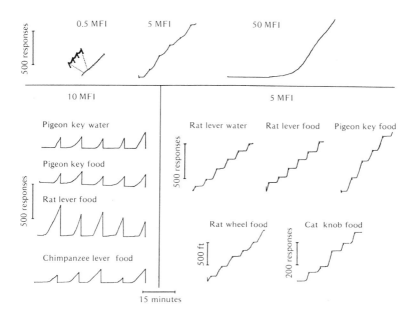

Fig. 1–5 Generality of characteristic fixed-interval performance, then acceleration to a maintained steady rate of responding. *Ordinate:* cumulative number of responses; *abscissa:* time. A fixed-interval schedule of presentation of food or water was in operation in all examples shown here. *Upper:* individual pigeon pecking a plastic key (food). Three different durations of the fixed interval (minute fixed interval, MFI) are shown; the general pattern persists despite the 100-fold change in the schedule parameter. Food presentations, ending each fixed interval, are marked by short diagonal strokes on the cumulative record. *Lower left:* performances under a 10-min, fixed-interval schedule. Food or water presentations, ending each fixed interval, are marked by the resetting of the recording pen to the baseline. *Lower right:* performances under a 5-min, fixed-interval schedule. The species, the type of switch recording the response, and the reinforcements presented are indicated above the records. The pigeon pecks a plastic key with its beak; the rat and chimpanzee press a horizontal lever with their paws; the cat depresses a rounded knob with its paw. The rat turns the wheel by running; only a turn of 180° is reinforced, but the cumulative distance the wheel turns is recorded directly. (Reproduced from Kelleher and Morse, 1968.)

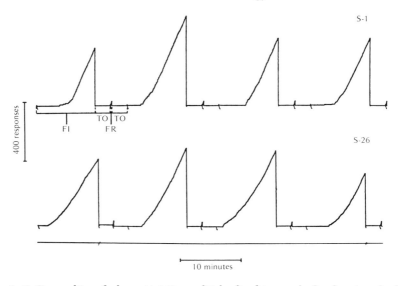

Fig. 1–6 Generality of characteristic multiple fixed-interval, fixed-ratio schedule performance in the squirrel monkey. The performances were maintained by food presentation (upper, monkey S–1) and by stimulus-shock termination (lower, monkey S–26). The sequence of visual stimuli and corresponding schedules was the same in the upper and lower records. At the beginning of the records, the FI 10-min schedule was in effect in the presence of a white light. At the termination of the FI component, the recording pen reset to the baseline. Following reinforcement, a pattern of horizontal lines was present for 2.5 min; during this time-out period (TO), responses had no programmed consequences. The next short diagonal stroke on the cumulative record indicates that the FR 30 component was in effect in the presence of a red light. Again the cumulative recording pen reset to the baseline at reinforcement and was followed by the 2.5-min TO component. This cycle was repeated throughout each session. At the bottom of the record for monkey S–26, the short diagonal strokes on the event line indicate electric shock presentations. The variation in the number of responses in fixed-interval components is normal. Note the similarities of the patterns of responding under these multiple FI/FR food and shock schedules. (Reproduced from Kelleher and Morse, 1964.)

within a narrow range of inter-response intervals is required, and a very high or a very low rate of responding reduces the reinforcement received. Such control is presumably behaviorally demanding, which probably explains why DRL performance takes a long time to stabilize and why it is so sensitive to physiological manipulation of the animal.

Equally precise high rates of responding are engendered by the differential reinforcement of high rates of responding (DRH), in which more than a certain number of responses are required during the inter-reinforcement time.

Avoidance of electric shock can also be programmed on a free operant schedule. Sidman gave his name to the procedure whereby a shock is programmed to occur regularly but is delayed by a fixed period every time a response is made. For example, shocks are given every 10 secs until a response occurs; following a response, there is a 10-sec delay until the next shock. Under such conditions, temporal discrimination develops and, as with DRL and DRH schedules, efficient behavior is achieved by responses occurring over a narrow range of inter-response intervals.

Multiple schedules. Multiple schedules are programmed by combining two or more schedules in a regular fashion. Alternation between two different schedules is most commonly used, for example, a multiple FI/FR schedule in which time and rate of responding alternate to determine reinforcement. A pattern of responding quickly develops, with the animal showing the characteristic scalloped pattern of responding during the FI component, followed by the high rate of responding during the FR component. Multiple schedules are of great value in studying drug effects, which are often partly determined by the ongoing rate of behavior. The stimulatory effect of amphetamine is one such example. It can be shown that the drug augments low rates of responding during the initial part of the FI components and depresses high rates during the FR components. To study a wider range of behavioral control, more than two components can be combined on a multiple schedule.

There are other interesting complex schedules that have not yet been much used in behavioral pharmacology. A compound schedule may reinforce a single response according to the requirement of two or more schedules of reinforcement simultaneously. CONJUNCTIVE FI/FR SCHEDULES are one such example; here a response is reinforced if a fixed interval of time has elapsed *and* if the fixed ratio of responses has been emitted. Another example are INTERLOCKING SCHEDULES; here a certain number of responses is required for reinforcement, but the absolute number varies with the time since the last reinforced response. The number may decrease or increase, and, under an increasing interlocking schedule, the demands of responding become so prohibitively large that reinforcement may never be obtained. Reynolds (1968) suggests that such a reinforcement principle operates in cumulative educational systems, where the requirements for success become increasingly large and where later success is precluded by an earlier lack of success. CONCURRENT SCHEDULES involve the reinforcement of two or more responses according to two or more simultaneous schedules. For example, pecking a red key may be reinforced on an FI, and pecking a separate blue key on an FR. Behavior is distributed between the keys in a complex manner, and a behavioral chain readily forms under these circumstances. If responding on one key happens to be reinforced when behavior is switched to that key, a chain of behavior is formed from the first key to the second key, which yields reinforcement. To prevent chaining, the schedule can be programmed so that behavior cannot be reinforced until a certain time after a switch, thus encouraging independent behavior under the two schedules.

In view of their relevance to most animal and human behavior, which is controlled by complex reinforcement contingencies rather than a single event, it is surprising that multiple schedules of this kind have not received more experimental investigation.

The most complex schedule so far discussed in this chapter involves no more than four simple schedules presented over a relatively short period of time. Experimental situations are now being explored in which the animal is controlled by programmed schedules for the whole day. Living environments are built in which dozens of different behaviors, their sequence, and their duration can be studied. The multi-operant repertoire represents an experimental effort to come to grips with this kind of complexity. Ferster (1966) has used a situation in which a pair of chimpanzees lived and worked in a semi-natural environment. They were free to work for food on certain cognitive problems, interact in a social environment, or sleep. Over a 5-year period, a remarkable orderly sequence of behavior was maintained with 4 to 6 hr of work and regular sleep. During the experiment, it proved necessary to replace the female animal, and this profoundly disrupted the behavioral stability of the male. Irrespective of responses to the new female, his work schedule was reduced, his appetite blunted. Experimental situations of this kind have an enormous potential for studying abnormal behavior and the ability of drugs to modulate such behavior. They offer the possibility of monitoring the whole output of behavior and the opportunity to manipulate experimentally the variables that control behavior.

Findley (1966) has pioneered such methods with humans, describing a situation in which the behavior of a 34-year-old male volunteer subject was studied over a 5-month period. This involved a chamber with eating, sleeping, and toilet facilities; a wide range of intellectual and physical activities could be enjoyed; and pleasant consequences of behavior, i.e. reinforcers like music and cigarettes were also offered. After 90 days, stress, which markedly influenced the distribution of behavior, was apparent—time spent on toilet facilities increased and intellectual activities decreased, while sleep occurred in more frequent, but shorter bouts. The potential of such methods for mimicking the total environment and for inducing abnormal behavior remains to be explored.

The value of multiple schedules in studying drug effects on behavior

With a multiple schedule it is possible to assess in a single subject, over a short period of time, a drug effect on behavior maintained by different reinforcers or different schedules of reinforcement, or by reinforcement as opposed to punishment, in signaled or unsignaled conditions. For example, Tye et al. (1977a) used a three-component multiple schedule to investigate minor tranquilizers. Rats were exposed to a sequence of three signal conditions, variable interval (VI) 30 sec for 10 min, followed by 4 min of time-out conditions, followed by 3 min on a conflict schedule (VI food plus shock). The sequence was repeated twice within a testing session. Response rates were high on the reinforced VI and low during time-out and punishment (Fig. 1–7). Minor tranquilizers, including chlordiazepoxide, increased punished responding, with little effect on food-reinforced behavior (Fig. 1–7, bottom). However, the response releasing effects seem to be specific in so far as equally low rates of responding controlled by time-out conditions were not increased to the same extent as punished responding. The possible permutations within the multiple schedule are enormous and many other examples of their use will appear later in the text. The use of multiple schedules avoids the need for independent groups of animals to assess drug effects on different aspects of behavioral control. The disadvantage is that the multiple schedule may introduce contrast effects between the various components which themselves may be affected by the drug.

Discriminative stimuli and sensory thresholds

If responses are emitted and reinforced in the presence of a stimulus, that stimulus is called a DISCRIMINATIVE STIMULUS, or an S^D, and subsequently has information value for the animal by indicating the reinforcing contingency in operation. An S^D sets the occasion for emitted responses to occur. Stimuli which indicate that reinforcement is not operating are termed S^Δ.

One may ask a number of questions about an animal's discriminative ability. For example, can one stimulus be distinguished from another? Free operant techniques using *rate* of responding or discrete-trial procedures are

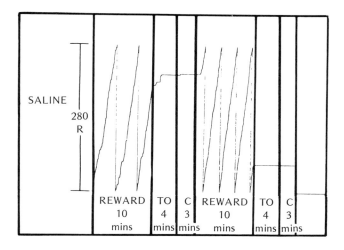

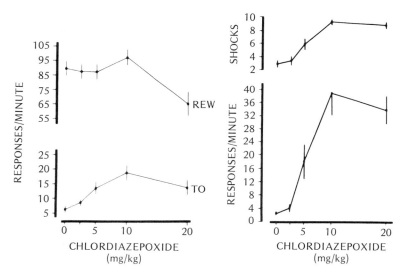

Fig. 1–7 Top: Control performance of rats on three-component multiple schedule involving 10 min VI 30 sec followed by 4 min time out and 3 min on VI food plus electric shock (conflict). Response rates were low during the TO and conflict components.

Bottom: Chlordiazepoxide increased rewarded and time out responding in a dose-related manner but increased punished responding to a much greater extent. (Modified from Tye, 1976; unpublished thesis.)

appropriate in this case. On a simple FI schedule, a house light may be the S^D; it is used to illuminate the testing chamber during the interval, but it is switched off immediately after the reinforcement, so that no light becomes the S^Δ. Light onset after the inter-trial interval signals the operation of the next FI. Similarly, in discrete-trial procedures the presence of the S^D in some trials and not in others indicates that a response is required. It may be important to know how precise the animal's idea of the S^D is, and in these circumstances a stimulus generalization gradient experiment provides the answer. An animal, for example, may be trained to respond in the presence of an S^D, e.g. a vertical line, and then be subsequently exposed to a range of lines tilted from vertical to horizontal. The rate of responding to the generalization stimuli indicates the strength of the original discriminative control (Fig. 1–8). If the animal noticed the training stimulus, a large number of responses are emitted when this stimulus subsequently appears. There is no response to unfamiliar stimuli. If, for some reason, the initial discrimi-

Fig. 1–8 Generalization gradients of tilt following training on a VI or a DRL schedule of reinforcement. Each group was composed of two subgroups, one trained with a vertical line as S^D (0°) and the other with a horizontal line as S^D (90°). The various stimuli presented during generalization testing are plotted on the abscissa in terms of the number of degrees they are from the S^D or CS (conditioned stimulus). (Reproduced from Hearst, Koresko, and Poppen, 1964.)

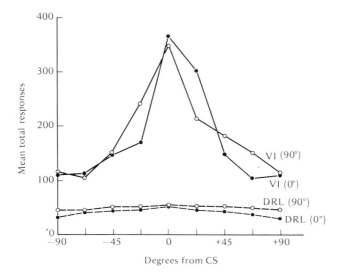

nation training is unsuccessful or if the animal has lost its discriminative capacity after training, stimuli presented during the generalization testing are responded to equally, and the gradient is said to be "flat." The generalization gradients produced in such experiments are "sharpened" if, during training, the animal is not reinforced for responding to a stimulus at one end of the range (the S^Δ), while being reinforced in the presence of the S^D, and if a reinforcement schedule that generates a high rate of responding is used during training.

Any sensory stimulus can theoretically acquire discriminative properties, although innate sensory capabilities and stimulus preferences determine the limits and priorities by which stimuli control behavior in any one species.

It may be important to know the limits of discriminability, the sensory threshold, within the sensory dimensions being studied. That is, for example, the smallest angle of tilt from the vertical that can be discriminated or the dimmest light that can be seen. These methods are derived from original studies of Blough (1966) describing titration methods for assessing thresholds. In a two-key situation pigeons were trained to peck key A when a light was visible and key B when it was not. A peck on A lowered the light intensity by a standard amount and a peck on B raised the intensity by the same amount. Thus, the pigeon titrated its visibility threshold by the distribution of pecks to keys A and B.

If a drug impairs discriminative performance, it may do so by impeding sensory processing or by altering the tendency of the animal to respond to the S^D. Performance on discrete trial procedures is amenable to analysis by signal detection theory (Appel and Dykstra, 1977) which, using rates of hit and false alarm responses on the discrimination task, makes it possible to distinguish changes in sensitivity, d^1, from changes in response bias, β.

Conditioned reinforcers

If a stimulus that has no innate reinforcing property occurs with one that has, the neutral stimulus acquires reinforcing properties and becomes a CONDITIONED or SECONDARY REINFORCING STIMULUS. A classical example would be the noise of the food magazine delivery system in a Skinner box. Once responding is established with food and the accompanying noise, it can be maintained by presentation of the noise alone, in the absence of the food reinforcement. The behavior extinguishes less quickly than when there is no food and no noise. In addition to retarding extinction, conditioned reinforcers, like unconditioned ones, increase the probability of the recurrence of the responses that produce them. Conditioned reinforcers may be associated with the occurrence of pleasant reinforcers or with the avoidance of unpleasant ones.

Although it is theoretically possible to separate discriminative stimuli and conditioned reinforcers, it is difficult to do so in practice. If an S^D is present throughout the FI and the final reinforcing event, it can theoretically also acquire conditioned reinforcing properties. Natural behavior consists of sequences or chains of responses under stimulus control, and the conditioned reinforcers of one response may be the discriminative stimulus for the next, and so on along the chain. For example, a pigeon is presented with a blue key, an S^D. Pecking changes the color to red; the key color change is a conditioned reinforcer (CR) for the response that produced it, and then the sustained color becomes the S^D for the next emitted response, a pedal press that changes the key color again. This chain of S^D and CR stimuli continues until a final response results in reinforcement. Key color change here is a conditioned reinforcer because, in the final segment of the chain, it is associated with food reinforcement. The conditioned reinforcing strength of a stimulus is in proportion to its distance from the unconditioned reinforcer, and the length of functional chains is limited for this reason.

There is considerable theoretical controversy about the mechanism of conditioned reinforcement that can be usefully investigated with chaining procedures. Traditionally, conditioned reinforcers were studied by pairing the potential conditioned reinforcers with an unconditioned reinforcing stimulus such as food and then assessing the ability of the conditioned reinforcer to maintain behavior in the absence of food. The behavior, thus, gradually extinguishes as the experiment progresses If, however, conditioned reinforcers are set up in chains, those not directly associated with the terminal food reinforcement maintain behavior in the early parts of the chain. Their properties and ability to maintain behavior can thus be assessed on a maintained behavioral baseline without extinction procedures being introduced.

Several competing theories have been proposed to explain how conditioned reinforcers come to control behavior. The most satisfactory explanation at present seems to be that the neutral stimulus becomes a reinforcing stimulus by classical conditioning between the unconditioned reinforcing stimulus and the neutral stimulus.

Extinction
If a strongly maintained behavior is suddenly no longer reinforced, extinction follows and the behavior gradually wanes. The characteristics of extinction depend on the schedule of reinforcement that originally maintained the

behavior. If every response had been reinforced (continuous reinforcement, CRF), then extinction is rapid. By contrast, if reinforcement has been irregular and generated a high rate of responding, as for example on a VR, extinction takes much longer, and bursts of responding are seen in the absence of reinforcement. It has been suggested that the rate of extinction depends on the ease with which the animal can discriminate the change in the reinforcement contingency. After CRF, extinction is immediately apparent, but, if reinforcement has been irregular, the change to extinction is much more difficult to discriminate.

Punishment
Concepts of punishment
The effects of aversive stimuli on behavior challenge behavior theory. As we have seen earlier, escape from or avoidance of such aversive stimuli as electric shock can act as a *reinforcing event* to increase the probability of the behavior that brought about the relief from shock. On the other hand, aversive stimuli presented under conditions where escape or avoidance are not possible clearly suppress ongoing behavior. First, it had to be established how escape from or avoidance of aversive stimuli could be fitted into reinforcement theory and, second, if punishment were a special case of reinforcement or an entirely independent means of manipulating behavior. Theorists have, in turn, either ignored these problems or have made them central to general theories of behavior. Many workers have focused on the aversive stimulus as being central to any theory of punishment and have considered the ways in which aversive stimuli can modify behavior. Given the procedure in operation, animals may, on the one hand, escape from or avoid shock, and, on the other hand, their behavior may be suppressed by shock. Observers of natural behavior might well characterize such defensive behaviors as flight and immobility. Theoretically speaking, flight is maintained by shock acting as a negative reinforcer. A negative reinforcer, like a positive reinforcer, increases the probability of responding (in this case, flight from the aversive stimulus). In contrast, responding may be suppressed by the presentation of shock, which is then considered to be a punisher. Despite the opposite influences on response probability of reinforcement and punishment, there have been continuing efforts to find a unitary explanation for the widely varying effects of aversive stimuli on behavior.

If we could convince ourselves that reinforcement was operating in all the procedures, we might be able to accommodate all the results of aversive stimuli into reinforcement theory. This was Skinner's attitude to punishment. He saw it as a special case of reinforcement, where avoidance of shock was mediated not by the observed reduction in responding, but by an increase in the probability of an internal and unobservable response in the animal. Thus, with punishment, as with reinforcement, a response probability (i.e. the response being not to respond) increases. This explanation is attractively parsimonious, but recourse to unobservable events for explanatory purposes does not produce an easily testable hypothesis. It would be convenient to encompass all the effects of aversive stimuli within reinforcement theory, but there is a strong current of opinion that maintains that a decrease in response probability to aversive stimuli (punishment) is a different process, which can be procedurally distinguished from the other varied effects of shock. There is also evidence that different neural systems underlie active and passive defensive reactions (McCleary, 1966) and that they are differentially affected by a variety of drugs (Kelleher and Morse, 1964). Thus punishment should be considered an independent behavioral contingency. In theoretical ferment of this kind, the existence of a confusing terminology is almost inevitable. We do not feel that it is relevant to consider the controversy in detail here, and punishment will be considered only in procedural terms.

Properties of punishment

A procedure described by Geller (1962) illustrates most directly the suppressive effects of punishment. A rat is trained to press a lever for food on a VI schedule. After high rates of lever pressing are induced, shock is introduced. The rat is shocked through the feet each time a response is made to the lever, and, although responses are still reinforced on the VI as well as punished, the overall rate of responding is severely depressed.

This procedure has been used very successfully in behavioral pharmacology to characterize drugs that counter the suppressive effects of aversive stimuli. For example, minor tranquilizers, such as the benzodiazepines, dramatically reinstate behavior suppressed by electric shock, and the use of this technique by Geller et al. (1962) provides the most specific test for this important group of drugs. Punishment programmed in this way is called IMMEDIATE punishment to denote the fact that it follows a response on a regular time relationship and to distinguish it from ADVENTITIOUS punishment, which occurs irrespective of the animal's responses. A rat, for example, could be shocked halfway through a VI period irrespective of whether the lever had just been pressed. The interval between response and shock would then be highly variable.

The difference between adventitious and immediate punishment would seem to be of considerable behavioral significance. One might suppose that punishment of known origin would be reacted to in a different way from punishment that apparently occurs randomly. But, in fact, since the distinction between the two kinds of punishment procedures has been recognized, this fascinating problem has not been adequately investigated.

Azrin and Holtz (1966) have provided a systematic description of immediate punishment. To be effective, immediate punishment must reliably follow responses. Foot shock has been found to be unreliable. The resistance of the animal, and particularly of the skin of the feet, varies and so does the effectiveness of the shock. The speed of leg withdrawal reflexes also determines the severity of shock actually received. To overcome these problems, Azrin implanted electrodes in various animals, so that shock was delivered directly to the body surface. Gold electrodes are implanted subcutaneously around the pubic bone of the pigeon, and skin electrodes are applied to the shaved tail of the squirrel monkey. In the pigeon, predictable relationships between ongoing food-reinforced behavior and immediate punishment can be demonstrated. The degree of suppression depends on (a) the severity of deprivation (Fig. 1–9A), (b) the strength of the punishing stimulus (Fig. 1–9C), (c) the schedule of reinforcement operating, and (d) the schedule of punishment (Fig. 1–9B).

It has been demonstrated that the delay between the response and the punishment is an important variable, and a graded effect with increasingly delayed punishment has been observed. There appear to be two factors involved in the suppression of behavior by punishment. One factor involves a specific suppression of the punished response by the association of punishment with the emission of behavior. Since associative learning depends upon the temporal relationship between the events to be associated, in-

---

Fig. 1–9 (A) Effect of food deprivation during fixed-ratio punishment of food-reinforcement responses. Every 100th response is being punished (160 V) at the moment indicated by the short oblique lines on the response curves. The food reinforcements (not shown) are being delivered according to a 3-min variable schedule. (B) Stable performance during fixed-ratio punishment at several fixed-ratio values from FR 1 to FR 1000. The oblique lines on the response curve indicate the delivery of a punishment (240 V). The food reinforcements (not indicated) are being delivered according to a 3-min variable interval schedule. (C) Effect of punishment intensity during fixed-ratio punishment. Every 50th response is being punished at the moment indicated by the oblique lines on the response curves. Each response curve represents the performance during the first 60 min of different sessions. The food reinforcements (not indicated) are being delivered according to a 1-min variable interval. (Reproduced from Azrin et al., 1963.)

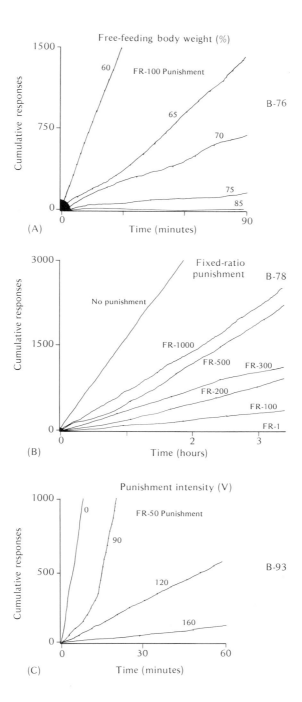

29

creasing delay of punishment would result in poorer learning, with a consequent reduction of the suppressive effects of punishment. The second factor involves a nonspecific suppression of behavior in the experimental situation, and this is relatively independent of the interval between the response and punishment. If the response–punishment interval is short, response suppression should occur because of the joint operation of these two factors. If punishment is delayed beyond the limits within which associative learning can occur, however, any suppression induced by punishment must be due solely to the non-specific effects of shock in the situation, and further increases in delay of punishment will have no further effect. A study of the suppression of worm eating in goldfish with electric shock gives such results (Myer and Ricci, 1968). Goldfish were placed in bowls for daily feeding sessions during which 20 small clusters of Tubifex worms were presented at 150-sec intervals. When the fish were reliably taking worms during the feeding sessions, shock was administered through electrodes immersed in the water on two sides of the bowls either when a fish seized a cluster of worms or 2.5, 5, 10, or 20 sec *after* the feeding response. At any particular delay, a suppression threshold was determined by increasing the intensity of the shock by 5 V each day until a criterion of 15 failures or more to feed on 3 successive days was reached. The amount of punishment required to suppress feeding was an increasing function of delay of punishment. The delay of punishment gradient increased sharply as the delay of punishment increased from 0 to 10 sec. Further increase in the response-shock interval had no effect on the suppression threshold. It is suggested that at very low intensities punishment was suppressive only if it was closely associated with the emission of the response. At longer delays (up to 10 sec) increased intensity of shock was required to suppress feeding. Increasing the delay from 10 to 20 sec presumably had no additional effect because the suppression exhibited was due entirely to the generalized suppressive effects of shock in the experimental situation, rather than to more explicit associative learning.

It is interesting that certain aversive stimuli do not appear to show such a gradient. Some rat poisons produce unpleasant effects in the animal long after ingestion, and yet the rats develop "bait shyness." This question has received experimental attention and Revusky (1968) finds that if rats are irradiated to induce radiation sickness 7 hr after drinking sucrose, the subsequent consumption of this solution is greatly reduced. Furthermore, aversion to food that has caused illness is associated with the taste and odor of that food and not its appearance. Garcia and Koelling (1966) report experiments in which rats drank lithium chloride (which causes a gastrointestinal disturbance) in the presence of a discriminative stimulus, a light-click stimulus. When subsequently offered, in the presence of the same discriminative stimulus, salt solution (which tastes like the lithium solution) and water, the salt solution was rejected and the water drunk, despite the fact that the visual and auditory discriminative stimulus associated with the lithium was presented during the test trials.

Punishing stimuli, like reinforcers, may act simultaneously as discriminative stimuli. This property of punishing stimuli interacts with their response-suppressing action and is the source of much of the confusion that surrounds punishment theory. Punishment may signal further punishing or reinforcing events. Dinsmoor (1952) randomly alternated fixed periods of time during which punishment was programmed, with periods of no shock. The rats quickly learned that a punished response meant further punishment, and the probability of responding dropped; in contrast, two unpunished responses meant no punishment, and response rates rapidly increased. In a pigeon experiment (Azrin et al., 1963), FR punishment was programmed. At first there was complete suppression, but, gradually, the pigeons learned that responses were never punished immediately after a shock, and responding reappeared at the start of each FR. Punishment may also signal reinforcement and can lead to increased rates of responding. Holtz and Azrin (1961) alternated periods of intermittent food reinforcement with periods of extinction, and all responses were punished during the periods of reinforcement. Here, again the occurrence of the punishing stimulus is used to detect reinforcement; this reveals a paradoxical effect of punishment—the rate of responding was higher in the presence of punishment than in the absence of punishment.

This effect of punishment is comparable to the use of a neutral stimulus, such as the click of a food magazine associated with food reinforcement. The click becomes a conditioned reinforcer, increasing rates of responding during extinction. In the Holtz and Azrin experiment (1961), a punishing stimulus is substituted for a neutral one, but procedurally speaking it is, nevertheless, a conditioned reinforcer. As with reinforcement, associated stimuli may be discriminative, they may act as conditioned reinforcers, or both; it is equally difficult to dissociate these properties of stimuli that become associated with punishment. To complete the correspondence of the two processes, as with conditioned reinforcement, conditioned punishment is being studied with chaining procedures. Furthermore, it is thought that neutral stimuli acquire their information value with regard to punishment by a classical conditioning process. On the Estes-Skinner (1941) procedure (see p.

36), the warning signal (CS) is paired with the shock (US) until the unconditioned response of anxiety or fear (UR) is elicited by the CS.

ABNORMAL BEHAVIOR
Introduction

Behavior is under the constant control of a wide range of internal and external stimuli. When the animal no longer responds to these controlling stimuli
in the usual way, we talk about maladaptive or abnormal behavior. In addition to its inherent scientific interest, behavioral science is of practical value
when it increases our understanding of the conditions that disrupt behavioral control and of the nature of the abnormal behavior. Unfortunately, the
complex nature of normal control makes it difficult to isolate and identify a
particular contingency that is disrupting behavior. Furthermore, there is a
very fine and ambiguous line between normal and abnormal behavior, and
often a behavior described as abnormal in one context is perfectly normal in
another. Aggression is one such example. Aggression includes threat and
attack and can be seen when an animal kills its prey, for example, rat killing
in the cat. It is also seen when animals fight over territory, but it can be
equally well induced in a pigeon if reinforcement is suddenly terminated in
an operant conditioning situation; is this aggression normal or abnormal?

It is essential to understand the control of normal behavior before turning
to the abnormal, and yet it is toward the abnormal that behavioral pharmacology should be turning, since much of its concern centers on drugs that
are used to modify or induce abnormal behavioral responses in man.

There is every reason to think that man's behavior is controlled by the
same basic contingencies as is behavior in the pigeon. The difference in man
is that his interaction with the environment is far more complex, and the
mosaic of controlling factors is accordingly much larger and more difficult to
identify. But progress can be made in understanding complex human behavior even by applying the comparatively simple principles gleaned from the
pigeon's behavior. Ferster (1966) draws analogies of this kind and says, "Animal experiments do not tell us why a man acts but they do tell us where to
look for factors of which his behavior is a function." He refers to the Estes-
Skinner procedure where behavior is suppressed when an animal comes to
anticipate a punishing stimuli after a warning signal; and Ferster draws an
analogy with the lack of behavior or abnormal behavior often seen in a den-
tist's waiting room or subjectively experienced when one is waiting to con-
sult a doctor about worrisome symptoms—a magazine scanned and not
read, conversation muted. Ferster maintains that when drugs are used to

ameliorate mental illness, they do not induce normality by creating behavior missing from the repertoire. Drugs can only influence the existing repertoire, modulating the complex relationship between controlling stimuli and behavioral responses.

Model systems for studying abnormal behavior

As we have seen, punishment provides the complementary force to reinforcement and, together, these events largely determine behavioral output at any one time. If we speak anthropomorphically, behavior is considered to be motivated on the one hand by the seeking and expectancy of pleasing events and on the other by the avoiding (or withdrawing from) and fear of unpleasant ones. It could be claimed that the emotional state of the organism reflects at any one time the balance of these motivating forces. The elation after reinforcement or the depression of behavior consequent to punishment should not be considered abnormal, but, clearly, the response to such events can become abnormally accentuated and markedly disrupt ongoing behavior.

In discussing normal behavioral control, we have tried to stress the fact that the way reinforcing and punishing events are scheduled is more important for our understanding of behavior than the nature of the events themselves. The same is true for behavior that appears to be abnormal. If such behavior is analyzed in sufficient detail, it is often possible to see that disordered behavior can be explained and that it has evolved from a particular combination and sequence of perfectly normal events (Sidman, 1960).

With regard to mental illness and abnormal behavior in man, there is a tendency to think that studies of social behavior, development, and maternal deprivation in animals are more relevant than the operant conditioning of simple responses. This may be so, but, until we have identified more fully the spectrum of controlling stimuli for these aspects of complex behavior, they do not provide useful experimental baselines. It remains a fact that, at present, some of the simple techniques for manipulating behavior with aversive stimuli are the most useful for illustrating how, under certain conditions, stimuli may induce abnormal behavior and how drugs can modify this relationship.

Historical view of experimental neurosis

Model systems for studying abnormal behavior have been developed, to a great extent, by manipulating unpleasant events to induce marked changes in the motivational and emotional state of animals. It was recognized that behavioral situations involving some conflict between the aspirations of the animal and the state of the environment were ideal for disrupting ongoing behavior, and there was a tendency to invoke anthropomorphic interpretations of the behavior in terms of motivational states. The term "experimental neurosis" introduced to describe such paradigms reflects this tendency.

Conflict during classical conditioning was studied first in Pavlov's laboratory. In 1921, Shenger-Krestovnikova classically conditioned a dog to salivate to a circle but not to an elipse. Finer and finer discrimination was required as the elipse was made more circular and, at the point where the dog could no longer discriminate, it became very excited and restless and so-called "neurotic" behavior emerged. Some years before, Terofeera had described similar phenomena, although their significance had not been appreciated. She conditioned salivation to an electric shock, which, after training, no longer gave rise to a strong defensive reaction. But, when she attempted to generalize the response to parts of the body that had not been originally stimulated by the shock, the defense reaction was restored and the dog showed general excitement. After Shenger-Krestovnikova's experiments, the importance of these observations became apparent to Pavlov, and the study of neurotic behavior came to dominate his experimental program. He became particularly concerned with the varying susceptibility of dogs to neurosis-inducing situations. He viewed nervous activity as a balance between excitation and inhibition and believed that dogs with a preponderance of excitation had a lower threshold for neurosis induction than those with a more strongly inhibited nervous system. Pavlov considered himself a physiologist, not a behaviorist, and this explains his concern with the interpretation of neurosis in terms of nervous activity and his lack of concern with behavioral details.

Complementary results were obtained by Liddell (1954) and his collaborators at Cornell in his classical studies of conditioned leg withdrawal in sheep and goats. The animals were placed in restraining harnesses, and front leg withdrawal was induced with electric shock. Leg withdrawal was conditioned to positive and negative stimuli, and a battery of physiological measures to assess respiration and cardiac function was taken as the animal responded. Liddell initially observed perfectly normal responses when the goat was given a limited number of trials per day, but when the number of trials in a session was increased to ten or twenty, aberrant behavior emerged. Persistent movement of the conditioned limb occurred between trials; the goat became unwilling to enter the laboratory and had to be forced onto the conditioning stand. Heartbeat and respiration became erratic. Sub-sequently, other modifications of the conditioning procedure were found to disrupt behavior; in order of importance they were discrimination between positive or negative stimuli, extinction of a positive conditioned response, and training on a rigid time schedule. Liddell's studies extended over many years, and he followed the social history of his subjects, their recovery, and the remission of their neurotic behavior. He reported that heartbeat in neu-rotic sheep is irregular under normal conditions, for example, while they are sleeping at night and, also, that they show marked frustration when mildly disturbing noises occur. Such neurotic animals also show themselves incapable of dealing with a situation of actual change in a realistic fashion. When dogs invaded the flock, it was invariably a neurotic sheep who was the victim. The animal's neurosis so damages its herd instinct that while other members of the flock escape together in one direction, the neurotic animal flees in panic in another. Clearly, both Pavlov and Liddell felt that their work on neurosis was relevant to human psychopathology.

In the next decade, Masserman (1943) took up the study of animal models of neurosis, using conflict in an operant conditioning situation. His interpre-tations had a strong psychoanalytical bias and as Broadhurst (1961) com-ments, "Masserman is avowedly anthropomorphic in a way which is rightly eschewed nowadays." His basic behavioral situation involved training a cat to make, in the presence of a discriminative stimulus, a box-opening re-sponse to obtain food. When the cat was well trained, box-opening attempts were accompanied by a strong puff of air and/or an electric shock. Such a procedure is essentially similar to the Geller immediate-punishment sched-ule. Masserman, however, was concerned with the behavior that emerged ·in this conflict situation rather than with the fact that box-opening was sup-pressed. Rating scales of enormous complexity (64 elements) were used to evaluate the neurotic profile, but it was found to be very difficult to disso-ciate the effect of drugs on neurosis with these methods; their value to be-havioral pharmacology was summed up by Masserman and Pechtel (1956) who decided that even with the data at hand "it is impossible to state the effects of any drug on any organism without considering the latter's genetic characteristics, past experiences, biological status, and perceptions, moti-vations toward and evaluations of its current physical and social milieu." As Weiskrantz comments, "If this were strictly true, no pharmacology textbook could ever have been written nor any anaesthetic given with confidence" (Weiskrantz, 1968, p. 81).

We believe that terms such as "emotion," "anxiety," and "neurosis" are sometimes convenient but can easily become misleading. The safest way to measure a behavioral phenomenon is to utilize a simple operant that is a part of the constellation but can be quantified. This explains our preoccupation in the rest of this chapter with *parametric* studies of how aversive stimuli change specified elements of conditioned or unconditioned behavior.

The use of electric shock to induce emotional behavior

Introduction

Shock can be used to sustain or suppress behavior. Its sustaining function on escape and avoidance schedules produces, as a corollary, facets of emotional behavior that have long been considered models of abnormal behavior. Since these procedures have been extensively discussed in the literature (Kimble, 1961), attention here will be given to punishment schedules as inducers of abnormal behavior.

A punisher is a stimulus that can suppress behavior preceding its presentation. The punishing stimulus, as discussed earlier, may either occur irrespective of the responses (adventitious or noncontingent) or it can be initiated by the animals' responses (immediate or contingent or response produced).

Adventitious shock

Several procedures involving adventitious punishment have been of continuing interest with respect to abnormal behavior. The general principle is to superimpose shocks on behavior maintained by some other motivation or state. A modification of this principle, devised originally by Estes and Skinner (1941), has been intensively studied for a number of years (Fig. 1–10). A rat is trained to respond for food reinforcement. A neutral stimulus, such as a colored light, is then introduced for regular periods during the operation of the reinforcement schedule, and, at the end of the S^D period, an unavoidable shock is given. Responding gradually changes so that, in the presence of the S^D, behavior is suppressed, and reinforced responding occurs only in its absence. The behavior during the S^D is the conditioned suppression produced by the shock. Its independence of ongoing responding is illustrated by the fact that, in entirely different behaviorial situations, the S^D is also able to suppress ongoing behavior that has never been associated with shock. The great interest in this procedure stems from the original hope that it would provide a model system of anxiety. The Estes-Skinner

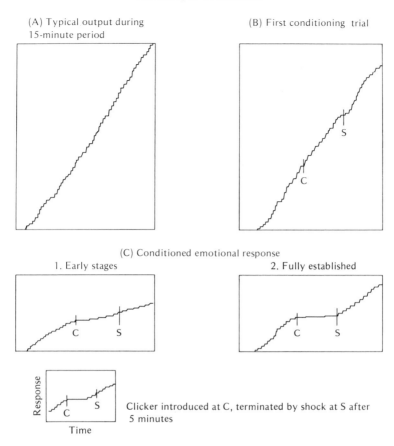

(A) Typical output during
15-minute period

(B) First conditioning trial

S

C

(C) Conditioned emotional response

1. Early stages

C   S

2. Fully established

C   S

Response

C   S

Time

Clicker introduced at C, terminated by shock at S after
5 minutes

Fig. 1–10   The conditioning of suppression during presentation of a preaversive stimulus. Typical VI performance reinforced by food is presented in (A). (B) shows the effect of a brief shock (S) on this VI performance. (C_1) and (C_2) illustrate early and late conditioned suppression with progressively fewer responses emitted during the clicks. (Reproduced from Hunt and Brady, 1951.)

procedure, however, turns out to be a complex and labile phenomenon. The presence of the S^D causes this procedure to differ from the most basic adventitious punishment procedure, where shocks would occur randomly irrespective of the animal's behavior and without warning. In the Estes-Skinner procedure, however, the interval between response and shock is variable, which is the central criterion of adventitious punishment. This procedure has been extensively studied for its own sake, and not surprisingly, the effect of the adventitious shock varies depending on the degree of motivation of the animal, the reinforcement schedule, the quality and intensity of the S^D, the shock level, and so on.

Strictly speaking, the Estes-Skinner procedure is a special example of adventitious punishment insofar as the S^D stimulus, which suppresses behavior, gains its controlling influence by being conditioned to the unconditioned aversive stimulus. Unpredictable shocks that occur without the presence of any overt discriminative cues will also produce marked changes in ongoing behavior. In natural situations, the source of aversive stimulation is often another organism, and the reaction is to engage in various species-typical aggressive and defensive behaviors. Azrin and his colleagues have recently studied such elicited aggression under laboratory conditions. Confined rats, when shocked, fight vigorously (O'Kelly and Steckle, 1939). The fighting behavior differs in wild and domesticated breeds of the same animal. If wild rats are used, the fighting involves attack. Ulrich, Hutchinson, and Azrin (1965) report, however, that, in laboratory-bred rats, the response is a form of "defensive" fighting, or boxing, and it may be that domestication has somewhat modified aggressive responses in such situations from attack to defensive behavior. Elicited aggression is influenced by the stimulus conditions under which it occurs. Rats paired with hamsters modify their boxing posture to suit the size of their adversary, or, when shocked in the presence of various inanimate objects, they attack some objects preferentially. Squirrel monkeys attack, by biting, any animate or inanimate object when their tails are shocked, but, again, stimuli vary in their ability to elicit biting. Given the choice of a rubber ball or metal box, the monkeys invariably attack the former. Biting after shock can be shown to be rewarding in that monkeys will learn to pull a chain to gain access to a rubber bite ball when shocked (Azrin et al., 1965). In several species, the intensity and frequency of biting attack varies with the intensity and duration of the shock (Hutchinson et al., 1968). Other aversive stimuli such as a heated floor with the rat and tail pinching with the monkey have been shown to elicit aggression.

The work on shock-elicited aggression has encouraged the view that there is some fundamental and unique relationship between pain and aggression. It is more likely, however, that moderate pain potentiates any active behavior that has a high probability of occurring. Rats in crowded living conditions show aggressive–defensive behavior, and if shock is added to the situation, these behaviors are even more likely to be released. Support for this interpretation comes from observations that other forms of behavior are potentiated by adventitious shock. Male rats were placed with receptive females and the frequency of copulation noted during several exposures (Barfield and Sachs, 1968). The males were then shocked in the presence of the females, and it was found that copulation occurred more often. Immediately after each shock, the female was paired and mounted, and the post-ejaculatory refractory period, when copulation does not occur, significantly decreased. A nonsocial behavior that has been studied in this way is eating. Ullman (1951) deprived rats of food and then studied their food intake during twenty 1-min sessions. During the first 5 sec of every minute, shock was administered, and, after several test days, it was observed that the greatest amount of eating occurred *during* these shock periods and the least in the 5 sec *after* the shock. In the nonsocial situation intense, unavoidable shock causes profound changes in behavior. Seligman (1975) has described such a procedure in dogs and rats. Dogs were strapped into a hammock and given 64 inescapable electric shocks (5 sec, 6.0 mA). The next day the dogs were placed in an escape/avoidance testing chamber, where on the presentation of a signal they could jump a barrier to avoid the shock. The dogs were found to be inactive and unable to learn this task.

The term "learned helplessness" was given to this behavior and at first it was compared to *reactive* depression in man and was considered a model with considerable potential in biological psychiatry. However, further work on the rat suggests that after repeated unavoidable shock, a form of conditioned immobility exists which is incompatible with the gross body movements required to successfully avoid shock by leaping a barrier. However, if an avoidance task is designed which requires minimal movement (e.g. protrusion of the nose through a hole), then animals that have received shock are able to learn to avoid further shocks, indeed learn at a faster rate than controls. This result puts the term "learned helplessness" in an ambiguous position and demonstrates how easy it is to jump to the wrong conclusions about grossly disturbed behavior patterns (Iversen, 1978b).

A comparison of immediate and adventitious punishment
in suppressing and disrupting behavior
Parametric studies of immediate punishment were described earlier (p. 28). As we have seen, adventitious punishment may, if given in certain situations, actually promote species-specific behaviors that are occurring or that may relate to the particular situation at hand. More commonly, if administered at certain intensity levels, and in situations where such relevant species-specific behavior as fighting or mating are not occurring, adventitious

punishment will produce responses incompatible with ongoing behavior. Shock does not have to be conditioned to a discriminative stimulus as in the Estes-Skinner procedure. Immediate punishment is more straightforward and effectively suppresses both operant and respondent behavior under all conditions. Solomon (1964) has suggested that consummatory responses are more readily suppressed by punishment than instrumental acts.

Some attempts have been made to compare the suppressive effects of the two shock procedures. Hunt and Brady (1955) trained rats to respond for food on a 1-min VI schedule during 12-min daily sessions; conditioning sessions were then introduced, and from the 4th to the 6th minute of the session a clicking sound was present. Some rats were shocked when they responded (immediate) during this period, and others received inescapable shocks (Estes-Skinner adventitious) at the end of the period. Lever pressing in the presence of the clicking sound was equally suppressed in both groups, but closer inspection of the overall behavior revealed interesting differences.

1. The adventitious group showed greater suppression when the conditioned stimulus was not present.

2. When, at the end of the experiment, sessions were given with the conditioned stimulus but no shock, responding in the immediate punishment group recovered more quickly than in the adventitious group.

3. During shock-induced suppression, the behaviors observed in the two groups differed; the adventitious animals displayed crouching and immobility, whereas the response-contingent group was more active and frequently made anticipatory responses to the lever. In the latter case, the suppressive effect of punishment seemed to be very closely tied to the lever-pressing response.

Azrin (1956) trained pigeons to peck a key for food on a 3-min variable-interval schedule. After responding was well established, the response key was alternately illuminated with an orange and a blue light every 2 min. The food reinforcement schedule remained in effect regardless of the color of the key, but a shock contingency was introduced in the presence of the orange light. Each animal was subjected to four different shock procedures, but shock-free recovery periods were interposed between the different procedures. Under the adventitious shock conditions, an inescapable shock was administered either a fixed or a variable time after the orange light came on. Thus, the orange light was a warning signal for an impending shock, regardless of the animals' behavior. Under the immediate punishment conditions, a shock was "due" some fixed or variable time after onset of the orange light but was not administered unless the pigeons pecked the key. If no response occurred between the time the punishment contingency came into effect and the end of the 2-min stimulus period, the color of the key was changed, and no shock was administered. There were variations in the pattern of responding in the presence of the orange light depending upon whether the shock occurred after a fixed or variable interval, but, with either schedule of administration of shock, there was much greater suppression of responding under the response contingent procedure than when shock conditions were independent of behavior.

Immediate punishment, unlike adventitious shock, will also suppress instinctive or consummatory behaviors. Mouse killing by certain strains of rats was studied by Myer (1966, 1968). Immediate punishment of the mouse-seizing responses dramatically suppressed the killing behavior, whereas similar adventitious punishment when the mouse was presented but had not been attacked did not suppress killing. These findings suggest that the suppression of attack behavior does not depend upon the association of shock with the stimulus that arouses attack, but rather on the association of shock with the attacking. Similar results have been obtained with dogs who were shocked either when food was presented or as eating started.

Brady (1958) extended his investigation of shock procedures to study the somatic consequences of adventitious punishment. He used intensive work schedules involving avoidance responding to eliminate shocks and produced a high incidence of such gastrointestinal lesions as ulcers. In his well-known "executive monkey" study, monkeys were yoked together so that they received an identical series of shocks, but one of the pair initiated the shocks by his responses, while the other passively received them at unpredictable times. The "responsible" animals, rather than the yoked controls, developed the lesions. The length of the work session was an important variable in these experiments; 6-hr avoidance–6-hr rest regimes produced ulcers, whereas alternated 30-min sessions were better tolerated. These results must be treated with caution, however, since the monkeys were not assigned to groups in a balanced order. The animals who learned the conditioned response first in this experiment became the "responsible" subjects. The study of Weiss et al. (1968) did not suffer from this defect and showed that, in the rat, the yoked subjects receiving adventitious shock lost weight, developed larger stomach ulcers more frequently, defecated more frequently, and showed a greater inhibition of drinking in the shock situation than rats who were able to avoid shock by their own actions.

Although there seems to be general agreement that conditioned responding is suppressed to a greater extent by immediate than by adventitious punishment, the picture is not so clear when unconditioned responses are monitored under these two conditions. More physiological and behavioral research is needed in this area, for we might suppose that the differences between self-initiated and adventitious punishment would be of great relevance to our understanding of the effects of aversive stimuli on human behavior.

Studies of aversive stimuli other than electric shock

Introduction
The preoccupation with shock as an aversive stimulus has had unfortunate theoretical implications. In his theory of avoidance behavior, Mowrer (1939) proposed that aversive stimuli induce fear, which is motivating, and that fear is always a conditioned response based on the association of some previously non-aversive stimulus with pain. There are, however, good grounds for questioning the assumption that all fears are conditioned responses of this kind. Many stimuli that are not painful or do not lead to painful consequences can be used as negative reinforcers or punishers and are highly aversive if their behavioral effects are observed. The termination of noise, for example, has been shown to reinforce escape behavior in humans (Azrin, 1958), monkeys (Klugh and Patton, 1959), cats, rats, and mice. Response-contingent noise suppresses responding in a similar range of species. Intense light will motivate escape learning and can serve as an unconditioned stimulus for avoidance learning. Forced swimming in cold water is highly aversive to rats (Glaser, 1910). Being touched by a hot or cold metal plate and blasted with air evoke active escape. Complex patterns of auditory and visual stimuli are apparently aversive in that they release typical patterns of defensive behavior in various species; ducklings, for example, freeze at the sight of a hawk. Bronson (1968) reviewed studies of the ontogenetic development of certain of these species-specific reactions to fear-arousing stimuli—particularly novel stimuli—and suggested how this kind of fear can disrupt behavior after normal development has been disrupted by isolation or maternal deprivation.

Novelty as an aversive stimulus
Bronson (1968) suggested that reactions to such nonvisual aversive stimuli as pain and loud noises should be called "distress reactions" and that these can be observed at a very early stage of development. He distinguishes

between these distress reactions and the fear of novelty, i.e. unfamiliar, visual stimuli, which develops later. A fair degree of stimulation at this stage of development appears to be a prerequisite for the maturation of normal responses to novelty. Levine's studies (1962) show that rats given excitatory stimulation associated with handling or electric shock are subsequently less fearful of novel situations than rats not given this experience. These kinds of experiments suggest that deprivation during development can markedly change responses to aversive stimuli. It could well be that partial deprivation occurs even when the mother is present, due perhaps to unusual characteristics of the infant or the mother. In either case, some early human psychopathology may have roots in disturbances beginning in the initial postnatal period.

Encoding the familiar is a prerequisite for the fear of novelty. Human infants must be capable of visual memory before a fear of visual novelty can develop. This seems to develop at about 2 months of age. Fantz (1964) found that before 2 months infants showed no difference in their reactions to new versus previously presented visual patterns, whereas after 2 months they spent less time gazing at "familiar" than at novel patterns. By 3 months, infants begin to smile less at strangers and from 6 months show attachment to a specific "mothering" person. Although physical contact seems to be paramount in allaying distress reactions, the mere presence of the mother within the child's visual field will allay tensions provoked by novel situations. It seems that infants begin to be disturbed by visual novelty at the time comfort is found in a visual awareness of the mother's presence. In monkeys, the fear of novelty and mother attachment occur at about 3 weeks of age (Harlow and Harlow, 1965). In the human, there is a gradual development of the ability to deal with novel visual experiences in the absence of the mother.

In view of such developmental evidence, it is not surprising to find that deprivation can permanently disturb the reaction to novelty. At the Yerkes laboratories, chimpanzees were separated from their mother at birth, and Davenport and Menzel (1963) reported that at 2 years of age such animals reacted by crouching, rocking, and swaying when presented with novel objects in their home cage. They made no attempt to withdraw from the objects, and the stereotyped behavior continued for several hours. The chimps seemed intensely fearful and did not approach and explore the objects. These mother-separated animals had been observed throughout the 2-year period, and it was clear that stereotyped behavior occurred even in the familiar environment of the home cage but was further intensified by novelty. Rhythmic rocking, swaying, or turning movements were seen as well as such repetitive activities as thumb-sucking and exaggerated chewing movements. Monkeys reared without a mother show similar behavior patterns. Comparable observations have been made in institution-reared infants (Bridges, 1932), and stereotyped rocking is characteristic of autistic (Hutt and Hutt, 1965) and schizophrenic (Bender, 1947) children. Autistic children seem to avoid visual novelty by their obsessive desire to maintain a familiar visual environment (Schopler, 1965), in their *eye-avoidance trait*, and in their preference for touch, taste, and smell rather than visual exploration. Similar symptoms have been described in 7- to 9-year-old schizophrenics.

Manipulation of reinforcement contingencies as an aversive stimulus

It is now clear that animals become very disturbed and aggressive, if, when they have been conditioned to receive reinforcers at a certain time and of a certain magnitude for a particular response effort, they are not rewarded in the expected manner.

Azrin et al. (1966) were the first to put this form of elicited aggression under experimental control. They described a procedure in which a pigeon was alternately rewarded ten times on a continuous reinforcement schedule for pecking a key and then was given a period of extinction. At the back of a cage, a suitably restrained "target" pigeon was positioned and the attack response to it recorded (Fig. 1–11). The attacks occurred during extinction and were most frequent at the start of the extinction period. Similar behavior has been observed in the squirrel monkey, when aggression was measured by the number of bites on a piece of hose pipe placed in the animal's cage (Fig. 1–12). Hutchinson et al. (1968) observed that the withdrawal of an intermittent reinforcement schedule produced more aggression than the termination of continuous reinforcement; several workers have gone on to show that fixed-ratio schedules will themselves induce aggressive responses even in the absence of any contrasting extinction period. Attack occurs with greatest frequency in the post-reinforcement pause. This has been very elegantly demonstrated by Cherek, Thompson, and Heistad (1973), who used a slightly modified Azrin apparatus. Pigeons faced two keys; pecks on one were reinforced on a 2-min fixed-interval schedule and pecks on the other "target" key were reinforced on an FR2 schedule with access to a live target pigeon. The birds responded on the target key in the early part of the FI period and vigorously attacked the target bird when it became accessible (Fig. 1–13). Schedule-induced aggression has been observed in rats, pigeons, and monkeys.

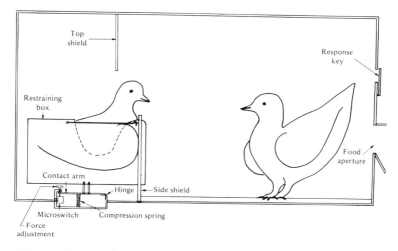

Fig. 1–11 A schematic drawing of the apparatus for measuring attack. The experimental chamber was 26 by 14 by 14 in. high. Plexiglas shields at the top and on the sides of the restraining box prevented the experimental pigeon from getting behind the target pigeon. (Reproduced from Azrin et al., 1966b.)

Falk (1972) has proposed that schedule-induced aggression is similar to an abnormal drinking behavior termed schedule-induced polydipsia. If water is freely available when rats lever press for 45-mg dry food pellets on a 1-min VI schedule, large quantities of water are consumed. During a 3.5-hr session, this can be three to four times the normal total daily intake. This does not occur with continuous reinforcement schedules but seems to appear when inter-reinforcement times exceed 30 sec.

Falk suggested that these be called "adjunctive behaviours," which he defines as "behaviour maintained at high probability by stimuli whose reinforcing properties in the situation are derived primarily as the result of schedule parameters governing the availability of another class of reinforcers." In the experiment of Cherek et al. (1973) the reinforcing effectiveness of the opportunity to attack depended upon the presence of a schedule of food presentation. Attack no longer occurred if the animal was not exposed to the intermittent schedule of reinforcement. Adjunctive behavior resembles the "displacement activity" classically described in the ethological literature.

Displacement behaviors are described as occurring when certain environmental events result in the interruption of some consummatory activity in an organism under high "drive" conditioning. These are exactly the condi-

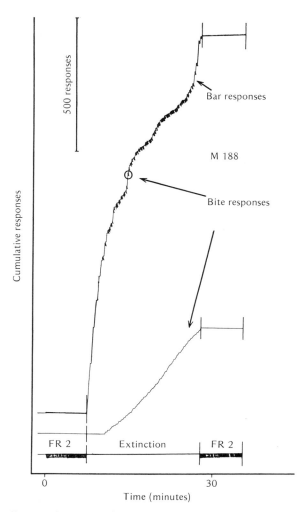

Fig. 1–12 Effect in the squirrel monkey of extinction on bar pressing and hose biting following FR 2. Bar pressing was recorded by the cumulative upward excursion of the pen in the upper curve. The response pen was reset to the baseline with each reinforcement. Hose biting was recorded by the brief downward deflections of the pen in the upper curve and by the cumulative upward excursion of the pen in the center curve. Food deliveries were recorded by the brief downward movement of the pen in the lower curve. (Reproduced from Hutchinson, Azrin, and Hunt, 1968a.)

tions that produce adjunctive aggressive behavior as defined by Falk. Aggression should not, therefore, be viewed as a behavior generated by a hypothetical internal state in the absence of eliciting stimuli, but rather as a behavior occurring in a *specific* situation—a situation in which another class of reinforcers is intermittently scheduled.

In addition to these effects of the schedule of reinforcement, sudden increases or decreases in the expected magnitude of the reward disrupt behavior. Crespi (1944) reported that if rats were trained in a runway to run to a goal box for a reinforcement of a certain size, they ran faster or slower if the size of the reward was unexpectedly increased or decreased in size. These sudden increases and decreases of ongoing behavior have been described as "behavioral contrast," and Baltzer and Weiskrantz (1970) have described a method for reliably generating these effects. Rats were trained on a 2-min VI schedule with one pellet per reward. Then small and large rewards (one or four pellets) were given on alternate daily sessions with different discriminative stimuli associated with the two conditions. After some days on the alternating procedure, daily sessions consisted of one reward condition associated with the appropriate discriminative stimulus. The effects of the intrusions within each session was assessed by the quotient

Fig. 1–13 Sample cumulative record for pigeon responding on FI 2-min food and FR 2 target presentation schedules. Simultaneous recording of food key, target key, and attack responding are represented. Following presentation of food, the stepper pen reset to the baseline (top). Attack responses are switch closures recorded when a force of at least 100 gm was exerted against the front of the restraining box (containing the target bird) by the experimental subjects during periods of fighting. The target bird was accessible for 15 sec following completion of an FR 2 requirement on the target key. (Reproduced from Cherek et al., 1973.)

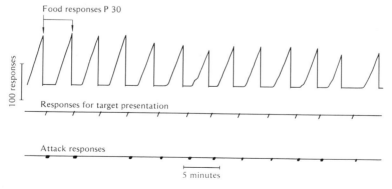

$$\frac{\text{rate during intrusion} - \text{rate before intrusion}}{\text{rate during intrusion} + \text{rate before intrusion}}$$

Behavioral contrast was assessed by comparing each animal's rate on the intrusion conditions with its rate on the baseline conditions during the immediately preceding day when responding was controlled by the small reward. Larger rewards tended to increase response rates and show positive behavioral contrast, whereas smaller rewards on a large reward baseline produced the opposite effect. The potential value of this technique, which generates behavioral states that could be likened to elation or depression, for characterizing the behavioral effects of certain drugs is mentioned later.

2. Basic Neuropharmacology

SOME BASIC PHARMACOLOGICAL PRINCIPLES
How drugs work and how their effects are measured

Most drugs interact in a specific manner with target sites in biological systems; such sites are pharmacologically defined as DRUG RECEPTORS. The drug–receptor interaction does not usually involve a covalent chemical linkage of the drug to the receptor, but rather a weaker interaction whereby the drug, because of its particular shape and charge distribution, can bind reversibly to a specific chemical site on the receptor and, in so doing, change the physiological reactivity of the receptor. The receptor, for example, may be an enzyme, and the drug may act to inhibit its activity. Alternatively, drug receptors may be specific membrane proteins in such excitable tissues as nerve or muscle, in which the drug–receptor interaction leads to a change in membrane permeability that, in turn, excites or inhibits the excitable cell. Not all drugs act by way of such specific receptor interactions; for example, many anesthetic drugs change the electric properties of nerves by dissolving in the lipoprotein membranes of such cells; this produces an overall change in the physiochemical properties of the membranes which inhibits excitation. The great majority of drugs, however, have more specific receptor interactions.

Drugs produce biological responses that are graded according to the amount of drug administered (DOSE). Such dose–response relationships are most conveniently plotted as biological response (on a linear scale) against log of dose, to yield an S-shaped (sigmoid) LOG DOSE–RESPONSE CURVE (Fig.

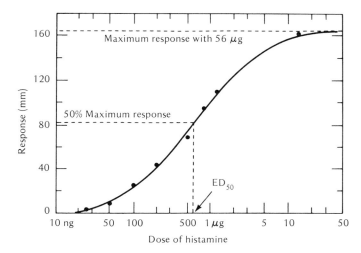

Fig. 2–1   Log dose–response curve for histamine acting on guinea pig ileum in an organ bath. Response magnitude (mm) is proportional to contraction of the ileum. Histamine dose added to a constant volume bath is shown on a logarithmic scale. (From Goldstein, Aranow, and Kalman, 1974.)

2–1). This is by no means the only way of expressing responses to drug, but it has several advantages over other graphical expressions. It allows us to depict drug responses over a wide range of doses, since the dosage scale is compressed by the log conversion. It is also found that, though the log dose–response is a sigmoid curve, an important portion of it (about 30 to 70% of the maximum response) approximates a straight line, thus making it possible to quantify and compare data in this dose-response range. Furthermore, a series of different drugs that produce the same response by interacting with a common receptor mechanism will give a series of parallel log dose–response curves. In such a series, the curve for the drug that interacts most strongly with the receptor will appear to the left of the others, since lower doses will be needed to produce the biological response. The PO-TENCY of drugs can thus be compared. The potency of a drug is often expressed as the dose required to produce one-half of the maximum response the drug is capable of eliciting; this is the ED_{50}. The shape of the log dose–response curve reflects the nature of the drug–receptor interaction. This interaction is analogous to the binding of substrate molecules to an enzyme. It is an equilibrium reaction, and the proportion of receptors occupied by the drug will depend on the affinity of the drug molecules for the receptors and the drug concentration at the level of the receptors. Since the number of receptor sites in a given tissue is finite, the drug–receptor interaction is a saturable relationship in which increasing the drug concentration (or dose) beyond a certain point cannot lead to further increase in drug binding, since all available receptors, or at least all those needed to produce a maximum biological response, are occupied.

Some drugs, known as AGONISTS, produce a direct measurable response by interacting with receptors, but other types of drugs alter the response normally elicited from the interaction of agonists with their receptors. Thus, ANTAGONIST drugs block the responses elicited by agonists. A simple, competitive antagonist, as the name implies, competes with an agonist drug for binding to the receptor sites. When receptor sites are occupied by the antagonist molecules, no response is produced, and the sites are not available to the agonist. Such competitive antagonism can be overcome, however, if the dose of agonist is increased. The actions of a competitive antagonist thus show up as a shift to the right in the log dose–response curve of the agonist drug (Fig. 2–2A). Noncompetitive antagonists block receptors in a way that cannot be overcome by increasing the agonist dose. The agonist log dose–response curve is again shifted to the right, but the maximum re-

Fig. 2–2   Analysis of receptor antagonist actions by log dose–response curves. Isolated cat spleen strips stimulated by norepinephrine (NEPI) at various concentrations at low and high concentrations of a competitive antagonists; (A) tolazoline, or a noncompetitive antagonist; (B) dibenamine. (From Goldstein, Aranow, and Kalman, 1974.)

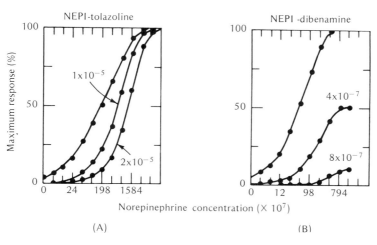

sponse is also depressed by the antagonist (Fig. 2–2B). Other drugs may increase the potency of an agonist, a phenomenon known as POTENTIATION which involves a shift in the agonist log dose–response curve to the left. Such potentiation is usually a consequence of more agonist drug being made available to interact with its receptors, rather than of any fundamental change in the properties of the receptors. Potentiation may occur, for example, by inhibiting the mechanisms normally responsible for removing an agonist from the environment of its receptors by metabolism or by tissue uptake mechanisms.

The use of log dose–response curves to assess the effects of drugs on behavior is no less desirable than in any other branch of pharmacology. Such a systematic approach allows us to compare the potencies of different drugs in a series of related compounds; at the same time it indicates whether these drugs act by way of a common mechanism. It also allows us to determine agonist/antagonist relationships and to compare the properties of drug receptors in the brain with receptors in the peripheral nervous system. There are several difficulties, however, in applying such an analysis to the effects of drugs on behavior. Classically, drug–receptor interactions are studied with simple isolated tissue systems (see Figs. 2–1 and 2–2), in which the concentration of drug to which the receptors are exposed is known and easily controllable and in which the drug interacts with only one type of receptor to produce a single type of response. Matters are never this simple in behavioral pharmacology. Behavioral responses are clearly of a far more complex nature than the contraction of a piece of smooth muscle in an organ bath. A behavioral response cannot always be easily quantified and measured on a linear scale, on which the magnitude of the response directly reflects the drug–receptor interaction. Apart from difficulties of measurement, one particular behavioral response may have complex effects on other behavioral responses, which, in turn, modify the response being measured; alternatively, the drug–receptor interaction may produce more than one type of response. Drugs often have multiple actions on different receptors in the brain, leading to a complex series of behavioral consequences that are not easily analyzed. Apart from these difficulties, there is the problem that the concentration of drug to which receptors in the brain are exposed is usually not known and cannot easily be controlled. For example, agonist drugs may have widely different potencies in eliciting a given behavioral response not because of any real difference in their potencies at receptor sites in the brain, but simply because some drugs penetrate more readily

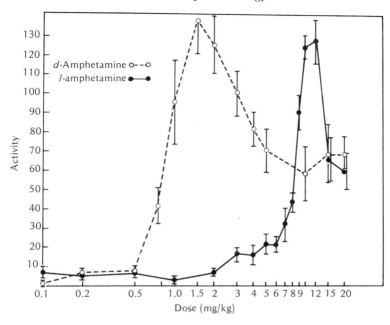

Fig. 2–3   Log dose–response curves for the effects of increasing subcutaneous doses of d- and l-amphetamine on locomotor activity in rats pretreated with iproniazid (150 mg/kg, i.p.) 16 hr earlier. Rats were placed in individual photocell activity cages, and locomotor activity was measured as the number of interruption of the photocell beam in a 30-min session. Each point is the mean and standard error for six determinations. (From Taylor and Synder, 1971.)

into the brain from the bloodstream than others. This problem is discussed in more detail below. Lest the reader be dismayed by the difficulties of the quantitative analysis of behavioral responses to drugs, it should be pointed out that such analysis is often possible, and the results can be valuable. For example, Fig. 2–3 shows an analysis and comparison of the motor stimulant effects of d- and l-amphetamine. The log dose–response curves are conventional in the sense that the lines from the two drugs are essentially parallel, but they differ from simpler responses in that the curves do not show simple plateaus at high doses of either drug, but rather bell-shaped curves in which the response falls off at very high doses. The result, however, clearly indicates that d-amphetamine is about ten times more potent than l-amphetamine in stimulating locomotor activity in the rat.

The penetration of drugs into the CNS
after peripheral administration

Drugs are most often administered systemically. This may be done by mouth (PER OS, P.O.) or by injection into the peritoneal cavity (INTRAPERITONEALLY, I.P.), into a large muscle (INTRAMUSCULARLY, I.M.), under the skin (SUBCUTANEOUSLY, S.C.), or into the bloodstream, usually by injection into a vein (INTRAVENOUSLY, I.V.). In all of these cases, the drug is distributed throughout the various tissues of the body after entering the bloodstream. The amount of drug entering peripheral tissues will depend on the rate at which blood flows through these tissues and on the ease with which the drug can escape from the bloodstream to enter the tissues. Most drugs escape readily from small blood vessels and equilibrate rapidly with the extracellular fluid space of peripheral tissues, from which a drug may then act on receptors on the external surfaces of cell membranes or may penetrate into the cells. The penetration of drugs from the blood into the central nervous system (CNS), however, is a special case. Drugs may enter the CNS either by direct penetration into the brain or spinal cord through brain capillaries or they may first enter the cerebrospinal fluid (CSF) from the blood and thence into the CNS tissue. In either case, the rate of penetration for most drugs is relatively slow compared to the rate of distribution of drugs into peripheral tissues. The brain has a very high blood flow, about 0.5 ml/gm/min compared with about 0.05 ml/gm/min in resting muscle, but drugs and other substances escape from the brain capillaries far less readily than from the capillaries in most other tissues. This is partly due to the special nature of the brain capillary walls, which lack the pores or fenestrations found in peripheral blood vessels. Substances passing out of brain capillary vessels have thus to pass through the endothelial cells of which the capillary wall is composed, rather than simply through the pores in the wall. In addition, the brain capillaries are wrapped tightly in a sheath of glial tissue made up of the processes of numerous astrocytes. This glial sheath is closely apposed to the surface of the capillaries and covers more than 80% of the exterior of the capillary. Finally, the CNS differs from most peripheral organs in that its cellular elements (neurons and glial cells) are tightly packed together, with only very small and tortuous clefts of extracellular space between them. Estimates of the volume of extracellular space indicate that it may be as little as 5–15% of the brain volume, compared with the 20–40% found in most other tissues. These unique anatomical features lead to a situation in which drugs and other water-soluble substances do not readily penetrate into the brain from the bloodstream. Most water-soluble substances penetrate the brain only after they have crossed the cell barriers of the capillary endothelium and its surrounding glial sheath, a process that is much slower than penetration through fenestrated capillaries into the extracellular space of the peripheral tissues. This unique relationship between blood supply and brain tissue has led to the concept of a BLOOD–BRAIN BARRIER, which describes the relatively slow penetration of many substances from blood into brain (Oldendorf, 1975). The term "barrier," however, is now generally accepted as a somewhat misleading description of the phenomenon, since there is probably no single anatomical feature that can be described as a barrier. Furthermore, the phenomenon is not so much that there is an absolute barrier to the penetration of substances into the brain, but rather that the *rate* of penetration is in general slower for brain than for most other tissues.

Penetration of drugs into the CSF occurs either by passage through the brain capillaries into the extracellular fluid of the brain—with which the CSF fairly readily equilibrates—or by passage through the blood vessels of the choroid plexus, the specialized, highly vascular structure in the ventricular system from which CSF is formed. In either case, the penetration of drugs into the CSF usually occurs no more readily than into the brain tissue. Once drugs have entered the CSF, however, they may leave the brain only slowly, since the CSF equilibrates only slowly with other body fluids.

The brain is not homogeneous in its blood–tissue permeability properties. Some regions of the CNS appear to lack any blood–brain barrier, and drugs and other substances penetrate readily; these include the pineal gland, the posterior lobe of the pituitary gland, and the area postrema, a small region situated on the roof of the fourth ventricle in the brainstem, which contains the chemoreceptors involved in the control of vomiting. The rate of penetration of drugs into other brain regions is not uniform. Regional blood flow varies considerably, with rates as high as 2.0 ml/gm/min in some cortical gray matter and as low as 0.2 ml/gm/min in most white matter. Consequently the distribution of drugs in the CNS is not even, and higher drug concentrations are reached—at least for short periods of time after drug administration—in regions in which gray matter predominates.

Since the blood–brain barrier poses such important problems for the interpretation of drug action on the CNS, it is worth considering some of the properties of drug molecules that are important in determining the rate at which they penetrate into the CNS after peripheral administration. Because of the cellular barriers involved in the penetration of drugs into the CNS from the bloodstream, the rules governing the permeability characteristics of the blood–brain barrier are similar to those governing the penetration of drugs or other substances across cell membranes, rather than through the usual capillary fenestrations in other tissues. The general principles involved are quite well understood and can be summarized as follows:

Binding to plasma proteins
Since only free drug molecules are available for passage across cell membranes, the extent of drug molecule binding to plasma proteins can be important. This binding reduces the plasma concentration of drug available for entry into the brain. In many cases, the proportion of circulating drug bound in this way can be very high; values of more than 90% are not uncommon.

Ionization of charged groups
Many drugs have ionizable groups, usually a weak acid or base, so that the ionization is incomplete at physiological pH values. The degree of ionization of such groups at physiological pH is a vital factor in drug penetration, since the permeability of cell membranes to the electrically charged ionized form of the molecule is usually very low compared to the much higher permeability of the same compound in the un-ionized (electrically neutral) form. The extent of ionization of these weakly acidic or basic groups on drug molecules at physiological pH is, in turn, determined by the chemical nature of the remainder of the drug molecule and can be estimated from the drug's pK value, the pH at which 50% of the drug molecules exist in the ionized form.

The importance of ionization in determining the penetration of substances from the blood into the brain is illustrated by the complete lack of penetration of such circulating organic amines as epinephrine (E), norepinephrine (NE), dopamine (DA), and acetylcholine (ACh) (see below). The pK of these substances is in the alkaline range, so that at physiological pH they exist almost entirely in the ionized form, with a positive electric charge. As an example, the CNS action of the cholinergic-blocking drugs, atropine, and its close analogue methylatropine can be compared (Fig. 2–13). These two drugs are of comparable potency in antagonizing cholinergic receptors in peripheral tissue, but the potency of atropine is many times that of its methyl analogue in the CNS. This is explained by the relative lack of penetration of methylatropine into the CNS, the methyl substituent converting

Table 2–1   Correlation of physical properties of drugs with their rates of penetration into the cerebrospinal fluid

Drug	Fraction bound to plasma protein*	Fraction un-ionized*	Partition coefficient n-heptane/ water of un-ionized form	CSF penetration†
Thiopental	0.75	0.61	3.30	1.4
Aniline	0.15	0.99	1.10	1.7
Pentobarbital	0.40	0.83	0.05	4.0
Barbital	0.02	0.56	0.002	27.0
Mecamylamine	0.20	0.02	400.0	32.0
Salicylic acid	0.40	0.004	0.12	115.0

(Modified from Goldstein, Aranow, and Kalman, 1974.)

*At pH 7.4.

†CSF penetration rates were recorded in dogs by measuring drug concentration in CSF at various times after drug administration. Results are expressed as the half-time (minutes) taken for the CSF concentration of drug to equilibrate with that in plasma.

the neutral drug atropine into a positively charged quaternary nitrogen compound.

Lipid solubility

The solubility of a drug in lipid is also of major importance in determining its rate of penetration into the CNS. Drugs that are quite soluble in lipid penetrate lipoprotein cell membranes far more readily than drugs that are relatively insoluble. A convenient assessment of lipid solubility is given by the partition of the substance between an organic solvent (such as benzene or heptane) and water; the proportion of drug in the water and in the organic solvent phase is measured after equilibrium has been reached (partition coefficient).

The role of these various factors in determining the rate of penetration of drugs into the CNS is illustrated by the results listed in Table 2–1, which compares the extent of protein binding, ionization, and lipid solubility of various drugs with the rates of penetration measured experimentally by the analysis of samples of CSF taken at various times after drug administration. Such drugs as thiopental and aniline penetrate into the CNS very rapidly because they are largely un-ionized at plasma pH and are soluble in lipids. Pentobarbital is much less soluble in lipid than is thiopental and penetrates more slowly. This correlates well with the almost immediate induction of anesthesia after an intravenous administration of thiopental, compared with the relatively slow induction after pentobarbital. Salicylic acid and mecamylamine are examples of drugs that penetrate into the CNS only poorly because they are very largely ionized at physiological pH. Though un-ionized mecamylamine is relatively soluble in lipid, the ionized form is not, and CSF penetration occurs only slowly.

Measurement of blood–brain barrier "brain uptake index"
A technique devised by Oldendorf (1971) has been widely used to assess the ability of naturally occurring substances and drugs to enter the CNS. The test substance, radioactively labelled with ^{14}C, is injected into a carotid artery and the amount entering brain is calculated from the amount of radioactive material remaining in venous blood sampled after a single passage through the brain capillaries. The "uptake index" is the percentage of radioactive substance remaining in the brain, which is compared to the corresponding percentage for tritium-labelled water, which penetrates cerebral capillaries freely. Results for a number of naturally occurring amino acids and for some neurotransmitter amines and related compounds are summarized in Table 2–2. Some amino acids, especially those which the brain cannot itself manufacture, penetrate readily from blood to brain, usually assisted by specialized membrane transport processes which are specific for the naturally occurring L-isomers. On the other hand, neurotransmitter amines and those amino acids with probable neurotransmitter function are almost completely excluded from passage into brain from blood; thus the brain is protected from circulating substances with high biological activity.

Alternative methods of administering drugs to avoid the blood–brain barrier

Because of the relatively poor penetration of many drugs into the brain following systemic administration, a number of alternative approaches have been devised to circumvent this problem (for review see Myers, 1975). The most direct approach is to administer the drug directly into the brain, and a number of ways of doing this are available. One can inject or infuse a solution containing drug into the CSF and observe its effects on behavior. To avoid performing the injection in an anesthetized animal, such administrations are often made through small tubes (cannulae) that have been surgically implanted under anesthesia. Such permanently implanted cannulae

Table 2–2. Brain uptake index—penetration of amino acids and neurotransmitter amines into brain

Compounds with good or moderate penetration		Compounds with poor penetration	
Tritiated water (reference)	100		
β-phenethylamine	67	Norepinephrine	4.5
Phenylalanine	55	Acetylcholine	4.5
Leucine	54	Dopamine	3.8
Tyrosine	50	Proline	3.3
Isoleucine	40	Glutamic acid	3.2
Methionine	38	Aspartic acid	2.8
Tryptophan	36	5-hydroxytryptamine	2.6
Histidine	33	Glycine	2.5
Valine	21	Epinephrine	2.4
L-dopa	20	GABA	2.2
Tryptamine	12.5	Histamine	1.6
Threonine	11.7		
D-Tyrosine	8.1		
Serine	7.5		
DL-5-hydroxytryptophan	7.4		
Alanine	5.7		

Data from Oldendorf (1971). The "brain uptake index" is the percentage of radioactivity remaining in the brain after one passage, compared to a tritiated water reference; amino acids are L-isomers except where noted.

are easily fitted through the skull of such small laboratory animals as the rat. Drug solutions injected into the CSF rapidly diffuse through the ventricular system, and drugs administered in this way gain ready access to many brain regions; there are, however, regional differences in the permeability of the lining of the ventricles, and some brain structures, which lie far away from the ventricular surfaces, may not be so readily exposed to the injected drug. In larger animals, several cannulae can be implanted in different parts of the ventricular system of the brain, so that drug solutions may be perfused through restricted areas of the CSF, thus exposing selected brain regions only. An even more selective exposure of brain regions to drugs is achieved by the microinjection of very small volumes of drug solution into a local region of brain tissue itself. This is done through very fine diameter needles or cannulae, the tips of which are precisely located in the brain by implantation with the aid of a stereotaxic apparatus and an appropriate brain atlas. Unless very small volumes are injected (less than 1 μl), however, the injected substance may still spread to regions up to 1 mm or more from the site of injection—a relatively large distance in such animals as mice and rats whose brains are quite small. The spread of the injected drug should ideally be determined by using radioactively labeled drug for test injections and examining the distribution of radioactivity at various times after injection.

An even more precise localization of administered drug can be achieved by the ejection of very small amounts of the drug from the tips of fine glass microelectrodes, using the passage of electric current through the electrode to move the charged drug molecules by iontophoresis. This technique has proved useful for studying the responses of single neurons in the CNS to a variety of test substances (see p. 79), but it seems unlikely to be of value for behavioral studies, since in order to evoke a measurable change in behavior it would probably be necessary to influence more than a small number of neurons. Also, the technique can be applied only to fully anesthetized animals at present.

At first glance, it might seem that the intracerebral administration of drugs would be the method of choice for studying drug actions on the CNS, since it avoids many of the difficulties outlined. One might think that this offers a method whereby the dose of drug applied to the brain could be precisely controlled and that a series of related drugs could thus be subjected to quantitative pharmacological analysis to assess their potencies in eliciting various forms of behavior. Although this may occasionally be possible, there are unfortunately a number of difficulties. The most important of these is that when drugs are administered intracerebrally they tend to leave the brain rather rapidly, and different drugs will leave at different rates. The rate at which substances leave the brain, largely by entrance into the bloodstream, is determined by factors similar to those previously described for the entry of substances from blood to brain. Thus, small uncharged molecules, which are very soluble in lipid, will disappear very rapidly, whereas water-soluble acids or bases may persist a much longer period of time. All substances administered in this way, however, will tend to escape relatively rapidly because the injection of a small amount of material into the brain or CSF means that there is always a large concentration gradient between the brain and the peripheral tissue, especially the relatively large volume of drug-free blood. Nevertheless, this technique has proved useful, particularly for drugs that hardly penetrate into the brain after systemic administration; these include the transmitter amines and amino acids, NE, DA, ACh, gamma-aminobutyric acid (GABA), and related compounds.

Another way of circumventing the blood–brain barrier is to observe the behavioral effects of systemically administered drugs in very young animals, in which the blood–brain barrier is not yet developed. For example, most substances penetrate readily into the CNS from the bloodstream in chicks, in which the normal blood–brain barrier is not fully developed until about 1 week after hatching. In mammals, such as the rat, a similar situation exists for the first few days after birth. This phenomenon has proved valuable in studying the CNS activity of otherwise impermeant substances, but this approach is, of course, limited by the fact that the brain is still highly immature in such young animals. They thus have neither the neuropharmacological nor the behavioral repertoire of the adult, and behavioral responses to drugs may not reflect the normal responses of the mature CNS.

It is sometimes possible to achieve exposure of the CNS to a drug by administering a precursor substance that penetrates into the CNS more readily than the drug itself and can be converted to the desired drug after it has entered the CNS. In the case of the transmitter amines, DA and 5-HT, for example, the precursor amino acids L-dopa and L-5-hydroxytryptophan enter the CNS after systemic administration, whereas the amines hardly penetrate the CNS (see Table 2.2). The amino acids are readily converted in the brain to the amines by aromatic amino acid decarboxylase. The amino acids probably enter the brain by way of special membrane transport systems, which the brain uses to obtain such substances as glucose or amino acids from the bloodstream. This approach has many virtues. In the examples cited above, the precursor substances themselves are virtually devoid of pharmacological activity and can be used in relatively large doses to load the CNS with active metabolites. Other examples include the metabolic conversion of the inactive drug chloral hydrate into the active CNS depressant trichlorethanol and the conversion of the weak cholinergic agonist tremorine into the more active oxotremorine (Fig. 2–13). Unfortunately, this approach is limited by the availability of suitable precursors that penetrate readily into the CNS.

Drug metabolism

Most drugs are metabolized in the body, and most of their metabolic products are both pharmacologically less active than the parent drug and more readily excreted. Generally, metabolism leads to a product that is more highly ionized than the parent drug. This product is then less readily reabsorbed from the renal tubules and is excreted more rapidly in the urine. By contrast, un-ionized, lipid-soluble substances readily diffuse back into the blood after filtration in the kidneys are thus less rapidly excreted in the urine. Drugs may be combined with such highly ionized substances as glucuronic acid, sulfate ions, and acetate, thus facilitating their excretion.

A wide variety of enzymes and many different types of chemical transformation are involved in drug metabolism, and a large literature on the subject now exists. The reactions usually involve oxidation, reduction, or hydrolysis. The major site of drug metabolism is the liver, but other sites include the kidneys, lungs, and blood plasma; some metabolism may occur within the CNS. An important series of enzymes involved in the metabolism of drugs is located in the membrane of the endoplasmic reticulum of the liver.

An important feature of the hepatic metabolizing enzymes is that the amount of these enzymes present in the liver can increase if the drugs that are metabolized by them are administered repeatedly. The repeated administration of such barbiturates as pentobarbital or phenobarbital, for example, gradually leads to an increase in the hepatic enzymes responsible for degrading these drugs. The result is that they are more rapidly degraded, and their action is progressively diminished upon repeated administration. Since the hepatic enzymes are relatively nonspecific, the metabolism of one drug may be influenced by prior administration of any other drug that can increase the enzymatic machinery of the liver. Differences in the activity of hepatic drug-metabolizing enzymes between different species, between male and female animals of the same species, or between individuals of different ages may also be important in determining the pharmacological response to drugs. These factors are illustrated in Table 2–3, for the sedative hexobarbital, for which the rate of drug metabolism is easily related to pharmacological effects, as measured by the average duration of sleep induced by the drug.

Tolerance and physical dependence

DRUG TOLERANCE is the term used to describe the diminished responsiveness of animals or man to a drug after previous administration of the drug or some related substance. PHYSICAL DEPENDENCE, sometimes associated with tolerance, is the term used to describe a state in which, after repeated drug administration, the organism may actually require the presence of the drug for normal functioning. Such a state of dependence or addiction is revealed by withdrawing the drug, which elicits a variety of physiological disturbances known collectively as the WITHDRAWAL SYNDROME. Virtually

Table 2–3. Species differences in metabolism of hexobarbital; changes with age

Species	Average sleeping time (min)	Hexobarbital half-life in plasma (min)	Liver enzyme activity (μg/gm hr^{-1})
Mice	12 ± 8	19 ± 7	598 ± 184
Rabbits	49 ± 12	60 ± 11	196 ± 28
Rats	90 ± 15	140 ± 54	134 ± 51
Dogs	315 ± 105	260 ± 20	36 ± 30
(hexobarbital dose in all species except dog, 100 mg/kg; dog, 50 mg/kg)			

	Average sleeping time (min)	Injected drug metabolized in 3 hours (%)	Liver enzyme activity (% added drug metabolized per hr)
Mice:			
1-day-old	>360	0	0
7-day-old	107 ± 26	11–24	2.5–3.5
21-day-old	27 ± 11	21–33	13–21
Adult	<5	—	28–39
(hexobarbital dose, 10 mg/kg)			

(From Goldstein, Aranow, and Kalman, 1974.)

all of the effects of the withdrawal syndrome are rapidly terminated if the drug is re-administered.

Tolerance and dependence are all too common features of psychoactive drug use. They arise by mechanisms that are largely unknown. One important mechanism that is fairly well understood is the induction of drug-metabolizing enzymes on repeated drug administration. At the least, this phenomenon can account for an important component of the tolerance that develops to such drugs as hexobarbital and pentobarbital upon repeated administration. Tolerance in such cases is due to an increased rate of metabolism of the administered drug, so that for a given dose the duration of effective exposure of the tissues to the active drug progressively diminishes as administration is continued. Even with the barbiturates, other less well understood mechanisms are involved in the development of tolerance. Rats given barbiturates repeatedly show progressively shorter periods of anesthesia following drug administration. That this cannot simply be due to a more rapid rate of drug metabolism is shown by the finding that the concentration of free drug in the brain at the time the animals wake up from the anesthesia progressively increases with repeated doses. Thus, the animals' threshold for anesthesia gradually increases. This is due to some cellular adaptation in the brain, whereby the receptors responsible for the drug action become less sensitive to the drug—a phenomenon sometimes called CELLULAR TOLERANCE.

Although tolerance develops to many psychoactive drugs, this is not always accompanied by the development of physical dependence. For example, tolerance to the hallucinogenic effects of lysergic acid diethylamide (LSD) develops rapidly in man, but there is no evidence of physical dependence. A similar situation holds for the amphetamines and the cannabis alkaloids. On the other hand, man and animals clearly show the development of tolerance and physical dependence after prolonged administration of alcohol, barbiturates, meprobamate, or the opium alkaloids. The latter group of drugs includes morphine, heroin, levorphanol, meperidine, and methadone (see p. 207). These drugs produce striking degrees of tolerance and dependence in animals and in man. Morphine addicts have been known to take daily doses of several grams, whereas such doses would almost certainly prove lethal to a naive subject. Rodents can be made tolerant to morphine by repeated administration of this or a related drug over a period of a few days (Fig. 2–4). The use of behavioral techniques to assess the development of tolerance and dependence to the narcotic drugs in animals will be discussed in more detail in Chapter 7.

Tolerance and dependence remain major problems in the use of many psychoactive drugs by man; they also present a formidable challenge to pharmacologists to understand the basic cellular mechanisms underlying these striking phenomena. Almost certainly, cellular changes in the biosynthesis of receptor molecules or of enzymes involved in the synthesis or breakdown of neurotransmitters or hormones are provoked by long-term drug administration, but the precise nature of these changes remains unknown.

THE ANALYSIS OF DRUG ACTION
ON THE NERVOUS SYSTEM
The neuron and the synapse—primary sites of drug action

The mammalian brain contains an incredibly complex collection of millions of nerve cells (neurons) with many billions of interconnections between

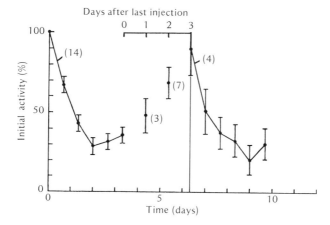

Fig. 2–4   Development of tolerance to morphine in mice. The effects of repeated doses of morphine (20 mg/kg every 16 hr) in stimulating running activity (measured with photocell cages) rapidly diminish. After six doses, drug treatment was stopped and some animals were tested with a single dose of morphine 1, 2, or 3 days later; note the reversal of tolerance during this period. When regular treatment was started again, tolerance again developed in a similar manner. (From Goldstein and Sheehan, 1969.)

them. The sheer numbers involved are difficult to imagine: 1 gm of cerebral cortical gray matter may contain 200 million neurons, and each of these on average makes contact with several thousand other neurons. When brain tissue is examined with an electron microscope, it presents an image of vast complexity (Fig. 2–5) including neurons, their many thin axonal and dendritic processes, and the specialized zones of contact between neurons known as synapses. Virtually all of the remaining space in the tissue is filled with the cytoplasm of the supporting cells, or neuroglia, of which there are several distinct varieties.

Although some synapses operate by direct electric communication between neurons, the great majority of synaptic contacts involve a process of chemical transmission, in which the arrival of a nerve impulse or an action potential at the terminal region of an axonal process leads to the release of a minute amount of chemical transmitter. This chemical messenger rapidly diffuses across the narrow cleft filled with extracellular fluid, that separates the nerve terminal from the dendrite or cell body of the neuron with which it communicates (the postsynaptic cell). The transmitter then acts upon spe-

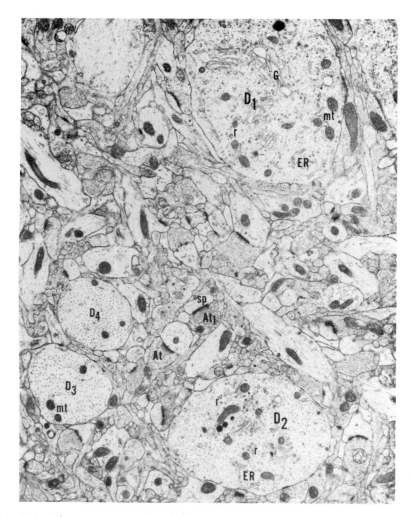

Fig. 2–5 Electron micrograph of the parietal cortex of the rat, layers II and III. The section is taken parallel to the surface of the cortex so that several apical dendrites (D₁-D₄) are seen in cross section. Note the tight packing of the neuropil. Sections through the base of dendrites contain Golgi apparatus (G), mitochondria (mt), endoplasmic reticulum (ER), ribosomes (r), and microtubules in their cytoplasm. Dendritic spines (sp) with axon terminals (At) synapsing on them can also be seen. Magnification, ×15,000. (From Peters, 1970.)

66

cialized receptor sites on the surface of the postsynaptic cell to trigger a rapid and short-lasting change in the permeability of the cell membrane. Depending on which transmitter substance and which type of receptor site are involved, this change in membrane permeability may either excite or inhibit the firing of action potentials by the postsynaptic cell. Excitation is usually accompanied by an increase in the permeability of the cell membrane to extracellular, positively charged ions, such as sodium, which then enters rapidly and momentarily depolarizes the postsynaptic cell. This, in turn, leads to the firing of a propagated action potential by the cell. Inhibitory synaptic transmission, however, is probably just as common as excitatory transmission in the mammalian CNS and is certainly just as important for the integrative functions of the neuronal network of the CNS, which would otherwise be in an uncontrolled and meaningless state of activity because of the rich interconnections between neurons. Inhibition is often brought about by a selective increase in the ionic permeability of the postsynaptic cell membrane to a negatively charged ion, such as chloride, which then enters to cause a hyperpolarization of the cell, making it relatively refractive to firing. In the mammalian CNS, most neurons receive a large number of synaptic inputs; large neurons in the cerebral cortex may have as many as 3000 to 4000 per cell. The inputs are both excitatory and inhibitory, so the activity of the cell from moment to moment is governed by the balance of these inputs. The neuron acts to integrate the excitatory and inhibitory synaptic inputs, which determine the rate of firing.

Although this simplified account might suggest that the CNS could function with only two transmitter substances—one for excitation and one for inhibition—this is not the case. At least 7 different amine and amino acid transmitter substances are known in mammalian CNS, with another 20 small peptides which may also function as neurotransmitters; and more probably remain to be discovered. The reason for this multiplicity of transmitters is not clear, but it may represent a mechanism for increasing the information content of the message transmitted across a synaptic junction, which may not simply be an "on" or "off" switch but may also involve more subtle long-term influences of the released transmitter on the postsynaptic cells. A multiplicity of transmitters may, in addition, control the firing of postsynaptic cells more flexibly, since the precise excitatory or inhibitory responses evoked by different transmitters are not the same, some producing, for example, inhibitory responses of very short duration (fractions of a millisecond), whereas others produce an inhibitory response of much longer duration (hundreds of milliseconds). The current list of established or candidate transmitter substances in CNS is given in Table 2–4; all of them are small, water-soluble molecules that diffuse easily. Most contain amine groups that are ionized at physiological pH, and the amino acid transmitters contain one or more carboxylic acid groups that are also ionized at physiological pH. Two of these substances, acetylcholine (ACh) and norepinephrine (NE) exist in the peripheral nervous system where they also act as transmitters, in this case mainly between neurons and a variety of effector tissues innervated by these neurons. Acetylcholine, for example, is the transmitter responsible for eliciting contraction from skeletal muscles in response to activity in the motor nerves innervating them. This amine is also released from both pre- and postganglionic parasympathetic nerves, mediating transmission between these two neurons in parasympathetic ganglia and between postganglionic parasympathetic nerves and the various muscle and glandular tissues of the viscera they innervate. Norepinephrine is the transmitter released by postganglionic neurons of the sympathetic nervous system; it elicits responses from the muscle and glandular tissues innervated by this system including heart muscle and the smooth muscle of the blood vessels, intestine, and urogenital system. The transmission of impulses from preganglionic sympathetic neurons to the NE-containing postganglionic neurons again involves ACh release from the preganglionic nerve terminals in sympathetic ganglia. Because ACh and NE were the first transmitters to be discovered, and because they can be studied easily in the readily accessible effector junctions and ganglia of the peripheral motor and autonomic nervous systems, a great deal of information is available about these two substances. The way in which they act on postsynaptic cells, the biochemistry of the mechanisms involved in their metabolism, release, and inactivation, and the actions of drugs on these systems are far better understood than are those for any of the other more recently discovered CNS transmitters. Fortunately, most of the knowledge gained from studies of cholinergic (acetylcholine) and adrenergic (catecholamine) mechanisms in the peripheral nervous system can be applied to those neuronal systems in the CNS that use these transmitters. A recent discovery is the unexpected finding that various small peptides are present in specific neuronal systems in mammalian brain (Table 2–4). Many of these peptides are already known to act as hormones or hormone-releasing factors in peripheral tissues and pituitary gland. Others are also found in the gut where they act as local hormones or modulators. The NEUROPEPTIDES seem likely to represent a new and diverse family of chemical messengers in CNS (Hughes, 1978; Emson, 1979).

Because many drugs that alter CNS function act primarily at the synaptic

Table 2–4. Neurotransmitter candidates in CNS

A. Amino acids and monoamines

Amines	Synonyms	Abbreviation	Transmitter status
Acetylcholine	—	ACh	OK
Dopamine	—	DA	OK
Norepinephrine	Noradrenaline	NE	OK
Epinephrine	Adrenaline	—	Probable
5-Hydroxytryptamine	Serotonin	5-HT	Probable
Histamine	—	—	Probable

Amino acids

Gamma-aminobutyrate	—	GABA	OK
Glycine	—	Gly	OK
Glutamate	—	Glu	Probable
Aspartate	—	Asp	Probable
Proline	—	Pro	Putative
Taurine	—	Tau	Putative

B. Neuropeptides (described in CNS at sites *other* than those related to endocrine or neuroendocrine functions)

Angiotensin II	—	—	?
Bombesin	—	—	?
Carnosine	—	—	Putative
Cholecystokinin	—	CCK	?
Corticotropin	—	ACTH	?
β-Endorphin	—	—	?
Leu-Enkephalin	—	—	Putative
Met-Enkephalin	—	—	Putative
Gastrin	—	—	?
Insulin	—	—	?
Luteinizing hormone releasing hormone	—	LHRH	?
Melanocyte stimulating hormone	—	α-MSH	?
Neurotensin	—	—	?
Oxytocin	—	—	?
Prolactin	—	—	?
Somatostatin	—	SRIF	?
Substance P	—	SP	Putative
Thyrotrophin releasing hormone	—	TRH	?
Vasoactive intestinal peptide	—	VIP	?
Vasopressin	—	—	?

level, the basic design and properties of synaptic junctions are worth considering in more detail. A typical CNS synapse is shown as it appears under
the electron microscope in Fig. 2–6, and in diagrammatic form in Fig. 2–7.
The synapse is an area of specialized contact between two cellular elements—the presynaptic nerve terminal and a small area of the surface of the
postsynaptic cell. The presynaptic element is often a "swollen" terminal of
one of the fine branches of the axons of the presynaptic neuron. In some
neurons, such synaptic swellings or *boutons* are not restricted to the axon
terminals but occur at many regions along the course of the axon, so that the
nerve fiber has a varicose appearance; each varicosity represents an area of
synaptic contact. Each nerve fiber can thus make contact with a large number of postsynaptic cells. This type of terminal arrangement is characteristic
of neurons using NE, DA, and 5-HT as transmitters. Such neurons appear
to release transmitter from numerous varicosities along their highly
branched nerve terminals—often without specialized synaptic contacts with
their target postsynaptic cells. The bouton or varicosity contains a store of
the transmitter, usually concentrated within the numerous small mem-
brane-enclosed spherical bodies known as SYNAPTIC VESICLES, which are
found in abundance in the cytoplasm of the presynaptic axon. The cytoplasm
of the bouton also contains mitochondria, all of the enzymes needed for
energy metabolism, and a special set of enzymes needed for the biosynthesis and metabolic breakdown of the transmitter. Each neuron normally
makes, stores, and releases only one type of transmitter from the many
branches of its axonal processes although some exceptions to this rule,
known as "Dale's principle," are now known to occur. The special enzymes
and other macromolecules needed for the storage and release of a particular
transmitter are found only in those neurons using that transmitter. Neurons
are thus biochemically differentiated, by virtue of the particular set of trans-
mitter-related macromolecules they contain, into "transmitter-specific"
types for the life of the animal. Although the bouton contains all this machinery, and can synthesize and store the transmitter locally, the macromolecules needed to catalyze these processes are synthesized in the cell body
or PERIKARYON of the neuron and must be transported down the length of
the axon as needed. This may explain why the transmitter and its related
enzymes are found throughout the neuron, including the perikaryon and
the preterminal axon, although they usually appear in much higher concentrations in the bouton.

The exact mechanism involved in the release of small amounts of transmitter from the presynaptic nerve terminal in response to waves of depolar-

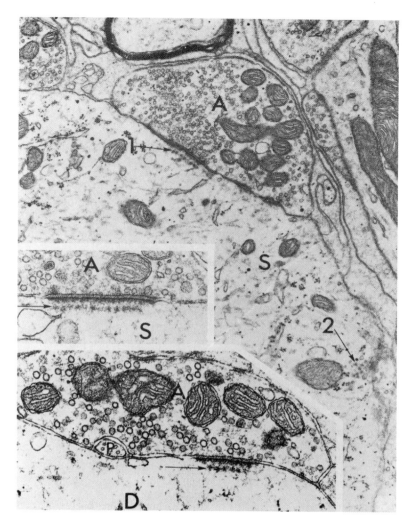

Fig. 2–6   Electron micrographs of synapses in cat oculomotor nucleus. A presynaptic terminal (A) makes synaptic contact with a large cell body (S), and under this synapse are a number of postsynaptic dense bodies (1). The insets show a similar synapse on a cell body and on a dendrite (D). Magnification, ×30,000 (insets, ×50,000). (From Pappas and Waxman, 1972.)

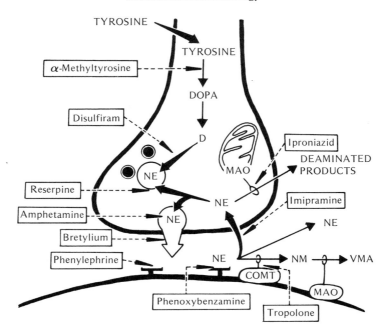

Fig. 2–7   A diagrammatic scheme indicating the multiple sites of drug action at a noradrenergic synapse. Some of the drugs that alter adrenergic transmission are shown; details of these actions are discussed in the text. COMT, catechol-O-methyl transferase; MAO, monoamine oxidase; NE, norepinephrine (noradrenaline); NM, normetanephrine; VMA, 3-methoxy, 4-hydroxymendelic acid; dopa, 3,4-dihydroxyphenylalanine. (From Rech and Moore, 1971.)

ization associated with the arrival of a nerve impulse at the terminal is not fully understood. The process has been most thoroughly studied at the neuromuscular junction. Here the arrival of a nerve impulse is followed by the release of ACh after a delay of about 0.3–0.4 msec. This burst of release of transmitter appears to occur as a consequence of the simultaneous release of the contents of several hundred synaptic vesicles. Shortly after the arrival of the action potential, these vesicles come into temporary contact with the external cell membrane of the nerve terminal, and areas of high permeability are formed in the neuronal membrane through which the vesicle contents are discharged to the exterior, a process known as EXOCYTOSIS. This process seems to be triggered by an inward movement of calcium ions from the extracellular fluid. Transmitter release in this and all other synapses is blocked if calcium is absent from the extracellular fluid. After the vesicles have discharged, they are apparently refilled by local biosynthesis of the transmitter.

The presynaptic nerve terminal is always separated from the postsynaptic cell by a gap, the synaptic cleft, containing extracellular fluid. The presynaptic terminal and postsynaptic cell, however, although separate, are tightly held together by fine threads of extracellular protein-mucopolysaccharide. In electron micrographs, the postsynaptic membrane appears thickened at the area of synaptic contact (Fig. 2–6), and sometimes a more complicated postsynaptic "web" structure may be seen. Most importantly, there are specialized receptor molecules in the postsynaptic membrane, which are so placed that the released transmitter diffusing across the cleft interacts with them to initiate the response of the postsynaptic cell. The nature of these receptors is still obscure, but recent studies suggest that they are proteins. Receptor molecules may be membrane proteins, which, in response to the transmitter, open or close pores known as IONOPHORES in the membrane, thus changing the membrane permeability to such inorganic ions as sodium, potassium, and chloride. Other types of receptor molecules may act by triggering reactions, catalyzed by membrane-bound enzymes; the end products of these reactions control membrane permeability by other mechanisms. For example, the production of cyclic AMP, which is apparently involved in synaptic transmission by some of the amine transmitters, is transmitter-stimulated.

Although each presynaptic terminal releases only one type of transmitter, the surface of the postsynaptic cell contains many different types of transmitter-receptor sites, since each cell receives inputs from presynaptic terminals using a variety of different transmitters, and receptors are transmitter-specific. It is even quite usual to find more than one type of receptor for a given transmitter; thus ACh interacts with two different types of receptor (see p. 87), which mediate quite different types of postsynaptic responses. Such receptors, however, usually occur on different postsynaptic cells. In skeletal muscle, only one type of cholinergic receptor exists, and these receptors are most dense in those regions of the muscle membrane immediately under the motor nerve terminals (the end-plate region). Whether transmitter receptors are similarly clustered under their appropriate nerve terminals in neurons in the CNS is not known.

Our knowledge of synaptic structure and function allows us to identify the various sites at which drugs may affect synaptic transmission. Drugs can act by altering the properties of (a) the presynaptic terminal and (b) the postsynaptic mechanisms. In the latter category are drugs that act directly on the transmitter receptors as agonists or antagonists of the naturally occurring transmitter. In this case, the "transmitter receptor" and the "drug receptor" are one and the same. There are also numerous sites at which drugs can act on the presynaptic machinery to alter the amount of transmitter released or to prolong its action after release. The possible roles of such drugs can be listed as follows:

Inhibitors of transmitter biosynthesis. Substances that inhibit one or another of the enzymes responsible for the normal replacement of transmitter in the presynaptic terminal. An alternative mode of action here would be to inhibit the uptake by the terminal of some precursor substance needed for transmitter synthesis.

False transmitters. Substances that are taken up and stored in presynaptic terminals and released in place of the naturally occurring transmitter. Such substances are usually less effective in stimulating the postsynaptic receptors and thus effectively depress synaptic transmission. This group also includes chemicals that can be converted by the normal biosynthetic enzymes into false transmitters.

Inhibitors of transmitter inactivation. Substances that potentiate and prolong the effects of the naturally occurring transmitter by inhibiting the normal mechanisms that terminate these effects at postsynaptic receptor sites. A degradative enzyme [e.g. acetylcholinesterase (AChE)], an "amine pump" mechanism, or both may be involved. For example, in monoaminergic neurons, the degradative enzyme monoamine oxidase (MAO) is present in nerve terminals that use catecholamine transmitters (NE and DA) or 5-HT and regulates the storage level of these amines, but these nerve terminals also possess specific uptake mechanisms that appear to terminate the effects of the amine transmitters. Inhibition of either mechanism tends to potentiate synaptic transmission in such neurons.

Depleting agents. The most widely used agent is the alkaloid, reserpine, which blocks normal storage of NE, DA, and 5-HT in synaptic vesicles and thus leads to a profound and long-lasting depletion of these three amines in the brain and to a block in synaptic transmission in neurons using these transmitters.

Displacing agents. Substances that effect the release of the endogenous transmitter onto receptor sites by displacing it from its neuronal storage sites. Such substances are themselves usually without direct affects on postsynaptic receptors but stimulate these receptors indirectly by releasing the endogenous transmitter.

Because neurons differ from other cells of the body in their biochemical machinery for transmission of nervous impulses, it is not surprising that many neuropharmacological agents act upon this machinery. Drugs that have this type of action are likely to act specifically on neurons, as opposed to other cells. Interference with other aspects of cell metabolism, such as protein synthesis or energy metabolism, is less likely *a priori* to selectively affect nervous system function.

Not all drugs act on the CNS at the synaptic transmission level. Some drugs affect the mechanisms involved in the propagation of nerve impulses in the neuronal membrane. Anesthetic drugs, for example, act to block propagation of the action potentials by changing the properties of the neuronal membrane; other more specific drugs selectively block membrane permeability channels for sodium and potassium, with the same result. The naturally occurring neurotoxins, TETRODOTOXIN (from the Japanese Pufferfish) and BATRACHOTOXIN (from the skin of a South American toad), act in this way. Such general interference with neuronal function, however, does not affect behavior in ways that can be studied, since such compounds are very toxic. Similarly, such drugs as the cardiac glycosides (e.g. ouabain) that block the active extrusion of sodium from cells and thus lead to depolarization of neurons and other excitable cells, or drugs that interfere with energy metabolism, do not affect behavior in ways that can be readily analyzed, since their action is so diffuse and undirected.

Having outlined some of the ways in which drugs can interact with the nervous system, we will briefly review some of the experimental approaches used by neuropharmacologists to determine how particular drugs work. These are broadly of two types: those measuring the effects of drugs on the electric activity of neurons in the CNS and those studying the effects of drugs by biochemical techniques.

Electrophysiological studies of drug activity in the CNS

Electrophysiology involves the study of electric neuronal activity, using sophisticated electronic equipment to amplify, record, and display the extremely small changes in current and voltage associated with such activity. There are two basic approaches: those that measure the overall electric activity of large populations of neurons and those that measure the electric activity of single neurons.

Neuronal population recording methods

Electroencephalography. This involves the recording of differences in electric potential (in microvolts) between different points on the surface of the brain; the waves thus obtained are amplified and recorded as an electroencephalogram (EEG). In animals, the relatively large electrodes used are usually placed on the surface of the brain, or inserted into the brain, through openings trephined in the skull; in man, the electrodes are placed on the scalp. Since EEG records are virtually the only form of electric recording feasible in human subjects, the method has been widely used in clinical studies.

Unfortunately, the EEG is a highly complex parameter, since it represents the resultant of electric changes in many thousands of neurons recorded by the electrodes. Nevertheless, the EEG is valuable in providing an overall index of the state of activation of such areas as the cerebral cortex. Characteristic changes in both the frequency and the amplitude of discharge of the EEG are known to be associated with different states of arousal and attention. Thus, for example, there are EEG changes typical of the various stages of sleep and of arousal, many of which can be mimicked by drugs. Barbiturates tend to produce an EEG pattern similar to that seen in normal slow-wave sleep; amphetamines, on the other hand, induce an EEG pattern characteristic of states of arousal (Fig. 2–8).

Evoked potentials. Evoked potentials are the electric changes, recorded from a relatively large electrode placed extracellularly, when a sensory pathway or remote brain area is stimulated. They represent the net result of complex firing patterns in the population of neurons affected by the stimulus. The pattern of a given evoked potential changes with states of arousal and sleep, and such changes can also be mimicked by certain drugs.

Single cell recording methods

Extracellular recording with electrodes. The activity of single neurons can be monitored in experimental animals by electrodes that usually consist of very fine diameter tungsten wire, insulated so that only the electrode tip records electric activity. By inserting such electrodes into precisely defined brain regions with stereotaxic manipulators, it is possible to record the discharge pattern of single cells in defined anatomical regions of the CNS. It may also be possible to identify the type of neuron from which the recording is being made by stimulating some remote brain region or a neuronal pathway from which the neurons are known to receive input or to which their axons project. For example, pyramidal cells in the cerebral cortex can be identified since they can be made to fire by stimulating the pyramidal tracts, thus evoking a flow of nerve impulses in the axons of these cells back to the

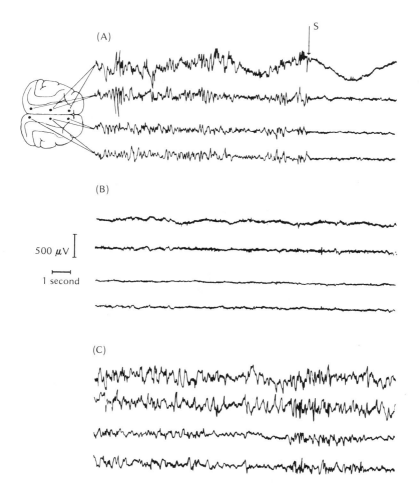

Fig. 2–8. Electroencephalographic records of electric activity in the cerbral cortex of an unanesthetized cat following administration of physostigmine and atropine. (A) Control record with an "arousal response" at S; (B) 10 min after 0.08 mg/kg physostigmine sulfate (i.p.); (C) 20 min after the subsequent injection of 3 mg/kg atropine sulfate (i.p.). (From Bradley and Elkes, 1957.)

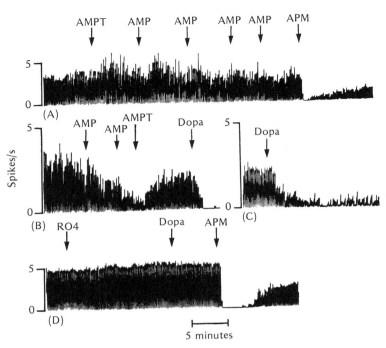

Fig. 2–9   Single cell recordings (rate meter trace) from dopaminergic neurons in the zona compacta of rat substantia nigra. In (A), treatment of animals with α-methyl-*p*-tyrosine (AMPT) 50 mg/kg prevented amphetamine (AMP) (1.0 mg/kg) inhibition of cell firing. Inhibition of firing by apomorphine (APM) (0.1 mg/kg) is, however, still seen. In (B), α-methyl-*p*-tyrosine reverses inhibition of cell firing by AMP given before the α-methyl-*p*-tyrosine. In (C), L-dopa inhibits cell firing similar to that seen after apomorphine. In (D), pretreatment with a large dose of dopa-decarboxylase inhibitor RO 4–4602 (RO4) (800 mg/kg) abolishes the inhibitory effects of L-dopa, although apomorphine inhibition still occurs. These results indicate that the effects of amphetamine and dopa on cell firing are indirect, involving in one case an induced release of endogenous dopamine and in the other conversion of L-dopa. (From Bunney, Aghajanian, and Roth, 1973.)

cell bodies in the cortex—in the reverse or "antidromic" direction to that in which the impulses normally travel. Figure 2–9 shows the results of an experiment in which amphetamine was found to alter the rate of firing of identified single neurons in that rat substantia nigra.

Extracellular recording with the iontophoretic application of drugs. The use of single cell recording in conjunction with a micromethod for the application of drugs to the immediate vicinity of the cell from which a recording is being made is one of the most powerful techniques of modern neuropharmacology. Application of drugs is by iontophoretic ejection of charged drug molecules from the tip of a finely drawn glass microelectrode. The rate of ejection of the drug can be controlled by regulating the current flowing through the electrode tip. The drug-containing electrode is part of a multibarreled electrode assembly in which one of the other electrodes is used to monitor the electric activity of the single cell. As many as four to six drug-containing electrodes together with a recording electrode can be used (Fig. 2–10), so that the effects of several drugs on the firing rate of a given cell can be measured (Fig. 2–11). Controls rule out effects due simply to change in pH, passage of electric current or diffusion of the drug to neighboring neurons. In addition, the amount of drug administered is generally proportional to the iontophoretic current applied through the microelectrode, so that it is possible to construct dose–response curves relating the graded effects of various amounts of drug on neuronal firing. A further refinement introduced in recent years is to study the effects of microiontophoretically applied drugs on physiologically identified neurons, using the methods for identifying single units described above. In this way, far more meaningful data on the pharmacological properties of neuron types in the CNS can be obtained. In much of the older literature, such techniques have not been

Fig. 2–10   Multibarreled microelectrode for application of chemicals by micro-electrophoresis.

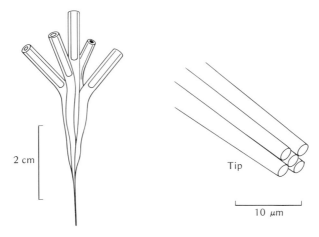

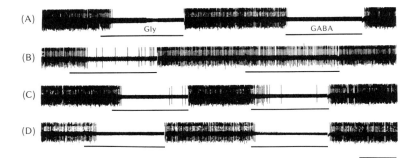

Fig. 2–11   The selective antagonistic action of bicuculline on the response of cuneo-thalamic relay neurons in cat brain to GABA. A continuous film records the firing of a touch cell whose discharge is maintained by constant iontophoretic release of glutamate. Cell responses to glycine and to GABA were tested alternately. The inhibitory responses at 14 nA of glycine and GABA in (A) were only just maximal, and bicuculline was relelased with a current of 168 nA, which began approximately 75 sec before the start of (B) and terminated between (B) and (C), which are continuous with each other and with (D). (Calibration, 5 sec.) (From Kelly and Renaud, 1973.)

applied to identified cell populations but simply to randomly selected neurons in a given brain area. Thus it is common to find that out of 100 cells tested with a given drug or transmitter 30% responded by excitation, 35% were inhibited, 25% did not respond at all, and the remaining 10% showed a mixed response with, for example, excitation followed by inhibition. When identified cell populations are tested, much more consistent results are usually obtained.

Despite the fact that iontophoretic application of drugs is a powerful tool for the direct investigation of drug action on receptor sites in the CNS, the technique has serious drawbacks. The electrode assemblies used are complicated, and the array of electrodes is fairly large. This means that drug application can rarely be restricted to single neurons, especially if they are small (see Fig. 2–10). Furthermore, the insertion of the electrode assembly into the brain necessarily produces some tissue damage in the region from which recordings are to be made. A difficulty in attempting to apply quantitative dose–response analysis to the effects produced by drugs administered iontophoretically is that there is no way of determining precisely what the concentration of administered drug is in the vicinity of the cell from which recordings are made, nor is it always known precisely how much drug is ejected from the microelectrodes by a given current. It is also necessary to use a very concentrated solution of the test drug to fill the drug electrodes, and this means that the test drug must be quite soluble in water; it must also, of course, carry a net positive or negative charge. Substances that are not readily water soluble or that lack ionized groups accordingly are not suitable for iontophoretic application. For such compounds a new technique involving the delivery of picoliter volumes of fluid from microelectrodes by a controlled pressure system is now becoming increasingly popular (Mc-Caman et al., 1977).

Intracellular recording techniques. The action of transmitters or related drugs on the membrane of postsynaptic cells can be analyzed most precisely when the tip of a very fine recording electrode can be inserted into the cells, while the test substance is administered to the external surface of the cell membrane through an extracellular electrode. This technique has been applied with considerable success to such peripheral synapses as the neuromuscular junction, but it has proved far more difficult to use in the CNS. It has, however, been possible to analyze the action of such CNS transmitters as NE, GABA, and glycine (Gly) in this way. The technique usually involves the construction of an assembly of glass microelectrodes as described above, but with the tip of the recording electrode set slightly in advance of the tips of the drug-containing electrodes. As the electrode assembly is slowly lowered into a brain region, large neurons may be impaled by the tip of the recording electrode, leaving the drug electrodes outside the cell. Because the recording electrode is very easily dislodged from its intracellular position, recording in this way is technically very difficult; a given cell can rarely be recorded from for more than a few seconds. Nevertheless, with such an arrangement, very sophisticated measurements of drug or transmitter action can be made. The test substance can be applied to the external surface of the cell, and changes in membrane potential and membrane resistance can be measured directly via the intracellular electrode.

The problems of intracellular recording from brain *in vivo* can be avoided by using thin slices of brain tissue incubated *in vitro*; such preparations offer stable conditions for intracellular recording, and neurons remain viable for several hours (Skrede & Westgaard, 1971). The *in vitro* brain slice preparation seems to offer considerable potential for detailed studies of drug and transmitter actions.

The biochemical analysis of drug actions on the CNS

In the last twenty years biochemical techniques have been applied with increasing frequency and success to the analysis of drug action on neuronal tissue. It is impossible to give more than a survey of the battery of tools now avilable for such studies and a broad outline of the types of approach possible with them. There are two levels at which biochemical analysis may be made: either by using an isolated preparation of brain slices, homogenates, or individual enzymes, receptor sites, etc., for the *in vitro* analysis of drug effects or by administering a drug to an animal and examining its effect on brain chemistry *in vivo*.

In vitro techniques

The various targets for drug action outlined in Fig. 2–7   can be isolated or dissected out and examined individually in various *in vitro* systems. For example, a drug that acts as an inhibitor or alternative substrate for enzymes involved in the biosynthesis or breakdown of transmitter substances can be studied directly in a test-tube system of the purified enzyme. Drugs that interfere with other aspects of metabolism, storage, uptake, or release of transmitters in presynaptic nerve terminals can be studied in *in vitro* systems containing presynaptic terminals isolated from brain homogenates. When brain tissue is disrupted by homogenization in an isotonic medium, the presynaptic nerve terminals tend to remain intact as "pinched-off" fragments, which round up to become membrane-bound spherical particles known as SYNAPTOSOMES.The synaptosomes can be harvested from brain homogenates by centrifugation techniques; they represent a useful system for studying drug effects, since they contain the machinery for transmitter metabolism and storage. Since synaptosomes take up and accumulate radioactively labelled transmitters, for example, they can be used to study drugs that inhibit such uptake, which probably represents the normal inactivation process for most transmitters in the CNS. Another widely used *in vitro* preparation is the brain slice. Thin slices of brain tissue remain metabolically viable for several hours if incubated in warm oxygenated saline solution, and they will take up transmitters or their precursors. These slices also release transmitters upon electric stimulation or application of transmitter-displaying drugs. They thus constitute a convenient system for studying the action of drugs on transmitter release processes and various other aspects of presynaptic neuropharmacology.

The analytical methods used for these *in vitro* studies, and for *in vivo* studies of transmitter metabolism, must be very sensitive since the concentration of any one transmitter substance in brain tissue is very low (micrograms per gram wet weight of brain). Such highly sensitive chemical techniques include measuring fluorescence or radioactivity of labelled transmitters or precursors.

A recent breakthrough in *in vitro* studies has been the development of methods that allow postsynaptic receptor mechanisms to be studied biochemically (Synder and Bennett, 1976; Yamamura, Enna and Kuhar, 1978). The most common approach involves the use of an antagonist or agonist drug that binds with a very high affinity and specificity to receptor sites. The drug is radioactively labelled, and its binding to intact tissues, to membrane fractions isolated from homogenates, or even to solubilized membrane proteins can be used to identify and quantify the receptor sites present. For example, the snake venom, α-BUNGAROTOXIN, binds with high specificity and affinity to cholinergic receptor sites on the surface of skeletal muscle—where it is a powerful antagonist—so that it can be used as a label to identify, count, and aid in the further isolation and purification of these receptor molecules. The specific receptor binding of a labelled antagonist drug to membrane fractions is defined by simultaneous incubation with a saturating concentration of nonradioactive agonists or antagonists of a given receptor and can be used as a biochemical index to identify and quantify drug and transmitter receptor sites in homogenates or slices of the mammalian CNS. Receptors for morphine and related opiate drugs, Gly, ACh, dopamine, NE, 5-HT, histamine, GABA, and neuropeptides (Table 2.5) have recently been studied this way.

In vivo techniques
One often-used approach has been to administer a drug to an animal and measure the changes in the concentration of transmitters or other chemical components of the brain. This technique was used to show that the alkaloid, reserpine, caused a profound and long-lasting depletion of catecholamines and 5-HT in the CNS. Changes in the steady-state concentration of chemical constituents of the cell in response to drug treatments, however, afford less information than dynamic changes induced by drugs in the release, resynthesis, or breakdown of the constituent being studied. Drugs may affect the rate of metabolic turnover of transmitters without necessarily changing the steady-state level. Transmitter turnover can be estimated by using a radioactively labelled transmitter or transmitter precursor and following the rate of appearance and disappearance of the labelled material in the brain. An index of the rate of turnover can sometimes also be obtained by measuring the concentration of transmitter metabolites present in the brain, since a more rapid breakdown of a transmitter (implying faster release and utilization in neuronal pathways) often leads to an accumulation of one or other of its degradative products. Homovanillic acid, for example, is the major metabolite formed during the breakdown of DA in the brain. The concentration

Table 2.5. Neurotransmitter receptor binding assays. Neurotransmitter receptors in mammalian CNS can be detected and studied by measuring the binding of radioactively labelled drugs

Receptor type	Radioligand(s)
Acetylcholine (muscarinic)	^{3}H-quinuclidinyl benzilate
	^{3}H-dexetimide
Acetylcholine (nicotinic)	^{125}I-α -bungarotoxin
GABA	^{3}H-GABA
	^{3}H-muscimol
Glycine	^{3}H-strychnine
Glutamate	^{3}H-kainic acid
Norepinephrine (α-adrenoceptor)	^{3}H-dihydroergocryptine
	^{3}H-prazosin
	^{3}H-clonidine
Norepinephrine (β-adrenoceptor)	^{3}H-dihydroalprenolol
	^{125}I-hydroxybenzylpindolol
Dopamine	^{3}H-haloperidol
	^{3}H-spiperone
	^{3}H-dopamine
	^{3}H-apomorphine
Opiate, enkephalin	^{3}H-naloxone
	^{3}H-dihydromorphine
	^{3}H-etorphine
	^{3}H-enkephalins
5-Hydroxytryptamine	^{3}H-5-hydroxytryptamine
	^{3}H-LSD
Histamine (H1 receptors)	^{3}H-mepyramine
Histamine (H2 receptors)	^{3}H-cimetidine
Angiotensin II	^{125}I-angiotensin II
Neurotensin	^{125}I-neurotensin

of this metabolite is increased under conditions in which DA release is accelerated, as is found after the administration of drugs that antagonize DA at its receptor sites in the CNS. Such receptor blockade causes a reflex increase in the rate of firing of dopaminergic neurons, which is interpreted as an attempt to counteract the effect of the drug. This is seen biochemically as an increase in DA turnover and an accumulation of homovanillic acid. The concept of "receptor feedback," as exemplified above, is useful in the analysis of agonist and antagonist drugs in the CNS, since antagonists generally increase the turnover of the transmitter whose receptors are blocked, whereas agonists tend to have the converse effect, selectively slowing turnover of the transmitter in question.

Other techniques are available that allow direct measurements of transmitter release to be made in intact brain preparations, although these usually involve the use of a fully anesthetized animal. Cannulae can be implanted into the CSF to perfuse the ventricular system or into the brain itself to perfuse a local region. Transmitter release can also be measured on the surface of the brain by means of a saline-filled collection cup placed there. The minute amounts of transmitter collected in such experiments often makes it necessary to prelabel the brain transmitter stores with radioactive transmitter or precursor in order to detect the material released. Techniques have been devised that allow such collection experiments to be performed on conscious animals by means of chronically implanted cannulae, thus permitting such studies to be undertaken during normal behavior. A promising new development makes use of chemically selective electrodes implanted in amine-rich areas of brain to monitor dopamine, NE, or 5-HT release by generating an electrochemical signal as these substances are oxidated at the electrode surface (Conti et al., 1978).

Neuropharmacology of individual neurotransmitter systems

Acetylcholine

Drug effects on metabolism (for review see Marchbanks, 1975). Acetylcholine (ACh) is synthesized from choline and the acetyl donor substance acetyl-coenzyme A (acetyl-CoA) in cholinergic nerve terminals; this reaction is catalyzed by the enzyme CHOLINE ACETYL TRANSFERASE (ChAc). Acetyl-CoA is formed during the metabolism of carbohydrates and fats in all living cells, but the choline needed for ACh synthesis depends upon a special membrane transport mechanism present only in cholinergic neurons. This uptake system has a very high affinity for choline and operates efficiently at external choline concentrations as low as 1 μM (Kuhar and Murrin, 1978). In the CNS, the biosynthetic enzyme ChAc is found only in cholinergic neurons; it is found in abundance in synaptosome fractions isolated from brain homogenates, which contain as much as 80% of the total tissue activity, indicating that most of the enzyme is localized in presynaptic nerve terminals. The biosynthesis of transmitter takes place in the cytoplasm of cholinergic terminals, but the resulting ACh is stored mainly within the synaptic vesicles in this cytoplasm. No drugs are known that act as specific inhibitors of ChAc, but one potent inhibitor of ACh synthesis is known. This is the compound HEMICHOLINIUM (HC3) (Fig. 2–12), which acts as a powerful inhibitor of the high affinity choline uptake system in the neuronal mem-

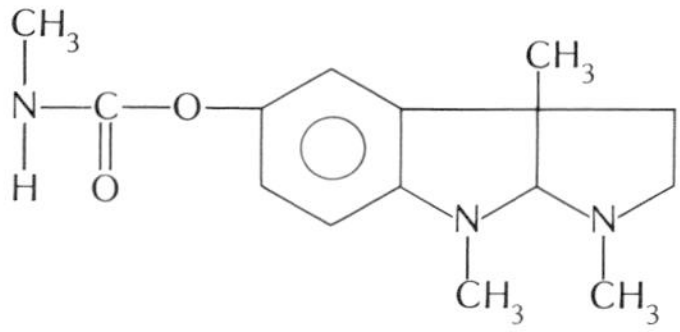

Physostigmine

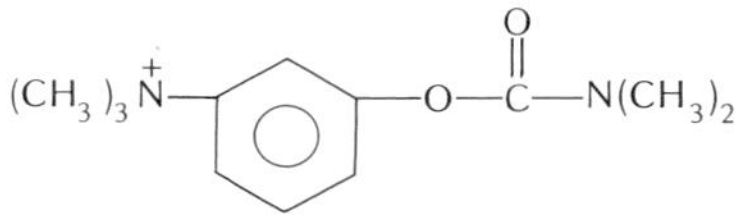

Neostigmine

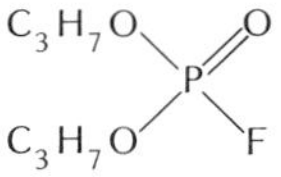

Diisopropylfluorophosphonate

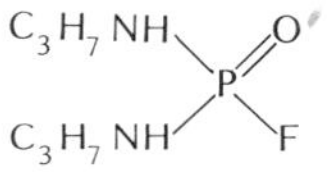

Mipafox

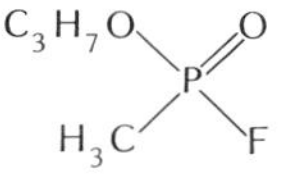

Sarin

(A) Inhibitors of Acetylcholinesterase

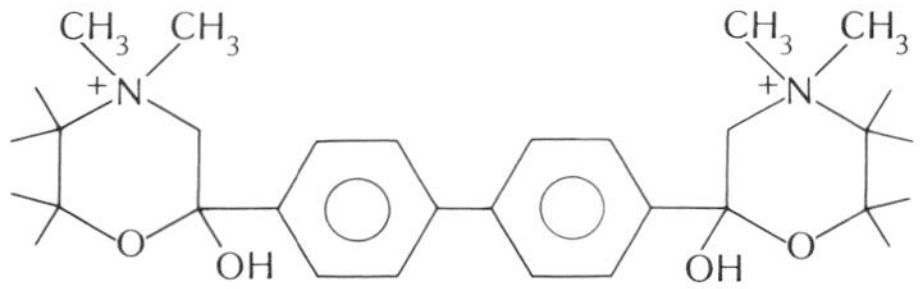

Hemicholinium (HC-3)

(B) Inhibitors of acetylcholine biosynthesis

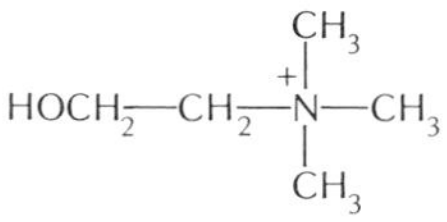

Choline

(C) Choline-precursor for acetylcholine biosynthesis

Fig. 2–12   Drugs that act on the synthesis and breakdown of acetylcholine.

brane, thus blocking the entry into the neuron of a vital precursor that cannot be synthesized locally within the cholinergic neuron. Unfortunately, HC3 does not penetrate readily into the CNS after systemic administration, although some penetration has been obtained by direct application on the brain or into the CSF.

Acetylcholine is metabolically degraded within cholinergic nerve terminals, and after its release from such terminals, by the enzyme ACETYLCHO-LINESTERASE, which hydrolyzes the transmitter to acetate and choline. The enzyme is present in or attached to the cellular and intracellular membranes of the presynaptic cholinergic neurons, but it is also present on the membrane of the postsynaptic or "cholinoceptive" cell. Acetylcholinesterase is an unusual enzyme in having an extremely high rate of catalytic action, a single molecule of enzyme being able to catalyze the breakdown of more than 100,000 molecules of ACh per minute. It is thus ideally suited for its main task, which is to inactivate ACh after release from cholinergic nerve terminals. This inactivation is by conversion of the transmitter to pharmacologically inert metabolites; since the enzyme is situated on the post- and pre-synaptic membranes, it has ready access to ACh in the synaptic cleft. In addition, AChE regulates the storage level of transmitter within the presynatic terminal by degrading any ACh synthesized in excess of the storage capacity of the synaptic vesicles. Numerous drugs are available that act as selective and potent inhibitors of AChE (Fig. 2–12). Not all of these compounds, however, penetrate into the CNS after systemic administration. PHYSOSTIGMINE and such organophosphorus inhibitors as DIISOPROPYL-FLUOROPHOSPHONATE (DFP) and SARIN have high CNS activity, whereas NEOSTIGMINE has little or no CNS activity owing to its poor penetration of the blood–brain barrier.

Few drugs are known that affect ACh storage or release. BOTULINUM TOXINS act specifically to block the release of ACh normally evoked by nerve impulses from cholinergic terminals, but they have little or no CNS application.

Agonist and antagonist drugs at cholinergic receptors. Although there are relatively few drugs that affect presynaptic cholinergic mechanisms, many drugs act as agonists or antagonists at postsynaptic cholinergic receptors. Two major categories of cholinergic receptor site are known, the MUSCAR-INIC and the NICOTINIC. In the peripheral nervous system, muscarinic receptors are found in all the postsynaptic cells innervated by the parasympathetic nervous system; the action of the vagus nerve in slowing the heart,

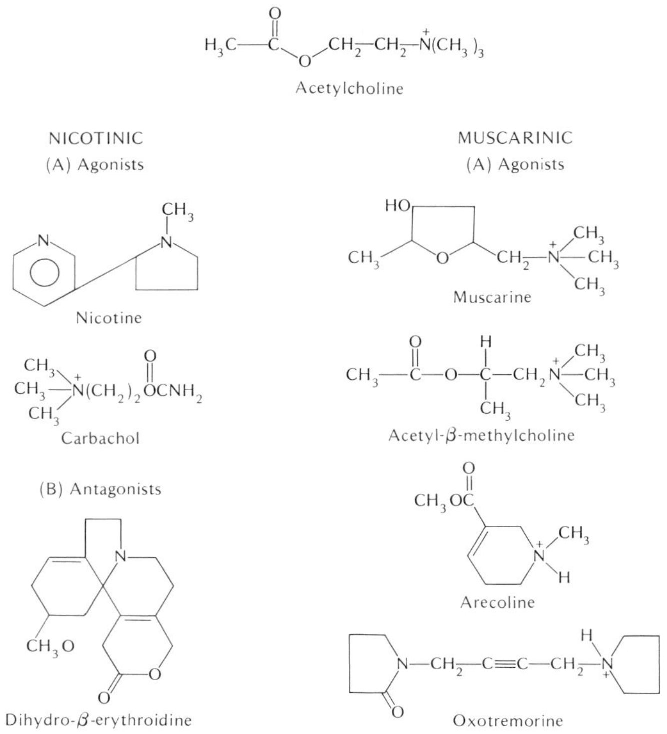

Fig. 2–13   Agonists and antagonists at cholinergic synapses.

for example, is mediated by such receptors. These are identified by the use of the drug MUSCARINE (Fig. 2–13), which mimics the actions of ACh on such receptor sites. Other agonists that are selective for muscarinic sites are ACETYL-β-METHYLCHOLINE, ARECOLINE, PILOCARPINE, and OXOTREMORINE. The latter substance has high CNS activity; as its name implies, it induces a Parkinson-like tremor in experimental animals. Acetylcholine itself and acetyl-β-methylcholine and arecoline penetrate only very poorly into the CNS after systemic administration.

ATROPINE is the classical muscarinic antagonist drug, and several related substances, such as HYOSCINE (SCOPOLAMINE) and BENZTROPINE, have similar effects; all three drugs act centrally. METHYL ATROPINE is a potent antagonist peripherally but does not penetrate the blood–brain barrier to any significant extent.

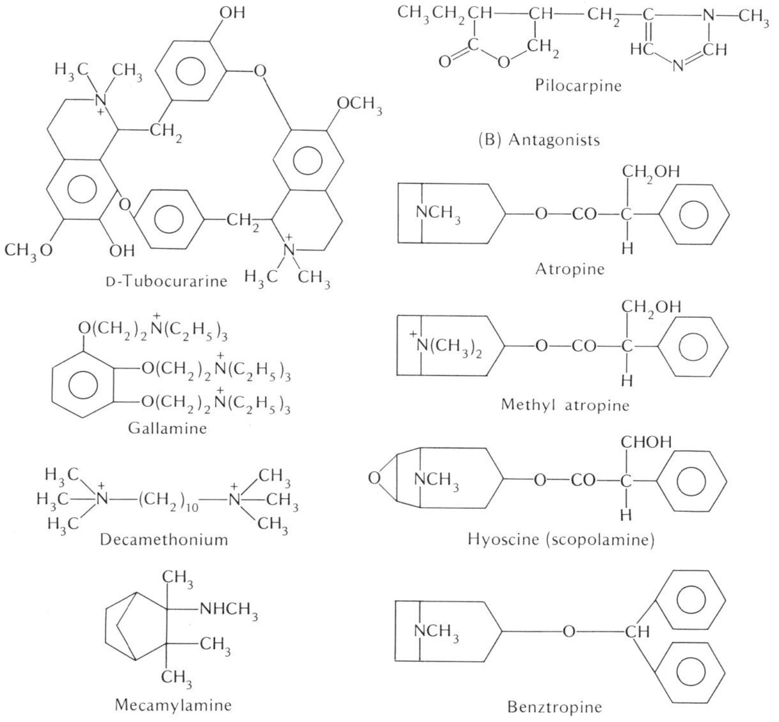

OH

CH_3CH_2CH——CH——CH_2—C——N—CH_3

Pilocarpine

H_3C CH_3

OCH_3

(B) Antagonists

CH_2

CH_3O OH

D-Tubocurarine H_3C CH_3

CH_2OH

NCH_3 —O—CO—C—

H

Atropine

$O(CH_2)_2\overset{+}{N}(C_2H_5)_3$

$O(CH_2)_2\overset{+}{N}(C_2H_5)_3$

$O(CH_2)_2\overset{+}{N}(C_2H_5)_3$

Gallamine

$\overset{+}{N}(CH_3)_2$ —O—CO—C—

CH_2OH

H

Methyl atropine

H_3C

H_3C—$\overset{+}{N}$—$(CH_2)_{10}$—$\overset{+}{N}$—CH_3

H_3C CH_3

Decamethonium

NCH_3 —O—CO—C—

$CHOH$

H

Hyoscine (scopolamine)

CH_3

—$NHCH_3$

—CH_3

CH_3

Mecamylamine

NCH_3 —O——CH

Benztropine

The nicotinic category of cholinergic receptor is so named because the action of ACh on such sites is mimicked by the drug NICOTINE. Two subcategories of nicotinic receptor exist in the peripheral nervous system, one on skeletal muscles mediating the effects of ACh on neuromuscular junctions, the other mediating the effects of ACh on autonomic ganglia. These two subcategories differ slightly in their sensitivity to drugs, and particularly to antagonists. All nicotonic receptors are selectively stimulated by the agonist drugs NICOTINE and CARBAMYLCHOLINE (CARBACHOL) (Fig. 2–14). The antagonists D-TUBOCURARINE, GALLAMINE, and DECAMETHONIUM act primarily on nicotinic receptors in muscle, whereas HEXAMETHONIUM, MECAMYLAMINE, PEMPIDINE, and CHLORISONDAMINE are selective ganglion-blocking drugs. None of these drugs penetrate the blood–brain barrier to any significant extent, although they can be used centrally if injected directly into the CSF or the brain.

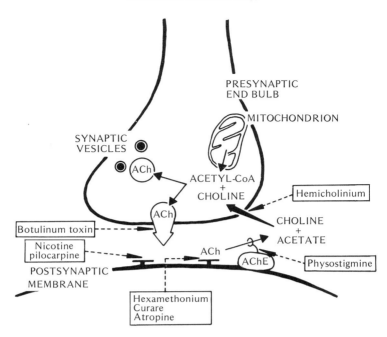

Fig. 2–14   Sites of drug action at a cholinergic synapse (cf. Fig. 2–7). (From Rech and Moore, 1971.)

In studying the molecular basis of nicotinic receptor action, the use of α-bungarotoxin has allowed progress to be made in isolating and purifying nicotinic receptors from skeletal muscle and from the electric organs of electric eels and fish; these latter are excellent sources for such receptors. The muscarinic actions of ACh in such peripheral organs as the heart, and possibly also the brain, have been found to be associated with increased production of the cyclic nucleotide cyclic-3'5'-guanosine monophosphate (cyclic GMP), suggesting that stimulation of muscarinic receptors by ACh leads to a stimulation of guanylate cyclase, the enzyme responsible for synthesis of this nucleotide. How cyclic GMP may then affect cell permeability to produce the characteristic tissue responses elicited by muscarinic stimulation is not yet known.

Cholinergic receptors in the CNS. The iontophoretic application of ACh evokes a response in a varying proportion of neurons in different brain regions. The response is usually excitatory, although some cells show only depression of firing and some may show excitation followed by depression.

There are only a few clearly defined systems in which cholinergic responses of known cell types have been analyzed. One of these is the Renshaw cell in the spinal cord. These cells are small inhibitory interneurons situated near large motor neurons in the ventral horn; they receive a cholinergic excitatory input from collateral axon branches of the cholinergic motor nerves as they leave the spinal cord. The Renshaw cells, in turn, send an inhibitory input to the motor neurons, thus constituting a self-damping feedback loop for motor neuron activity. The effects of ACh on Renshaw cells have been extensively studied; the cells can be easily identified, since they are excited when motor nerves are stimulated antidromically. Iontophoretically applied ACh mimics the normal excitatory synaptic potentials of these cells; ACh activity appears to be mediated mainly by nicotinic receptors, i.e. the effects are mimicked by nicotine and carbachol and blocked by dihydro-β-erythroidine and d-tubocurarine, whereas atropine blocks the effects only weakly. In contrast, cholinergic responses in most supraspinal regions of the CNS, such as the hypothalamus, basal ganglia, and cerebral cortex, appear to be predominantly muscarinic in character. The action of ACh iontophoretically applied to physiologically identified pyramidal Betz cells in the cortex has been especially thoroughly studied. A high proportion of these cells are excited by iontophoretically applied ACh; muscarine rather than nicotine mimics this action, and atropine rather than dihydro-β-erythroidine blocks it.

Catecholamines

The catecholamines DA and NE are present in specific neuronal pathways in the mammalian CNS, where they almost certainly act as transmitters. Epinephrine is formed from norepinephrine but is present in mammals mainly as an adrenal medullary hormone, occurring only in small amounts in the CNS. Although DA and NE are present in different neuronal pathways in the CNS, and serve independent transmitter functions, the basic pharmacological and biochemical properties of the two types of adrenergic neuron are so similar that the effects of drugs on the presynaptic adrenergic terminals will not be considered separately.

Drug effects on metabolism. The catecholamines are synthesized from the amino acids L-phenylalanine and L-tyrosine by a multi-enzyme pathway in adrenergic neurons (Fig. 2–15). The enzyme TYROSINE HYDROXYLASE catalyzes the hydroxylation of phenylalanine to tyrosine and the further hydroxylation of tyrosine to the catechol amino acid L-dopa. This is decarboxylated by AROMATIC AMINO ACID DECARBOXYLASE (sometimes called DOPA-DECAR-

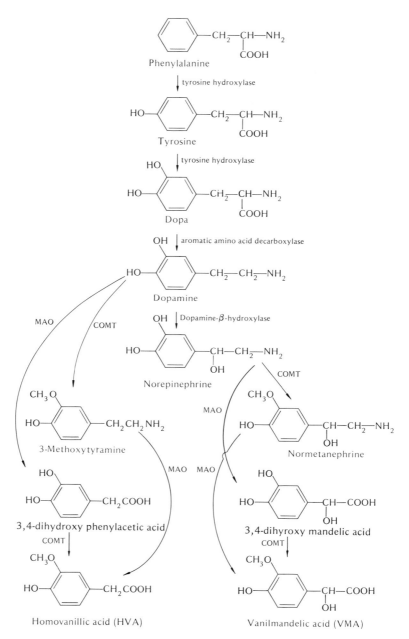

Fig. 2–15 Synthesis and metabolism of the catecholamines. MAO, monoamine oxidase; COMT, catechol-*O*-methyl transferase.

BOXYLASE), and the produced DA is converted to NE by another hydroxy-lating enzyme DOPAMINE-β-HYDROXYLASE. Dopaminergic neurons lack the latter enzyme, and DA is thus the end product of biosynthesis in these cells. The other two enzymes are present in both types of adrenergic neuron, and, in each case, tyrosine hydroxylase has a much lower activity than aromatic amino acid decarboxylase, thus catalyzing the slowest step in the pathway and governing the overall rate of catecholamine synthesis. The tyrosine hy-droxylase reaction is regulated by a series of complex mechanisms to adjust the rate of catecholamine synthesis to meet the moment-to-moment de-mands for transmitter release. Tyrosine hydroxylase and aromatic amino acid decarboxylase are present in the cytoplasm of the adrenergic nerve terminals, whereas dopamine-β-hydroxylase is strictly localized to the membranes of synaptic vesicles in noradrenergic terminals. Since tyrosine hydroxylase is the rate-limiting enzyme for the overall pathway, drugs that inhibit this enzyme are the most effective in limiting the overall rate of catecholamine biosynthesis. The most commonly used inhibitor of tyrosine hydroxylase is the amino acid α-METHYL-p-TYROSINE (Fig. 2–16), which is an effective inhibitor of the enzyme *in vitro* and *in vivo*. After administration *in vivo*, this compound causes a near total inhibition of DA and NE synthesis in all parts of the body, which lasts for 6 to 8 hr. Because α-methyltyrosine is not very soluble, the methyl ester, which is more soluble in water, is often used for *in vivo* administration; this compound is converted to α-methylty-rosine in the body.

It is possible to inhibit the synthesis of NE without affecting that of DA by using drugs that act as inhibitors of dopamine-β-hydroxylase; these in-clude DISULFIRAM (DIETHYLDITHIOCARBAMATE) and FLA-63 (Fig. 2–16). Although these components are effective inhibitors of NE synthesis *in vivo*, they are, unfortunately, not very specific, since they both act by forming complexes with copper, which is present as an integral part of the enzyme dopamine-β-hydroxylase. These drugs thus tend to inhibit a variety of other copper-dependent enzymes and are more toxic and less specific than one would wish for drugs that are used in behavioral studies.

Another way in which drugs can interact with the catecholamine biosyn-thetic pathway is as substrates for one or another of the enzymes involved. Thus, L-DOPA is a useful substance for systemic administration, since, unlike the catecholamines, it penetrates the blood–brain barrier and is converted in the CNS to DA and, to a lesser extent, NE. A related amino acid, 3,4-DIHYDROXYPHENYLSERINE (DOPS), also enters the CNS and is converted by decarboxylation directly to NE. The NE formed after DOPS administra-

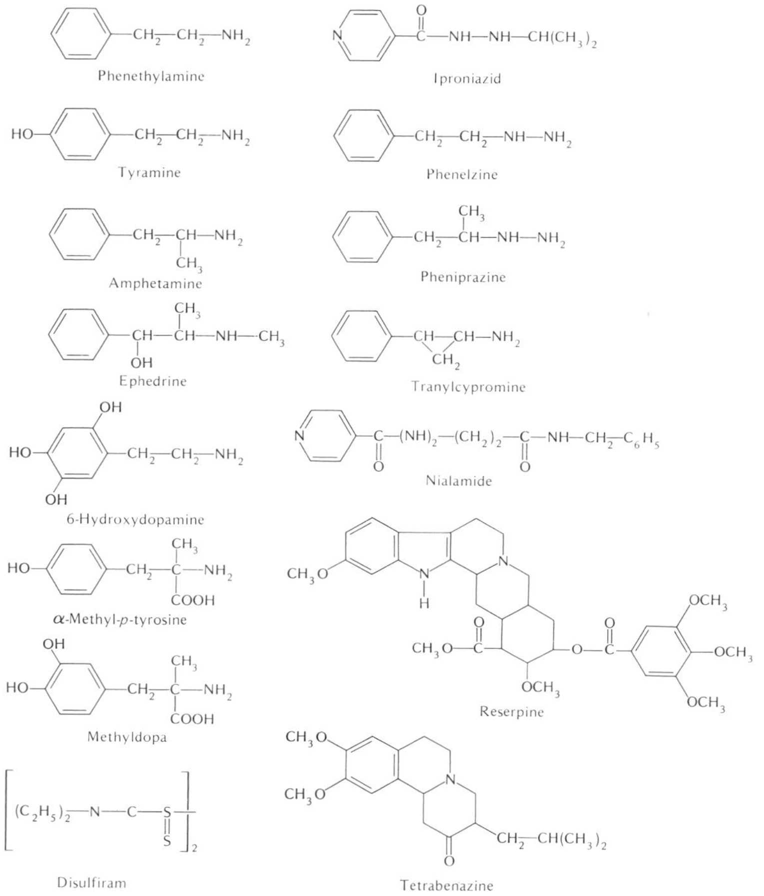

Fig. 2–16   Drugs that act at adrenergic synapses.

tion may not necessarily be in appropriate cellular locations, however, since the amino acid can be decarboxylated by aromatic amino acid decarboxylase in DA and 5-HT neurons as well as in noradrenergic neurons. The amino acids α-METHYLDOPA and α-METHYLMETATYROSINE also enter the brain and can be metabolized to the amines α-methyltyramine, metaraminol, α-methyldopamine, and α-methylnorepinephrine. These amines can be stored and released from adrenergic neurons, and their effects are generally less potent than those of the normal catecholamines; they thus act as "false transmitters," diluting and diminishing the effectiveness of the naturally oc-curring transmitters.

Metabolically, NE and DA are degraded by similar pathways involving two enzymes: catechol-O-methyltransferase (COMT) and monoamine oxi-dase (MAO) (Fig. 2–15). These two enzymes, unlike AChE, are not local-ized at adrenergic synapses, but are widely distributed in neurons and glial cells of the CNS and peripheral tissue. Both enzymes, however, are present in adrenergic neurons, with COMT localized in the cytoplasm and MAO in the mitochondria. The latter enzyme in particular seems to play an im-portant role in regulating the steady-state storage level of NE and DA in adrenergic neurons. Inhibitors of COMT include the simple aromatic compounds CATECHOL and PYROGALLOL and the more potent ISOPROPYLTROPOLONE (THUJAPLICIN). Numerous inhibitors of MAO are known, and many of these compounds are used clinically in the treatment of depression (Fig. 2–16); they include such hydrazine analogues of the cate-cholamines as IPRONIAZID, PHENELZINE, and PHENIPRAZINE and such non-hydrazines as PARGYLINE and TRANYLCYPROMINE. All of these compounds can produce a marked and long-lasting inhibition of MAO *in vivo*, the effects of a single dose persisting for several days. After administration of an MAO inhibitor, the concentrations of DA and NE in the CNS and peripheral tis-sues are increased, often by more than 100% over normal steady-state con-centrations. Neither COMT nor MAO are specific for the catecholamines; COMT will catalyze the methylation of a variety of substrates that have a catechol grouping in the molecule, and MAO will oxidatively deaminate many different amines. Substrates for MAO include the indolamine trans-mitter 5-HT (see p. 102) and various phenylethylamine and indolamine drugs related in structure to the catecholamines or to 5-HT. Drugs that have an α-methyl substituent adjacent to the amine group, however, are not sub-strates for MAO. Thus, the false transmitter amines α-methyldopamine and α-methylnorepinephrine are not degraded by MAO, and this is one factor contributing to the persistence of these substances in adrenergic neurons after administration of their precursors.

Drug effects on other aspects of presynaptic adrenergic mechanisms. There are various other sites of drug activity at adrenergic terminals (cf. Fig. 2–7). The catecholamines are inactivated after their release mainly by processes of reuptake, whereby released amines are taken up from the extracellular fluid by high-affinity transport systems located in the axonal membrane of the presynaptic terminals. The uptake systems in dopaminergic and noradrenergic neurons in the CNS are similar in their basic properties, but they differ in their sensitivity to drug inhibition. Thus, although some substances such as AMPHETAMINE and COCAINE, act as potent inhibitors of both systems, other drugs are more potent inhibitors of one rather than the other. The most striking difference in drug sensitivity is the effects of such tricyclic antidepressants as IMIPRAMINE and AMITRIPTYLINE, and their derivatives. These substances are very potent inhibitors of the uptake system in NE-containing neurons, acting at concentrations as low as 0.01 μM, but they are one hundred to one thousand times less potent as inhibitors of the DA uptake system in dopaminergic nerve terminals. Conversely, some drugs, notably the anti-parkinsonian drug BENZTROPINE (see Fig. 2–13), are more potent inhibitors of DA than of NE uptake; benztropine is approximately thirty times more effective in the former system. Benztropine has already been described as an anticholinergic drug of the atropine type; its potent effects on DA uptake sites illustrate the common finding that drugs may have multiple sites of action in CNS tissues—a fact that always makes interpretation of drug effects on behavior in neuropharmacological terms extremely difficult. Hardly any drugs have completely specific, single neuropharmacological sites of action, and yet we must argue from the known pharmacological effects of drugs to interpret their mode of action in eliciting behavioral changes. One partial solution to this problem is to test many drugs on a given system. If a given behavioral syndrome is always associated with drugs having a particular neuropharmacological site of action, a more convincing case for the existence of a causal relationship between these phenomena may be established, since other secondary pharmacological activities of a group of drugs are unlikely to be similar.

The storage of catecholamines at adrenergic nerve terminals involves complex chemical mechanisms within the synaptic vesicles, whereby very high concentrations of catecholamine are maintained inside these vesicles by the formation of a complex with the nucleotide adenosine triphosphate (ATP). These storage mechanisms also represent a target for drug action. The alkaloid RESERPINE (Fig. 2–16) and some of its derivatives and TETRABENAZINE and its derivatives act to block the vesicle amine storage system; these drugs can severely deplete catecholamines and 5-HT in adrenergic neurons in the brain and peripheral nervous system. The amine is released from its normal storage sites and degraded by MAO within the adrenergic terminals and no massive release of catecholamine outside the nerve terminal occurs after reserpine administration; the resulting depletion is very long lasting. It may take 1 or 2 weeks for the CNS concentrations of DA and

NE to return to normal. Tetrabenazine has a similar mode of action, but its effects are of much shorter duration, with amine concentrations returning to normal within 24 hr. Another important group of drugs also affect catecholamine storage sites, but they act by displacing the catecholamines and promoting their release into the extracellular fluid, thus mimicking the effects normally produced by adrenergic nerve activity. These compounds are all structural analogues of NE and DA and belong to a large group of phenylethylamine compounds that have pharmacological activity similar to that of the catecholamines; they are known as the SYMPATHOMIMETIC AMINES. Drugs that mimic catecholamine actions by displacing NE and DA from their normal storage sites are termed "indirectly" acting sympathomimetics, in contrast to directly acting sympathomimetics that mimic amine actions by functioning as agonists at adrenergic receptor sites on postsynaptic tissues (see below). Some of the sympathomimetic amines may show both types of activity, acting directly as an agonist and also displacing catecholamines from adrenergic terminals. The activity of such purely indirectly acting sympathomimetics as β-PHENETHYLAMINE, OCTOPAMINE, TYRAMINE, and AMPHETAMINE is easily distinguished, since their sympathomimetic effects disappear when the adrenergic terminals are destroyed surgically or by chemical sympathectomy or when catecholamine stores are depleted with reserpine or by the synthesis inhibitor α-methyl-p-tyrosine.

Certain drugs affect adrenergic nerve terminals because they are substrates for the amine uptake mechanisms; they are thus selectively concentrated within adrenergic neurons as opposed to other tissues of the body. The compound 6-HYDROXYDOPAMINE (Fig. 2–16) is taken up by adrenergic nerve terminals; there it reacts to produce a permanent degeneration. 6-Hydroxydopamine acts on both dopaminergic and noradrenergic neurons in the CNS, provided it is directly introduced into the brain or CSF, and it can cause a permanent and near total loss of the catecholamine nerve terminals in the brain and spinal cord in experimental animals. It has proved a most useful research tool for investigating the activity of drugs thought to exert effects via the above pathways.

Agonists and antagonists at catecholamine receptors. As is the case for ACh, the actions of NE are mediated by two categories of receptor site, the α- and β-ADRENOCEPTORS. α-Adrenoceptors, for example, mediate the action of NE in causing contraction of vascular smooth muscle cells and are thus important in controlling blood pressure by regulating peripheral resistance. β-Adrenoceptors mediate the action of NE in stimulating the contraction of heart muscle or in causing relaxation of smooth muscle cells in the intestine and bronchi. These two types of receptor are thus not simply excitatory or inhibitory, but are distinguished rather by the fact that they have different agonist and antagonist specificities, as are nicotinic and muscarinic cholinergic receptors. Both types of receptor respond to the catecholamines norepinephrine, epinephrine (E), and ISOPROTERENOL, but the order of potencies of these agonists on the two receptors is quite different, being, for α-adrenoceptors, NE = E> ISOPR and, for β-adrenoceptors, ISOPR> E = NE. There are also different antagonist drugs that selectively block one or the other of the receptor types (Fig. 2–17). Among the α-adrenoceptor antagonists are PHENOXYBENZAMINE, DIBENAMINE, PHENTOLAMINE, TOLAZOLINE, and YOHIMBINE, all of which can act centrally. β-Adrenoceptor antagonists include DICHLOROISOPRENALINE, BUTOXAMINE, and PROPRANOLOL.

Both the α- and β-adrenoceptors can be further divided into subtypes, known as α1 and α2 and β1 and β2. These can be distinguished by the existence of selective agonist and antagonist drugs which act only, or preferentially, on one of the subtypes, whereas the majority of α- and β-adrenoceptor drugs act with comparable potencies on each receptor subtype. The recently described α2-adrenoceptors are a special type which is located on the nerve terminals of adrenergic nerves. NE released from such nerves acts on the α2-receptors to inhibit its own release, and these so-called AUTORECEPTORS thus represent a negative feedback control system which acts to dampen transmitter release. Similar autoreceptor mechanisms are known to exist on cholinergic, dopaminergic, and other transmitter-specific neurons. The α2-adrenoceptors are selectively blocked by certain antagonists, such as yohimbine and stimulated by selective agonists such as CLONIDINE (Table 2–6). α1-Adrenoceptors are the conventional type located postsynaptically on smooth muscle and other effector tissues. Selective antagonists are PRAZOSIN and WB-4101 and agonists are PHENYLEPHRINE and METHOXAMINE.

β-adrenoceptor subtypes, β1 and β2 occur postsynaptically and different tissues contain different proportions of the two types. Thus β1 receptors predominate in heart and fat tissue and mammalian brain, while β2-receptors are found in uterus and tracheal smooth muscle and in bird or frog brain. Selective antagonists and agonists are listed in Table 2–6.

There is little evidence that dopaminergic neurons exist outside the CNS in mammals, so the pharmacology of DA receptor sites is less clearly understood than that of NE receptor sites, which have been studied mainly in peripheral tissue preparations. Studies of DA receptor sites in the CNS, however, suggest that APOMORPHINE and related derivatives and PIRIBEDIL

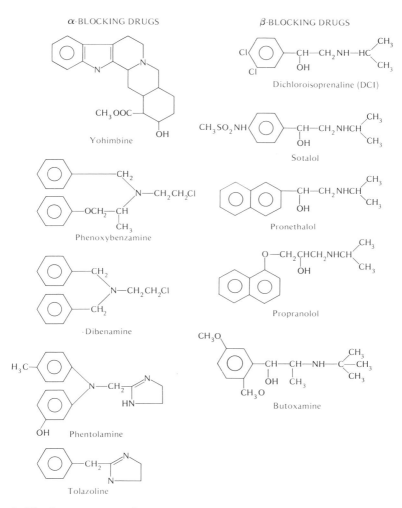

Fig. 2–17   Antagonists at adrenergic receptors.

(ET495) can act as selective agonists, whereas antagonists include the neu-roleptic drugs CHLORPROMAZINE and related PHENOTHIAZINES, HALOPERI-DOL and related BUTYROPHENONES, PIMOZIDE, and CLOZAPINE (see Figs. 10–1, 10–2). Some of these drugs, notably chlorpromazine, are also quite potent antagonists at α-adrenoceptors, and, in addition, have other proper-ties as local anesthetics. Nevertheless, an overlapping specificity between dopaminergic and noradrenergic receptor sites might be expected in view

Table 2–6. Multiple receptor subtypes for catecholamines

| | Norepinephrine | | | | Dopamine | |
| | Alpha | | Beta | | | |
	α1	α2	β1	β2	D1	D2
Example of cellular location	vascular smooth muscle	NE nerve terminals	Heart	Trachea	Retina	Anterior pituitary
Nonselective agonists	NE,E	NE, E	ISOPR, E,NE	ISOPR,E,NE	DA, apomorphine (partial)	DA apomorphine
Selective agonists	Methoxamine Phenylephrine	Oxymetazoline Clonidine Tramazoline	—	Carbuterol Salbutamol Terbutaline	—	Piribedil Bromocriptine
Nonselective antagonists	Phentolamine	Phentolamine	(—)Propranolol	(—)Propranolol	Chlorpromazine Fluphenazine	Chlorpromazine Fluphenazine
Selective antagonists	Phenoxybenzamine Prazosin, WB-4101	Yohimbine Mianserin Piperoxane	Practolol, Atenolol Tolamolol	H35/25	cis-Flupenthixol cis-Piflutixol	Haloperidol Spiperone Metaclopramide Sulpiride
Selective radioligand	^{3}H-Prazosin	^{3}H-Clonidine	—	—	^{3}H-Flupenthixol	^{3}H-Spiperone

References: Berthelson and Pettinger, 1977 (α-adrenoceptors); Clark, 1976 (β-adrenoceptors); Kebabian and Calne, 1979 (dopamine receptors).

of the close structural similarity between DA and NE. There is sufficient evidence that the receptor sites for DA do belong to a separate category that is distinguishable from either α- or β-adrenoceptors.

As with the NE receptors, DA receptors can be further categorized into D1 and D2 subtypes (Kebabian and Calne, 1979). The D1 type is characterized by its coupling to cyclic AMP formation, and is found in all dopamine-rich areas of brain and in retina. The D1 receptors are potently antagonized by many neuroleptic drugs (see Chapter 10) but only weakly by those of the butyrophenone series. D2-receptors are also found in most brain areas and on cells in the anterior pituitary, where dopamine acts to inhibit the release of the hormone prolactin. D2 sites are not cyclic AMP coupled, and are potently inhibited by butyrophenones such as haloperidol and spiperone. Bromocriptine and related ergot derivatives are potent agonists of D2 receptors, but act only as antagonists at D1 sites (Table 2–6).

Catecholamine receptors in CNS. Understanding the actions of catecholamines in the CNS is not made easier by the fact that all six catecholamine receptor subtypes (α1, α2, β1, β2, D1, and D2) appear to exist in brain. Biochemical studies, using radioligand binding assays and measurements of cyclic AMP changes elicited by NE and DA, show unequivocally that all of the receptor subtypes occur in mammalian brain, with different proportions of the various receptors in different brain regions and in different species. While DA receptors occur only in those regions of brain (and retina) that normally contain DA neurons, NE receptors appear to be widespread in all brain regions. In view of the multiplicity of catecholamine receptors in CNS and lack of knowledge of their detailed cellular locations, it is perhaps not surprising that neurophysiological studies of catecholamine actions in brain have yielded complex results (Moore and Bloom, 1978; 1979). Thus, although iontophoretically applied NE evokes inhibitory responses in many neurons to which it is administered, excitatory responses can also be evoked in some cells. The proportion of neurons in a given brain region that are excited by NE is sensitive to various features of the experimental design, such as the anesthetic employed and the pH of the iontophoretic solution. Inhibitory responses to NE, nevertheless, appear to represent the predominant form of response, and such effects are blocked by β-adrenoceptor antagonists. As in the periphery, β-adrenoceptors in CNS appear to be linked to an adenylate cyclase mechanism, and cyclic AMP increases elicited by NE and other β-adrenoceptor agonists are blocked by β-adrenoceptor antagonists. Inhibitory response to NE, in Purkinje cells of cerebellum, for example, can also be mimicked by direct iontophoretic application of cyclic AMP, and responses to both cyclic AMP or NE are enhanced by inhibitors of phosphodieseterase, which normally breaks down cyclic AMP (THEO-PHYLLINE, PAPAVERINE) (Moore and Bloom, 1979).

5-HT

5-HT-Containing neurons exist in the CNS and probably also in the intestine. We know far less about the properties and pharmacology of such neuronal systems, however, than we do about ACh and the catecholamines, probably because 5-HT has not been clearly established as a neurotransmitter at any peripheral synapse.

Drug actions on metabolism and other presynaptic mechanisms. 5-HT is synthesized from the plasma amino acid L-tryptophan in a two-step pathway involving hydroxylation by TRYPTOPHAN HYDROXYLASE and decarboxylation of the product (L-5-hydroxytryptophan) by AROMATIC AMINO ACID DE-CARBOXYLASE (Fig. 2–18). It appears that the latter enzyme is the same as that responsible for decarboxylating L-dopa in adrenergic neurons. Tryptophan hydroxylase is susceptible to inhibition by the amino acid L-*p* CHLO-ROPHENYLALANINE (PCPA), and this is one of the effective inhibitors of 5-HT biosynthesis available for *in vivo* studies. A single dose of PCPA can inhibit 5-HT synthesis for many hours. The rate of 5-HT biosynthesis is sensitive to the availability of L-tryptophan in blood and brain, since the normal concentration of the precursor amino acid seems to be below the threshold for saturation of the biosynthetic enzyme tryptophan hydroxylase. In catecholamine biosynthesis, on the other hand, the concentration of L-tyrosine is less important, since normal tissue concentrations are well above the saturation point for tyrosine hydroxylase. 5-HT synthesis in the CNS can thus be increased by the administration of the precursor L-TRYPTO-PHAN and inhibited by the administration of amino acids, such as LEUCINE and VALINE, that compete with tryptophan for transport into the brain from plasma. 5-HT synthesis in the CNS can also be stimulated by the administration of L-5-hydroxytryptophan, which, like L-dopa, penetrates the blood–brain barrier.

5-HT is degraded metabolically by MAO, which is also found in adrenergic neurons. This appears to be the only important metabolic route for 5-HT breakdown in the CNS, leading to the formation of the metabolite 5-HY-DROXYINDOLEACETIC ACID (5-HIAA) (Fig. 2–18). All the inhibitors of MAO described above are also effective in preventing 5-HT breakdown in the

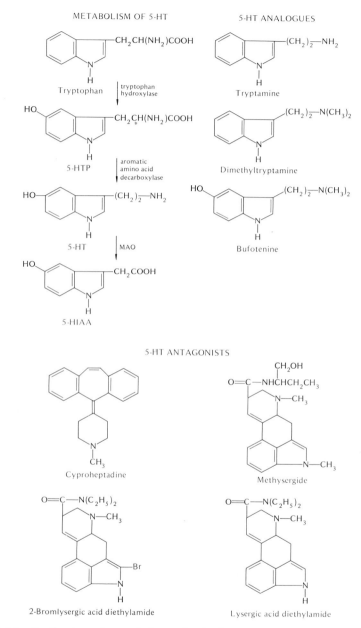

Fig. 2–18 Synthesis and metabolism of 5-hydroxytryptamine (5-HT) and some drugs that affect tryptaminergic mechanisms.

brain. Like the catecholamines, however, free extracellular 5-HT appears to be removed not by metabolic breakdown but by a reuptake mechanism located in the membranes of 5-HT-containing nerve terminals. This uptake system is a high-affinity mechanism with a high specificity for 5-HT. It is inhibited by various indolamine analogues of 5-HT, such as TRYPTAMINE, α-METHYLTRYPTAMINE, and α-METHYL-5-HT. 5-HT uptake is also inhibited by many of the tricyclic antidepressants drugs, which act as potent inhibitors of NE uptake sites. But the exact structure-activity relationships for inhibition of 5-HT and NE uptake by these compounds are not the same (cf. Table 7–1). For example, NE uptake sites are inhibited by the imipramine analogues, DESIPRAMINE and CLOMIPRAMINE, but the order of potency is desipramine > imipramine > clomipramine, whereas the order of potency of these drugs as inhibitors of 5-HT uptake is reversed. Recently, more selective inhibitors of 5-HT uptake have been developed, which have only very weak effects on NE uptake; these include ZIMELIDINE, FLUOXETINE, and CITALOPRAM (Iversen and Mackay, 1979). The 5-HT analogues 5,6-DIHYDROXYTRYPTAMINE and 5,7-DIHYDROXYTRYPTAMINE are selectively accumulated by 5-HT-containing neurons and act as specific neurotoxins, as 6-hydroxydopamine does for catecholamine neurons.

5-HT storage sites in tryptaminergic neurons are sensitive to RESERPINE and related drugs, as are the sites in adrenergic neurons, another point of similarity between 5-HT and catecholamine-containing cells.

Drug actions on 5-HT receptors (see Aghajanian, 1975). Receptors for 5-HT have not been well defined, even in peripheral tissues. In the intestine two types of 5-HT response have been described: one antagonized by METHYSERGIDE and CYPROHEPTADINE, the other not. Recent biochemical studies in brain also suggest that multiple receptor subtypes exist for 5-HT, as for the catecholamines. Peroutka and Snyder (1980) suggested that one type (5-HT$_1$) binds ^{3}H-5-HT with high affinity, and is antagonized potently by D-LYSERGIC ACID DIETHYLAMIDE (D-LSD), the 5-HT analogues BUFOTENIN and 5-METHOXYTRYTPAMINE acting as potent agonists; this receptor appears to be coupled to cyclic AMP formation. A second type (5-HT$_2$) binds the neuroleptic drug ^{3}H-SPIPERONE (which also binds avidly to CNS dopamine receptors) with high affinity, is not adenylate cyclase coupled, and is potently antagonized by D-LSD and by METHYSERGIDE, CYPROPHEPTADINE, and CINANSERIN. This, however, remains a hypothetical scheme and further clarification of the pharmacological specificity of 5-HT receptors in CNS and peripheral organs is needed. The fact that a number of compounds structur-

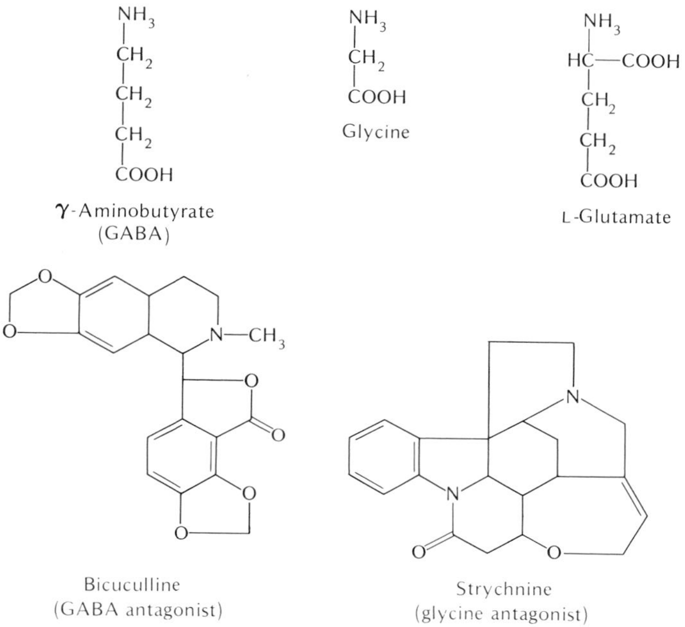

Fig. 2–19   Amino acid transmitter candidates and related drugs.

ally related to 5-HT, such as D-LSD, bufotenin, PSILOCIN, and N-DIMETHYL-TRYPTAMINE are powerful hallucinogens makes it tempting to speculate that these properties are connected with the ability of such drugs to interact with CNS 5-HT receptors, but this remains to be established.

GABA, glycine, and glutamic acid (Fig. 2–19) (for review see Roberts et al., 1976)

GABA is now generally recognized to be the most commonly used inhibitory transmitter in the mammalian CNS. It is found in all regions of the brain and spinal cord and probably is the transmitter in as many as one-third of all synaptic terminals in the brain. Glycine has a more circumscribed function, since its inhibitory transmitter role is restricted to the spinal cord, the lower brainstem, and, possibly, the retina. Glutamic acid is not yet firmly established as a transmitter, but it seems likely that it is a major excitatory transmitter in the mammalian CNS.

Drug effects on metabolism. Few specific inhibitors of the biosynthesis of any of these amino acids are available. Certain pyridoxal phosphate antagonists, such as THIOSEMICARBAZIDE and ISONIAZID inhibit GABA biosynthesis, and this action may be related to the convulsant effects induced by these and related hydrazides, although they are also likely to affect many other metabolic pathways that use pyridoxal phosphate as a cofactor. A more specific inhibitor of GABA biosynthesis is the compound β-MERCAPTOPROPIONIC ACID, which is also an effective convulsant *in vivo*. The metabolic breakdown of GABA by transamination can be inhibited by the compounds AMINOOXYACETIC ACID, β-HYDRAZINOPROIONIC ACID, GABACULINE, and γ-VINYLGABA, all of which are effective *in vivo* inhibitors, and lead to substantial increases in brain concentrations of GABA. No selective inhibitors of glycine or glutamate metabolism are known, and such compounds would in any case be unlikely to affect only those neurons using these amino acid transmitters since, unlike GABA, glycine and glutamate exist in all cells and are metabolized as part of the free amino acid pool needed for protein synthesis. Specific, high-affinity uptake processes exist in the CNS for all three amino acid transmitters, but so far no selective and potent inhibitors of these uptakes are available.

Drug effects on amino acid receptors. Although the receptors for the amino acids are not well characterized, since they exist only in the CNS, some selective drugs are available. The convulsant alkaloids, STRYCHNINE and BICUCULLINE (Fig. 2–19), are selective antagonists of glycine and GABA receptors, respectively. Various compounds have been reported as potential glutamate antagonists, including NUCIFFERIN and GLUTAMIC ACID DIETHYLESTER.

The alkaloid MUSCIMOL acts as a potent agonist at GABA receptors and QUISQUALIC and KAINIC ACIDS are potent agonists at glutamate receptors. Kainic acid exerts a unique neurotoxic effect: when administered by local microinjection into various brain regions it causes an extensive destruction of all neurons at the injection site, leaving axons and terminals of remote neurons and glial cells intact.

Other possible transmitter substances
Even if the three amino acids described above are accepted as neurotransmitters, it is likely that there are still other CNS transmitters to be discovered. For example, the nature of the excitatory transmitter released by neurons in any of the primary sensory nervous pathways remains unknown.

Thus, we do not know the transmitter in peripheral sensory nerves or in the optic nerve. Among possible candidates for transmitters in these and other CNS pathways are the amino acid ASPARTIC ACID (which has an excitatory action similar to that of glutamate), the amine HISTAMINE (which exists in small amounts in specific locations in the CNS), small peptides such as SUB-STANCE P (which are known to be present in dorsal roots and other sensory nerves), ENKEPHALINS and numerous other neuropeptides (see Table 2–4) (Emson, 1979).

CHEMICAL PATHWAYS IN THE BRAIN
Introduction

The concept of chemical transmission in the CNS is a relatively new one. We are only beginning to define the "chemical pathways" in the CNS, in the sense of describing neuroanatomical pathways of neurons with known transmitters. This information, insofar as it is currently available will be summarized for the amine, amino acid, and putative peptide transmitters.

In some instances, our understanding of such chemical pathways has progressed rapidly following the development of histochemical techniques for selectively staining neurons that contain particular transmitters. A fluorescence technique pioneered by Hillarp and his colleagues has been used successfully for staining NE-, DA-, and 5-HT-containing pathways. With such methods, the neuron perikarya and fibers with their terminal vesicular stores of specific chemical transmitters can be visualized and their distribution plotted throughout the CNS. Immunohistochemical staining methods, involving the use of specific antisera, are now being applied widely to map the distribution of peptide-containing neurons in CNS. Such methods can also help to map the distribution of neurons containing amine or amino acid transmitters, using antisera directed against enzymes involved in their biosynthesis, such as tyrosine hydroxylase (NE and DA), dopamine-β-hydroxylase (NE), and glutamic acid decarboxylase (GABA).

There is still no direct staining technique for ACh, and knowledge of its distribution rests largely on the indirect approach of staining the ACh-hydrolyzing enzyme AChE. In the case of GABA, the evidence for distribution is based on immunohistochemical staining of the biosynthetic enzyme glutamic acid decarboxylase, and on autoradiography. Brain tissue is incubated with radioactively labeled GABA, which is selectively taken up by the GABA-containing neurons. The density of radioactivity in autoradiograms of the tissue identifies these neurons. At present, however, there are no com-

plete maps of the distribution of GABA- or other amino acid-containing neurons in the CNS.

The distribution of NE, DA, and 5-HT

Formaldehyde condensation to form fluorescent derivatives was first used
by Eränko to visualize catecholamines in the adrenal medulla, but Falck and
Hillarp saw the tremendous potential of the technique and were the first to
use the highly fluorescent condensation products to plot amine pathways in
the brain (Fig. 2–20).

Both NE and DA form tetrahydroisoquinoline derivatives that yield green
fluorescence on exposure to ultraviolet light. The NE fluorophore, however,
has a labile hydroxyl group and, after treatment with hydrochloric acid, its
emission peak shifts slightly. This small change can be detected microspec-
trofluorimetrically. Alternatively, pharmacological treatments, which interfere with one or another of the catecholamines,can be combined with fluorescence histochemistry to visualize NE and DA independently.

Such indolamines as 5-HT also form fluorescent condensation products
when exposed to formaldehyde gas, but in this case the yellow fluorescence
color is easy to distinguish from the greenish products produced from NE
and DA.

Dahlström and Fuxe (1964) were the first to use these techniques to demonstrate the distribution of CNS cell bodies, axons, and terminals that contain NE, DA, and 5-HT. Ungerstedt (1971) extended such studies and added
more details of the terminal distribution of the NE and DA pathways. The
development of a new technique, involving condensation of the catecholamines with glyoxylic acid rather than formaldehyde, further increased the
sensitivity and resolution of fluorescence histochemical techniques, and allowed the description of previously unknown catecholamine-containing systems in CNS (Lindvall and Björklund, 1974; 1978; Moore and Bloom, 1978;
1979).

Distribution of NE pathways (see Lindvall and Björklund, 1978; Moore and
Bloom, 1979).
Norepinephrine terminals in all areas of brain originate from small groups
of neurons whose cell bodies are located in the pons and medulla, which
have been designated cell groups A1, A2, A4, A5, A6, and A7 (Dahlström
and Fuxe, 1964). The neurons of the locus coeruleus (A6) have multipolar
axons, one branch innervating the Purkinje cells of the cerebellum and others forming a "dorsal bundle" of NE fibers, which terminate in the cortex,

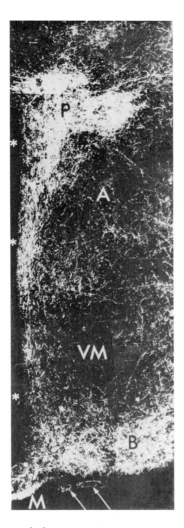

Fig. 2–20   Fluorescent catecholamine-containing nerve terminals in the rat hypothalamus adjacent to the third ventricle, visualized in the fluorescence microscope after exposure of the tissue section to formaldehyde vapor. Magnification ×200. P = periventricular nucleus, A = anterior hypothalamus, VM = ventromedial nucleus; B = basal hypothalamus, M = median eminence. (From Hokfelt and Ljungdahl, 1972.)

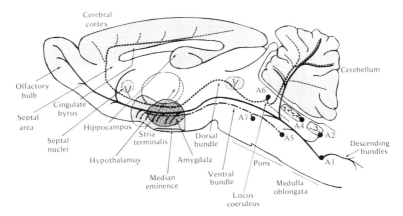

Fig. 2–21 Distribution of norepinephrine-containing pathways in rat brain. (From Livett, 1973.)

thalamus, and hippocampus. The remaining cell groups contribute axons mainly to a "ventral bundle," which innervates the hypothalamus, basal forebrain, and parts of the limbic system. Some of the cell groups, especially A1, also produce descending fibers to the spinal cord, where they terminate mainly in the lateral column in the region of the preganglionic sympathetic neurons.

At the level of the diencephalon, the ascending NE fibers in the dorsal and ventral bundles merge in the medial forebrain bundle, and the fibers then separate to make their discrete terminal innervations (Fig. 2–21).

The dopamine systems (see Lindvall and Björklund, 1978; Moore and Bloom 1978).

The DA-containing neuronal systems lie principally in the midbrain anterior to the NE cell bodies. Cell groups A8 and A9 are located in the substantia nigra, and their fibers form the nigrostriatal pathway, which projects together with the NE fibers into the medial forebrain bundle at the diencephalic level. The dopamine fibers leave the medial forebrain bundle more anteriorly to innervate the corpus striatum (caudate nucleus and putamen) and globus pallidus. Cell group A10, which is medial to the substantia nigra, produces an ascending fiber system innervating the nucleus accumbens, amygdala, the olfactory tubercle, and some areas of cortex (Fig. 2–22). Cell group A12 is contained within the arcuate nucleus of the hypothalamus, and the short axons of these neurons innervate the median eminence. Also, DA-containing neurons are found in the amacrine cell layer of the retina.

The contribution of the fluorescence histochemical method to our knowledge of neuroanatomy is well illustrated by the discovery of the nigrostriatal DA pathway. Although this neuronal system contains about three-quarters of all the DA in the brain, the fibers are extremely small, and their existence had not been detected with classical silver-staining histological methods. After the histochemical demonstration of this pathway with fluorescence, more refined modifications of the Nauta silver-staining techniques were used to demonstrate fibers from the substantia nigra to the striatum. Experiments also indicate that this major chemical pathway has an important role to play in motor integration (Ungerstedt, 1971); it is doubtful whether it would have been discovered without this sophisticated chemical mapping approach.

Distribution of 5-HT (see Azmitia, 1978)

The location of 5-HT neurons and their fiber and terminal systems in the rat brain were described initially by Dahlström and Fuxe (1964). In succeeding years, the 5-HT system received less attention by anatomists than the NE and DA systems.

In the rat, the 5-HT containing neurons are located in the nuclei of the raphe system situated dorsally near the midline of the brainstem. They ex-

Fig. 2–22 Diagrammatic representation of the distribution of dopamine neurons in rat brain. Fiber pathways (solid black lines) originate from dopamine neuron cell bodies in substantia nigra (SN) and ventromedial tegmentum (A10) and project in medial forebrain bundle (MFB) to striatum (S), nucleus accumbens septii (AS), olfactory tubercle (OT), frontal cortex (FC), anterior cingulate cortex (ACC), entorhinal cortex (EC), and amygdala (AMY). From Lindvall and Björklund (1978.)

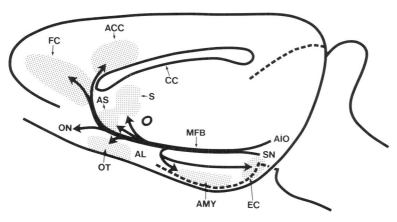

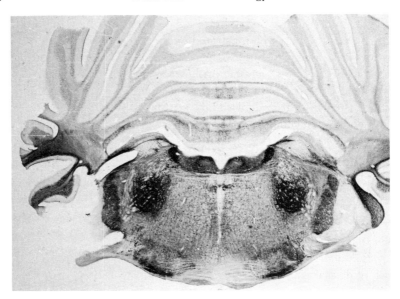

Fig. 2–23　Section of rat brainstem stained for acetylcholinesterase. Note intense staining of oculomotor nuclei in the brainstem and the relatively weak staining of the overlying cerebellum. (Kindly supplied from unpublished results by Dr. P. Lewis, Physiological Laboratory, University of Cambridge.)

tend from the raphe pallidus nucleus in the caudal medulla to the raphe dorsalis nucleus in the caudal mesencephalon. Some 5-HT cell groups are located more laterally in the paragigantocellularis nucleus and in the ventral part of the area postrema. At least some of the ascending 5-HT fibers to the forebrain travel in the medial forebrain bundle. The terminals of the 5-HT axons innervate the pontomesencephalic reticular formation, hypothalamus, lateral geniculate nuclei, amygdala, pallidum system, hippocampus, anterior hypothalamus, and preoptic area and cortex. The raphe 5-HT neurons also send descending fibers to the spinal cord.

Distribution of cholinergic neurons

Although cholinergic neurons were among the first to be studied in CNS, surprisingly little is known about their detailed anatomical distribution. This is largely due to the lack of a specific histochemical staining procedure for such neurons. Most studies have made use of staining reactions for the en-

zyme AChE: in this technique the brain is perfused *in vivo* with formaldehyde and then sectioned on a freezing microtome. Alternate sections are
incubated with butyrylthiocholine (a substrate for nonspecific cholinester-
ases) or acetylthiocholine together with a pseudocholinesterase inhibitor to
demonstrate true AChE. The sections are then treated with copper sulfate
and sodium sulfide, which stain enzyme sites black (Fig. 2–23). Since AChE
is distributed throughout the neuron, it is impossible to determine from any
given section whether stained axons are afferent or efferent to a given brain
structure. Shute and Lewis (1967), however, discovered that AChE actively
changes in different ways on the two sides of a cut axon. The enzyme accu-
mulates on the cell body side of the cut and disappears on the terminal side.
The combination of selective lesions with the AChE staining technique
helped in their detailed mapping of AChE-positive neurons in brain. So did
biochemical assays of the biosynthetic enzyme, choline acetyltransferase,
which is an exclusive marker for cholinergic neurons. Following lesions to
a cholinergic pathway, the activities of AChE and choline acetyltransferase
fall in a parallel manner. Clearly, a histochemical staining technique for choline acetyltransferase would be an ideal method for identifying cholinergic
neurons, and progress is being made in the development of immunohistochemical methods based on the use of antibodies against the purified enzyme. Meanwhile, the detailed information available on the distribution of
AChE-positive cells in CNS has to be viewed with some caution. For example, Shute and Lewis (1967) showed clearly that a number of cell groups
in the mesencephalon were AChE-positive and that their axons projected to
forebrain regions, including cerebral cortex, as part of the "ascending reticular activating system." Subsequently, however, it has become apparent that
some of these neurons are in fact monoamine-containing, e.g. the dopaminergic neurons of substantia nigra and ventral tegmentum, the noradrenergic neurons in locus coeruleus, and the 5-HT neurons in raphe nuclei
(Butcher, 1978). This association of cholinesterase with monoamine-containing neurons remains unexplained, but it indicates the hazards of using a
nonspecific marker such as AChE to identify cholinergic neurons (for review
see Lehmann and Fibiger, 1979).

   Nevertheless, the combination of AChE staining with lesions and measurements of choline acetyltransferase has made it possible to identify some
cholinergic neuronal pathways. For example, long-axoned cholinergic pathways extend from neurons in the septum to the hippocampus, and from
neurons in habenula nucleus to the interpeduncular nucleus, which has the
highest density of cholinergic terminals in any CNS region. There is also a

large ascending cholinergic projection from forebrain nuclei to all areas of cerebral cortex. The cholinergic neurons forming this cortical projection are located in a single continuous system of cells in the nucleus of the diagonal band, the medial and lateral preoptic nuclei, the nucleus basalis, and the entopeduncular nucleus (Emson and Lindvall, 1979).

Distribution of GABA and other amino acids

There are as yet few histochemical methods that allow direct visualization and mapping of neurons which use GABA and other amino acid transmitters. However, such neurons can be identified by autoradiographic techniques after exposure of brain tissue to labelled amino acids; recently, an immunohistochemical method was developed for the GABA biosynthetic enzyme, glutamic acid decarboxylase, which is exclusively localized in GABA neurons (Roberts et al., 1976). Thus, rapid progress may be expected in understanding the detailed neuronal distribution of this and related amino acids.

GABA (see Fonnum and Storm-Mathisen, 1978)

GABA is probably the most common inhibitory transmitter in mammalian CNS. Autoradiographic studies show that about one-third of all nerve terminals in CNS become labelled after exposure to labelled GABA, and are thus presumptively GABAergic in nature. In most CNS regions GABA is found in local inhibitory interneurons having short axons. For example, much of the GABA in cerebral cortex, cerebellar cortex, hippocampus, and spinal cord is present in such local interneurons. There are only two known GABA-containing neuronal pathways involving long axonal projections from one region of the brain to another: the Purkinje cells of the cerebellum and their various projections to cerebellar and vestibular nuclei, and a system of neurons whose cell bodies lie in corpus striatum with axons projecting to substantia nigra. The latter region of brain contains the highest known concentration of GABA; more than half of all the nerve terminals in substantia nigra may be GABAergic and GABA appears to be an important inhibitory input to the dopaminergic cells of this brain region.

Other amino acids

Glycine acts as an important inhibitory transmitter in spinal cord, but not in supraspinal regions of CNS. In the spinal cord it appears to be localized to small interneurons located in the medial gray matter having short axons

Table 2–7. Distribution of neuropeptides in CNS

Peptide	Spinal cord and brainstem	Basal ganglia	Hypothalamus	Median eminence	Amygdala	Hippocampus	Cerebral cortex	Peripheral nerves
TRH	+	+	++0	+++	+	–	–	–
LHRH	–		+0	+++	+	–	–	–
Somatostatin	++	+	+++0	+++	++0	+0	+0	+
Substance P	+++	+++0	++0	+	++0	–	+	+
Cholecystokinin-like	+++	+	+	–	+	+++0	+++0	+
VIP	+	+	+	–	+	+++0	+++0	+
Enkephalins	+++0	+++0	++	++	++0	–	+	+
ACTH/β-endorphin	+	–	+0	+	+	–	–	–
Neurotensin	+++	+	+++0	+++	+++0	–	+	–

Based on immunohistochemical results, using antibodies directed against the various neuropeptides.
+ = low density; ++ = moderate density; +++ = high density of peptide-containing nerve terminals present;
0 = presence of peptide-containing nerve cell bodies; ; – = no detectable peptide-containing nerve terminals or cell bodies.
References: Hökfelt et al. (1978); Emson (1979).

projecting to motor neurons and other cells in the ventral horn. Glycine neurons possess a specific high-affinity uptake process for glycine, and can thus be visualized autoradiographically after radiolabelling.

Glutamic acid-containing neurons can similarly be visualized after labelling with glutamic acid, but this approach is complicated—as in the case of GABA—by the extensive labelling of glial cells which also occurs when brain tissue is exposed to labelled glutamate. Nevertheless, this approach is being successfully used (Storm-Mathisen and Iversen, 1979), and glutamate remains likely to prove one of the most common excitatory transmitters in mammalian CNS. It has been suggested as a prime candidate for the role of sensory transmitter in large-diameter sensory afferent fibers in all primary sensory pathways; it also occurs widely in interneurons within CNS. Its role as an excitatory transmitter in the hippocampus has been particularly well studied (Storm-Mathisen, 1979).

Neuropeptides
A great deal of interest is currently focused on the numerous peptides that have been found in CNS (see Table 2–4). The extensive use of immunohistochemical techniques, using antisera raised against the various peptides, has led to rapid progress in mapping their neuronal distribution in brain and spinal cord (Hughes, 1978; Hökfelt et al., 1978; Emson, 1979). In each case, the immunohistochemical results have shown that the peptides are present in highest concentrations in small nerve terminals, but are also detectable in the cell bodies of the neurons from which such terminals originate. Although mapping studies are still in progress, several distinct neuronal pathways can already be described and some of this information is summarized in Table 2–7. Some peptides, such as substance P, and somatostatin are found in primary sensory fibers as well as in intrinsic pathways of neurons within CNS. The opioid peptides, the enkephalins and β-endorphin, are widely distributed in CNS both in regions in which their function can be associated readily with control of pain pathways and in other regions (e.g. globus pallidus, hypothalamus) where no such connection obviously exists (Fig. 2–24). It seems likely, as in the case with amine and amino acid transmitters, that each peptide occurs in many different neuronal pathways, involved with a variety of different physiological functions. What the biological advantage was for such a bewildering array of different chemical messengers to have evolved in the mammalian CNS remains completely unknown.

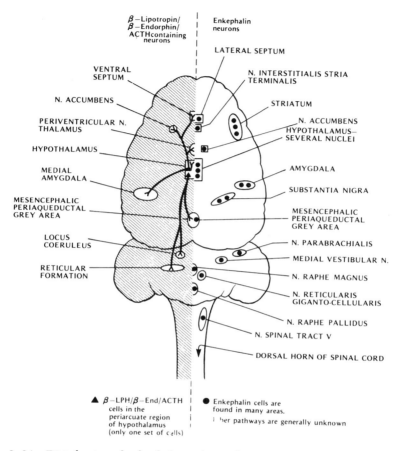

IMMUNOCYTOCHEMISTRY OF THE ENKEPHALINS
β ENDORPHIN, β –LIPOTROPIN AND ACTH IN RAT BRAIN

β –Lipotropin/
β –Endorphin/
ACTHcontaining
neurons

Enkephalin
neurons

LATERAL SEPTUM

VENTRAL
SEPTUM

N. INTERSTITIALIS STRIA
TERMINALIS

N. ACCUMBENS

STRIATUM

PERIVENTRICULAR N.
THALAMUS

N. ACCUMBENS
HYPOTHALAMUS–
SEVERAL NUCLEI

HYPOTHALAMUS

MEDIAL
AMYGDALA

AMYGDALA

SUBSTANTIA NIGRA

MESENCEPHALIC
PERIAQUEDUCTAL
GREY AREA

MESENCEPHALIC
PERIAQUEDUCTAL
GREY AREA

LOCUS
COERULEUS

N. PARABRACHIALIS

MEDIAL VESTIBULAR N.

RETICULAR
FORMATION

N. RAPHE MAGNUS

N. RETICULARIS
GIGANTO-CELLULARIS

N. RAPHE PALLIDUS

N. SPINAL TRACT V

DORSAL HORN OF SPINAL CORD

▲ β –LPH/β –End/ACTH
cells in the
periarcuate region
of hypothalamus
(only one set of cells)

● Enkephalin cells are
found in many areas.
ther pathways are generally unknown

Fig. 2–24   Distribution of enkephalin and β-endorphin in separate neuron systems
in rat brain. The endorphin-containing neurons also show positive immunostaining
reaction for β-lipotropin and ACTH which may coexist in such cells. Neuron cell
bodies depicted as circles or triangles, fiber pathways as solid lines—no long fiber
pathways are known for enkephalin. From Watson et al. (1979).

3. Determinants of Drug Action

DOSE-RESPONSE RELATIONS AND MODE OF ADMINISTRATION

It is not adequate in behavioral pharmacology to study the effect of a single dose of a drug on a complex behavior. As the dose of drug is increased, a point is reached where any behavior is depressed. At doses below this point, the drug may stimulate or disorganize the ongoing behavior, but, in many cases, the effective dose range producing this effect is narrow and easily missed unless a wide range of doses is studied. This is a hard lesson to learn because, when one considers many of the classical pharmacological systems for quantifying drug action, such as isolated smooth muscle (cf. Fig. 2–1), the response varies in a graded manner with increasing dosage. In such preparations, the dose-response curves tend to be simple, and, since there is only a single variable (e.g. contractility) to be influenced by the drug, interpretation of the results is easy. Other physiological responses, however, are, like behavior, determined by several interacting variables. For example, if the activity of drugs that change blood pressure is to be understood, their effects on all the interacting variables must be considered. Of course, it is only a matter of technical competence to investigate the effects of various doses of a drug on a variety of behavioral parameters; the more difficult task is to select the parameters to be studied.

In studying psychoactive drugs, there is a tendency to think that all behavioral effects are mediated by effects of the drug on the brain. Systemically injected drugs may, however, have pronounced peripheral as well as central effects, and the possibility that behavioral effects are secondary to changes in peripheral physiology should be considered. For example, iso-proterenol is an agonist at β-adrenoceptors. Intravenous injections of small doses of isoproterenol (4 μg) induce drinking behavior. The drug releases renin from the kidney, which promotes the formation of angiotensin in the blood, and this peptide passes the blood–brain barrier and induces drinking by stimulating a site in the preoptic region of the hypothalamus. In the rat, the injection of 40 μg of isoproterenol into the preoptic region induces drinking, and this result has been used to support the hypothesis that there are β-adrenoceptors in the brain involved in the induction of drinking. It is probable, however, that after such a large intracerebral injection a sufficient amount of isoproterenol could leak from the brain to the systematic circu-lation to induce renin release and that drinking was a result of this periph-erally mediated effect rather than of any direct action of isoproterenol on the brain. This is supported by the observation that surgical removal of the kidney abolishes isoproterenol-induced drinking irrespective of the route of drug injection. Peripheral drug effects may also serve as discriminative stimuli for behavior. Cook et al. (1960) describe experiments in which dogs were set up in restraining harnesses and their respiration, heart (EKG) and intestinal activity, and leg withdrawal recorded. *l*-norepinephrine (10 μ/kg), or ACh (20 μg/kg) were infused intravenously, and, 30 sec after the injec-tion, the leg was shocked and the withdrawal reflex observed. Leg with-drawal within 30 sec of the injection prevented the shock. No other stimuli preceded the shock, and, yet, after a certain number of training trials, suc-cessful avoidance occurred with all the injected substances.

ONGOING BEHAVIOR AS A DETERMINANT OF DRUG ACTION
Schedule of reinforcement

Reinforcing events are the major determinants of ongoing behavior, and a given drug can produce very different effects depending on the precise na-ture of such reinforced behavior. Drugs that increase behavior show these effects most clearly. Dews (1955a) was the first to recognize the schedule of reinforcement as the most important determinant of drug action. He re-ported that the behavioral effects of the barbiturate, pentobarbital (1 mg), in pigeons depended on the operating schedule of reinforcement. For ex-ample, fixed-interval responding was markedly reduced by this dose of the drug, whereas FR 50 responding was increased (Fig. 3–1). At this dose of pentobarbital, there is no obvious physical disability, and, yet, "by use of these techniques a behavioral effect of a drug can be detected."

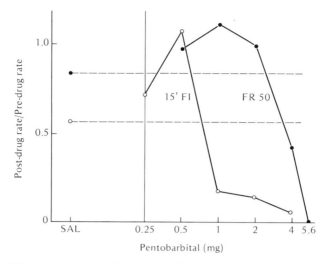

Fig. 3–1   Effect of pentobarbital on pecking behavior of pigeons. Log dose–response curves. Each point represents the arithmetic mean of the ratios for the same four birds at each dosage level on each schedule. Open circles, mean effects, birds working on 15′ FI; solid circles, birds working on FR 50; dotted lines, control response levels; SAL, after saline injection. (Reproduced from Dews, 1955a.)

In a subsequent study, Dews (1958) compared pentobarbital with three stimulant drugs, methamphetamine, *d*-amphetamine, and pipradol. Again pentobarbital further increased the already high rates of FR responding in addition to VI and FI responding, while depressing FR 900 performance. The amphetamines, however, gave the opposite pattern of results, markedly increasing FR 900 and FI 15′ responding and barely increasing the FR 50 or VI 1′ baselines.

Multiple schedules provide a powerful technique for demonstrating schedule control of drug effects. Instead of studying FI and FR performance independently, a multiple schedule can be used in which a fixed-ratio requirement alternates with a fixed-interval condition. Distinctive visual stimuli signal which component of the multiple schedule is operating at any one time. Using such a baseline, the effects of amphetamine and pentobarbital can be clearly dissociated. Amphetamine increases FI and decreases FR responding, whereas pentobarbital depresses FI responding and leaves FR performance intact.

It is possible to use yet more complex multiple schedules. Cook and Kel-

leher (1962), for example, described a four-component schedule under the
discriminative control of four visual stimuli. A 10-min FI followed by 2.5
min timeout with no reinforcement; a FR 30 followed that, and the cycle
ended with another 2.5 min time-out (Fig. 3–2). Such schedules can be
used to demonstrate the considerable specificity of drug action. The minor
tranquilizer, meprobamate, at a dose of 50 mg/kg increased terminal rates
of responding during the FI component without increasing FR rates or inducing responses during the time-out. Discrimination between the conditions and of the temporal relationship within the FI were normal. At 100
mg/kg of meprobamate, however, although discrimination between the four

Fig. 3–2   Effects of meprobamate on a squirrel monkey's behavior maintained by a
multiple schedule of food reinforcement, including FI-10 (a), FR-30 (c), and TO-2.5
(b and d) components. The recording pen reset to the bottom of the record when
reinforcement occurred. (From Cook and Kelleher, 1972.)

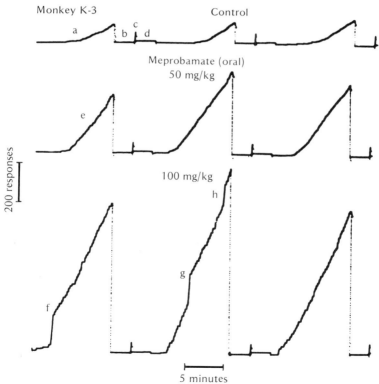

elements remained, discrimination within the FI was disrupted, and bursts of high responding occurred at random times during the interval and often in the initial segments when response rates are normally very low.

The nature of the reinforcer

It is commonly assumed that the nature of the reinforcer maintaining behavior is the most important determinant of any effect drugs may have on that behavior. Contrary to this belief, there is a growing realization that, first, relationships between stimuli and their reinforcing potential are not rigid, and, second, the important thing is not the nature of the event that follows behavior but rather the way the event is programmed in relation to behavior.

Food and water reinforcement are most commonly used in behavioral pharmacology, but intracranial self-stimulation (which in some way mimics the cues associated with natural reinforcement) and heat (Weiss and Laties, 1961) can also be used to maintain identical patterns of responding. It is not difficult to accept the common behavioral property of positive reinforcers, but it is important to realize that negative reinforcers also share this common behavioral property. For example, shock is called an aversive stimulus, but when programmed on an avoidance or escape schedule, it increases rates of responding.

It is striking that the reinforcers food and shock can be programmed to produce indistinguishable patterns of responding. To illustrate this point, Kelleher and Morse (1964) presented cumulative records of lever pressing in squirrel monkeys maintained either on a multiple FI/FR for food or for shock-escape (see Fig. 1–6). It is well known that amphetamine increases FI and reduces FR responding for food, and, despite the opposite direction of the behavioral changes, the anorexic effect of the drug has been used to explain the depression of FR responding. The observation that FI/FR responding for food or shock-escape is changed in an identical manner by amphetamine undermines any motivational interpretation of the action of the drug (Fig. 3–3).

Chlorpromazine also affects behavior maintained under the two conditions of motivation in an identical manner. As far as studies of the major classes of psychoactive drugs are concerned, the schedule of reinforcement rather than its nature is the more important determinant of drug action. If the generated pattern of responding is identical, so is the drug response.

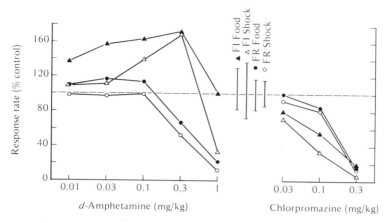

Fig. 3–3   Effects of *d*-amphetamine sulfate and chlorpromazine hydrochloride on rates of responding under multiple FI-FR food and shock schedules. Three monkeys were studied on each multiple schedule. Each drug was given intramuscularly immediately before the beginning of a 2.5 hr session. At least duplicate observations were made in each monkey at each dose level; thus, each point is based on six observations or more. Summary dose–response curves for the four-component schedules were obtained by computing the means of the percentage changes in average response rates from control to drug sessions. The dashed line at 100% indicates the mean control level for each component. The vertical lines in the middle of the figure indicate the ranges of control observations expressed as a percentage of the mean control value. Note the general similarity of the pairs of dose-effect curves for fixed-interval and fixed-ratio components. (Reproduced from Kelleher and Morse, 1964.)

Discriminative stimuli as determinants of drug action

A discriminative stimulus is one in the presence of which an animal is reinforced (S^D) or not reinforced (S^Δ). Such stimuli can be used to modulate responding in very specific ways, and certain drugs have been shown to selectively modify this control. Many classes of drug have an effect on discriminative control, but, in most cases, this effect is only one of a wide spectrum of behavioral effects and, therefore, does not characterize the drug. As we shall see, however, the phenothiazines are an exception to this rule. Their effect on discriminative control has proved valuable both in differentiating phenothiazines from other drugs such as reserpine, that also have a generally depressant effect on behavior, and in differentiating among the various phenothiazines (Cook and Kelleher, 1962).

Discriminative stimuli may be exteroceptive (e.g. visual or auditory stimuli) or interoceptive (e.g. autonomic responses, time cues). Interoceptive cues have not received much attention. This in unfortunate because there is every reason to suppose that these cues are extremely important in determining drug responses; they are after all the autonomic and, therefore, invariant stimulus corollaries of drug action. Particularly important is the possibility that interoceptive cues associated with drug injections may be as important in determining the behavioral response to the drug on that *and subsequent* occasions (Overton, 1966) as any specific effects it may have on the CNS. By comparison, the external stimulus environment is somewhat arbitrary. The blood pressure response to epinephrine is invariant, although the environmental conditions under which the drug is taken may vary each time.

Dews (1955b) first reported the significance of exteroceptive visual cues and how drugs could modify the control exerted by such discriminative stimuli on schedule-controlled responding. Pigeons were trained to peck an illuminated key on a VI 1-min schedule. During the 30-min session, S^D (S + and S^Δ (S −) periods alternated. The response key was illuminated with one of four different colored lights, and the house light in the testing chamber was either on or off. These stimuli could be combined to form eight discrete discrimination stimuli, and six of them were used as the S^D and S^Δ stimuli. Four schedules were studied; on three of them single S^D and S^Δ alternated; on the fourth the stimuli were conditional, e.g. the house light was either combined or not combined with red for S^D and S^Δ stimuli, and, in addition, none of the stimuli were repeated within the session (Fig. 3−4). Phenobarbital was one of the drugs studied, and it was found that a dose of 3 mg/kg

---

Fig. 3−4   (A) Diagram showing sequence of stimuli in the various schedules used. R, B, Y, and W indicate that the red, blue, yellow, and white lights, respectively, were on behind the key. (B) Effect of pentobarbital on performance on schedule 1. Ordinate and abscissa scales have been superimposed on an original record. The short diagonal lines on the original record show when the rewards occurred. Below the record is a key showing the nature of the stimuli throughout the run. The conventions in the key are the same as those of Fig. A. Note the almost complete absence of responding in the S − periods and lack of effect of 3 mg pentobarbital (PB) on performance on this schedule. (C) Effect of pentobarbital on performance on schedule 4. Note the almost complete absence of responding in the S − periods before the drug, but the large number of responses in the second S − period after the drug. Performance in the S + periods is not obviously affected by this dose of pentobarbital. (Reproduced from Dews, 1955b.)

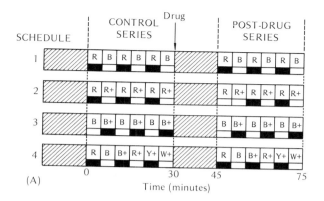

(A)

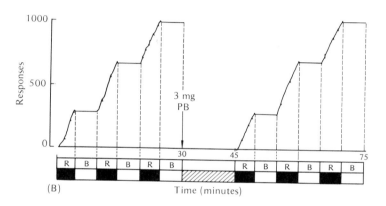

(B)

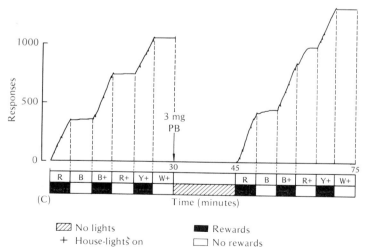

(C)

had no effect on S^Δ responding on schedules 1–3 but markedly increased S^Δ responding on schedule 4. Dews concluded that the more complex the discriminative control the more likely it is to be disrupted.

Chlorpromazine is a drug that alters discriminative control regardless of the complexity of stimulus control. On a simple FI/FR schedule, chlorpromazine results in a flattening of behavior control. The scalloped FI pattern becomes a steady low rate throughout the interval, and the characteristic high FR rates are reduced. These changes are often considered to reflect a loss of discriminative control, but, on this basic schedule, such a loss cannot be differentiated from the general depressant effects of chlorpromazine on all response patterns. The same criticism can be applied to the study of Blough (1957), in which pigeons were trained on a conditional discrimination to peck the darker of two keys when a vertical bar between the keys was illuminated, and the lighter key when it was not. Two measures of performance were observed: the total response output and the accuracy of the discrimination. Chlorpromazine lowered both, although the finding that the effect on discrimination lasted longer than the general depression of responding suggests that the two effects may be dissociable. Vaillant (1964) achieved such a dissociation by using a more complex discrimination schedule with pigeons.

The specificity of stimulus control can be demonstrated with stimulus generalization methods (see Fig. 1–8). Use of this method is limited to stimuli that belong to identified physical continua. When an animal is under the control of more complex stimuli, such as visual patterns, or, more importantly, the whole constellation of environmental cues encountered under normal conditions, the experimenter is at a loss to know how to vary the stimuli systematically. Stimulus generalization and discrimination methods provide a potentially powerful way of finding out exactly how a stimulus appears to an animal under the influence of a drug, although as yet these methods have not been fully exploited in behavioral pharmacology. In the studies reported to date, several drugs have been shown to modify generalization gradients, but in no case has this proved to be a unique effect of the drug class in question. Hearst (1964), who pioneered these studies, reports that d-amphetamine, scopolamine, and caffeine all modify generalization gradients to a range of lights varying in brightness.

Terrace (1963) discovered another important feature of stimulus control when he observed that the method of acquiring a discrimination influenced its susceptibility to drug action. Pigeons learned a horizontal/vertical discrimination where they were exposed to the S^D and S^Δ throughout training or when the S^Δ was introduced initially as a weak physical stimulus and only gradually achieved equal intensity with the S^D. In the former condition, errors were made to the S^Δ during learning; in the latter, the tendency to respond to the S^Δ was very weak, and learning, therefore, occurred without error. Imipramine and chlorpromazine had no disruptive effect on discrimination achieved by errorless learning but had a marked effect if errors had been made during acquisition. When given the drug, the birds made a high number of erroneous responses to the negative pattern.

As far as interoceptive cues are concerned, the most attention has been given to the role of temporal cues as discriminative stimuli. Sidman (1956) was one of the first to recognize the value of differential reinforcement of low rates of responding (DRL) schedules for studying timing cues. In the DRL procedure, an animal must space his responses in time. For example, on 20-sec DRL, a lever press produces a reinforcement only if 20 sec or more have elapsed since the preceding response. If a response occurs too soon, the DRL timer is reset, and the timing interval begins anew. The frequency distribution of time intervals between successive responses (inter-response times) illustrates the accuracy of timing that develops on DRL schedules.

Amphetamine increases the frequency of short inter-response times, and this disrupts DRL performance; with appropriate methods of analysis, it can be shown that any disruption of temporal control is secondary to the more basic response-stimulating effect of amphetamine. By contrast, it can be shown that the effects of chlorpromazine on schedules involving temporal discrimination are much more closely tied to sensory control (Weiss and Laties, 1964a). Pigeons were trained on an FI 5-min schedule. Then, on alternate intervals, an external visual "clock" was superimposed, and discrete form stimuli appeared on the response key during successive segments of the FI (Fig. 3–5). When the clock stimuli were present, the pigeons achieved even better controlled scalloped response patterns on the FI. Under amphetamine only the "no clock" FI performance was disrupted; in the presence of the clock, the disruptive influence of the drug was attenuated. Chlorpromazine, however, disrupted the pattern of responding under both conditions, suggesting that neither intero- nor exteroceptive cue could control behavior in the presence of this drug. Specific evidence of an effect of chlorpromazine on the discrimination of interoceptive cues comes from a study of Cook et al. (1960), in which dogs no longer showed conditioned leg avoidance to injections of NE after a dose of 50 μg/kg of this phenothiazine.

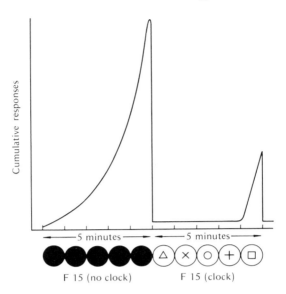

F 15 (no clock)   F 15 (clock)

Fig. 3–5   Symbols used during the clock and no-clock conditions. During the no-clock condition the key was illuminated by a red light. The cumulative records above the symbols represent typical performance during the two conditions. (Reproduced from Weiss and Laties, 1964a.)

Punishing procedures as a determinant of drug action

If an unpleasant stimulus, such as a shock, is unavoidable, the effect on behavior is quite different from that seen if the same shock is used as a negative reinforcer. Punishing stimuli that are programmed to occur following responses suppress behavior severely, and *immediate punishment* procedures of this kind have been very useful in characterizing drug effects. The Geller procedure, a concurrent VI for food, with every response simultaneously punished, can be used to illustrate the fact that, although certain psychoactive drugs are insensitive to the nature of the reinforcer, they are influenced by whether reinforcement or punishment is operating. Amphetamine, for example, which invariably increases reinforced responding, further decreases punished responding regardless of how the punishing stimulus is scheduled. Another example is provided by such minor tranquilizers as chlordiazepoxide, which strongly increases the rate of punished responding although it has weak rate-increasing effects on behavior maintained by reinforcers (Geller and Seifter, 1960; Geller et al., 1962).

On the Geller-Seifter procedure, the responses of the animal initiate the punishment stimuli. If these stimuli are programmed to occur irrespective of the animal's behavior, suppression is less complete. There is some evidence that the tranquilizing drugs, which release shock-suppressed behavior, act less potently if such adventitious punishment has been used.

One of the punishment procedures most extensively used in behavioral pharmacology is the Estes-Skinner procedure. Different studies have produced a confusing array of results with this procedure, and these results would not, on their own, have revealed how crucial punishment is in determining drug action. Reserpine, morphine, and meprobamate have been claimed by some to restore responding during the preshock stimulus and by others not to. The results with this procedure illustrate the necessity of defining the operating behavioral variables in any procedure before using it to characterize drugs. Further study of the Estes-Skinner procedure itself has shown that, under certain conditions, responding may increase during the preshock stimulus, and, even when suppression occurs, its degree depends on: (a) the duration of the preshock stimulus, suppression being greatest with short stimuli; (b) the schedule of reinforcement used to maintain responding; (c) the experimental history of the animal.

Since these variables are themselves determinants of drug action, irrespective of their interaction with response-suppression, it is not surprising to find that the Estes-Skinner procedure has yielded conflicting results.

Rate and pattern of ongoing behavior as determinants of drug action

Dews drew attention to the importance of rate of responding as a determinant of the action of certain classes of drugs. In the study referred to earlier, in which four different schedules of reinforcement were studied (Dews, 1958), amphetamine increased responding where the baseline activity was low and had no effect on or decreased high baselines. This was interpreted in terms of drug effects on inter-response times.

Analysis of the changing response rate during FI performance provides another way of getting at this problem. FI reinforcement generates an escalating response rate over the time interval: a low rate immediately after the reinforcement and a high rate as the next reinforcement approaches. This cumulative record of FI performance is therefore "scalloped"; under amphetamine, the scallop becomes a linear increase. Several workers have measured response rates in the consecutive segments of the FI, and an analysis of the effect of amphetamine shows a clear relationship to the different baseline rates during the various segments. Kelleher and Morse (1968) have analyzed the effect of amphetamine in this way on FI/FR shock avoidance behavior in the squirrel monkey. Amphetamine illustrates the rate dependency most clearly. Barbiturates also show rate-dependent effects on low-response baselines (Fig. 3–6) but reduce high rates of responding less dramatically than amphetamine (Dews, 1964). The minor tranquilizers, meprobamate and chlordiazepoxide, are more like amphetamine but have not been intensively studied.

This important principle of rate dependency is not widely referred to, and, yet, a cursory inspection reveals that it is obeyed with amphetamine-induced stimulation when ICS, food, water, temperature presentation, postponement of electric shock, termination of loud noise, and termination of shock are used to maintain *low* rates of ongoing behavior. Similarly, irrespective of the reinforcer, high rates of responding are insensitive to amphetamine.

Multiple schedules that juxtapose low and high rates of responding demonstrate this very clearly. Using FI/FR multiple schedules of food or shock-escape reinforcement in the squirrel monkey, Kelleher and Morse (1964) show that 0.3 mg/kg d-amphetamine almost doubled response rate on FI while almost halving FR responding (Fig. 3–3). In the rat, Clark and Steele (1966) used a three component schedule: a 4-min period with no reinforcement followed by a 4-min FI, in turn followed by three reinforcements under an FR 25 schedule. After amphetamine they consistently found increased responding in the first two segments and decreased responding in the third segment.

Punishment as we have seen, also generates low rates of responding, but

---

Fig. 3–6   Dependence of the effect of amobarbital (AB) on the predrug rate of key pecking in the pigeon. *Abscissa:* log of rate as responses per session (total of 500 sec, since each 25-sec period occurred once in each of 20 cycles); *ordinate:* change in log rate following amobarbital, intramuscularly. Since the 500-sec interval was divided for recording purposes into 20 periods of 25 sec, there are 20 points on each graph, 10 representing periods when the light was on (circled triangles) and 10 representing periods when the light was off (triangles). The line through the points was calculated by least squares from all points. On the ordinate are plotted all points where the mean rate of responding was 1 or less response/500 sec; this arbitrary assignment makes possible the logarithmic plot. Exclusion of these indeterminate points would not appreciably affect the regression line. (Reproduced from Dews, 1964.)

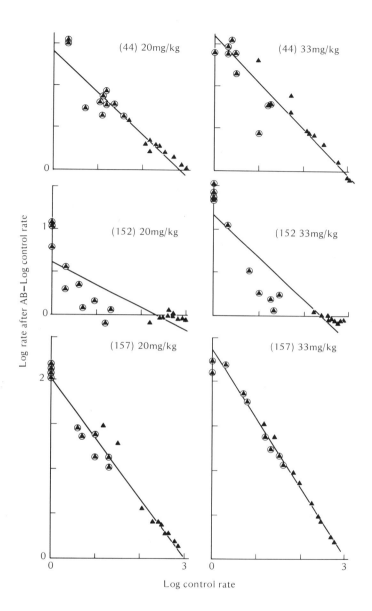

it seems that the releasing effect that such drugs as the minor tranquilizers have on punishment are not entirely explicable in terms of rate-dependency. If matched rates of responding are generated by a multiple FI food, FI punishment schedule, chlordiazepoxide and meprobamate increase responding more in the VI punishment segment than in the food-reinforcement segments, indicating a unique relationship between tranquilizers and punishment, which is independent of their rate-increasing effects (McMillan, 1973a).

Further perspective—how far do schedules of reinforcement predict drug effects?

The first part of this chapter described studies which support the view that under a wide variety of conditions the behavioral effects of drugs are determined by the ongoing *rate* and *pattern* of schedule-controlled responding in the absence of the drug. It has become widely accepted that, given such information, drug responses can be predicted. Particular emphasis has often been given to the fact that the *nature* of the controlling event is unimportant for such predictions. If two different events maintain characteristic responding on a fixed-interval schedule, then a given drug will affect each behavior pattern in the same way. Food presentation and shock avoidance or escape would be two such events, and, as we have seen, amphetamine increases low rates of responding in the early part of the fixed interval in a similar manner under these two conditions. It has been stressed that such observations undermine the value of describing the controlling events in motivational terms. Intuitively, one would suppose that the motivational response to a rewarding and an aversive stimulus would be different. Yet the behavioral baselines both stimuli control are influenced in an indistinguishable manner by drugs. Thus, the nature of an event (i.e. whether it is pleasant or unpleasant) is not a good predictor of how it will control behavior.

To illustrate this point, experiments can be cited in which a pleasant event, food presentation, suppresses behavior; that is, acts as a punishing event. Azrin and Hake (1969) reported that in rats responding was maintained under a variable-interval schedule of food or water presentation. A stimulus (relay clicks, 6/sec) was presented occasionally, and its termination was paired with the response-independent presentation of food or water or with electrical brain stimulation. They found a reduction in responding in the presence of the stimulus, just as in earlier experiments suppression of responding had been seen during the preshock stimulus on the Estes-Skinner procedure. Furthermore, McKearney (1968a) showed that in certain circumstances strong electric shock could maintain high rates of responding, that is, its control of behavior is indistinguishable from that of a traditional reinforcing event. Squirrel monkeys were first trained on shock avoidance. The schedule was then modified so that the first response after 10 min now produced a shock. Scalloped patterns of responding emerged on this concurrent 10-min fixed-interval schedule. When the avoidance contingency was finally removed, the remaining shock presentation every 10 min maintained patterns of responding indistinguishable from those seen with schedules of fixed-interval shock avoidance reinforcement. How shall we define the shock in this experiment: as a reinforcer or a punishment, as pleasant or aversive? It is clear that a naive animal exposed to such a shock would show a marked suppression of behavior, yet after a certain experimental history, the same stimulus is able to maintain high rates of responding. This example illustrates *par excellence* that the nature of an event will not reliably predict how it will control behavior, or, by extension, how that behavior will respond to pharmacological manipulation.

Thus, it is fair to say at present that knowledge of the nature of an event controlling behavior is of less predictive value than the schedule of presentation of that event and the consequent pattern and rate of responding maintained by it. This view has been strenuously advocated by Kelleher and Morse in a number of scholarly reviews (Kelleher and Morse, 1968; Morse et al., 1977).

Since the publication of the first edition of this book, however, a few bold experimenters have sought to test the generality of these dicta. One outcome of this work has been a growing list of exceptions to the general principles. An excellent survey of some of these studies is to be found in McKearney and Barrett (1978) who state: "The eager search for general principles must proceed with a corresponding regard for the complex and multiple ways in which behavior is determined. . . . Schedule factors are of tremendous importance, but not to the exclusion of the profound influence of the total environmental context and of the individual's past experience. Full appreciation of these complexities is a prerequisite to meaningful understanding of either the environmental control of behavior or of the behavioral effects of drugs."

In support of this statement, the final section of this chapter seeks not to question the established and important general principles, but to explore the exceptions and to place behavioral control mechanisms in a broader biological context. To do this a few questions will be posed, the answers to which include reference to the most recent areas of investigation on the schedule control of behavior. The results of these investigations cast doubt on some of the earlier predictive relationships described between drug action and behavior. Whereas much of the earlier work was concerned with behavior maintained by traditional reinforcers, the newer work has focused on the control of behavior by aversive events.

1. Is the nature of the controlling event always irrelevant?

Further research on schedule control of behavior has uncovered a wide range of factors that are influential, and comparisons of the effects of different drugs on these new baselines have been made. Of particular importance has been the introduction of shock presentation as a means of sustaining patterned rates of responding. We have seen that patterns of fixed-interval responding for shock avoidance or escape and for food presentation are modified in a similar way by a number of drugs. We have also seen that food presentation and shock presentation maintain indistinguishable patterns of responding on fixed-interval schedules, but these patterns are not always affected by a given drug in the same way.

Morphine, for example, increases responding for shock presentation, while reducing responding for food presentation. Alcohol, chlordiazepoxide, and pentobarbitone also have different effects on responding maintained in these two different ways, decreasing responding for shock while markedly increasing food-maintained responding. The task now is to determine why identical baselines are differentially affected by drugs. Perhaps the differential motivational properties of food and shock are more important determining factors than absolute response output. But just as it is dangerous to interpret drug action on the basis of a single dose effect, so it is premature to undermine the central role of schedule control before the different controlling events have been studied in a parametric fashion.

2. Are there exceptions to the rate-dependency principle?

Is it always the case that when drugs have rate-increasing effects, low rates are affected more than high rates? The rate-dependency relationship, as we have seen, has received much support, but we are now concerned with exploring the exceptions to the rule and assessing how far such exceptions undermine the generality of the relationship originally demonstrated between the rate of ongoing behavior and its modulation by certain drugs. First, it is not the case that the lower the baseline the greater the rate-increasing effect. There is a rate of responding below which drugs are no longer able to stimulate. It has been shown that normally effective doses of methamphetamine do not increase responding when control rates of responding are low because behavior has no consequences or when responding is poorly developed in early stages of training on a schedule. McMillan (1973a) has reported similarly poor rate-increasing effects of d-amphetamine on the lower rates of responding seen in the very early segments of fixed-interval schedules. If rates of responding are low because of the powerful control exercised by discriminative stimuli, then rate-increasing relationships of the predicted value are also not observed.

For example, McKearney (1970) has tested pigeons on various modifications of a paradigm first described by Dews (1964) in which two different discriminative stimuli alternate during successive 1-min segments of a 10-min fixed-interval schedule of food presentation. During odd-numbered minutes of the fixed interval an S^Δ condition prevailed (S^Δ being defined as a stimulus in whose presence food was never presented). Responding during even-numbered minutes in the presence of S^D (a stimulus in whose presence food was presented) showed the usual pattern of positive acceleration; responding during S^Δ was similarly graded, but rates were much lower. In agreement with Dews' (1964) earlier findings, the response rate-increasing effects of amobarbital were inversely related to control rates of responding, regardless of whether S^Δ or S^D rates were considered. When S^Δ was a change in key-light color or a change from a darkened to a brightly illuminated chamber, the increases in S^Δ responding were considerably less than would be predicted on the basis of the effects on S^D responding. But when S^Δ was a change from a darkened to a dimly illuminated chamber (i.e. when the change in stimulus intensity was less), increases in S^Δ responding after amobarbital were considerably greater, and of the approximate order expected on the basis of control rate. Such increases were systematically related to the intensity of the S^Δ stimulus; that is, the less intense the stimulus the greater the increase after amobarbital, even though *control* rates of responding themselves were observed to change little as S^Δ intensity was decreased. Thus, the dependence of drug effects on control rates of responding can be modified when behavior is under the control of powerful discriminative stimuli.

Punishment generates low rates of responding and one might suppose that this paradigm, like the fixed interval, would provide a model baseline for studying rate dependency. Again, however, there are a number of exceptions. Amphetamine, an archetypal drug for demonstrating rate dependency on food-reinforced baselines, is unable to stimulate, in the same manner, equivalent low rates of punished responding. A range of results have been obtained with amphetamine on baselines of punished responding. Amphetamine has been reported to decrease further punished responding, or to release it to a degree, or as we have seen to produce large increases in certain contexts. Clearly, although we have identified a number of factors influencing the interaction between amphetamine and punishment, there must remain a crucial variable that has not yet been discovered.

Despite this intriguing exception, punished responding does provide good evidence for rate-dependency in the case of those drugs which reliably release punished responding, notably the barbiturates and benzodiazepines. Although the minor tranquilizers (including barbiturates) generally stimulate behavior in a rate-dependent fashion, it can be shown with multiple schedules that their effect is greater on punished than on unpunished responding. By contrast, under similar schedule conditions the rate-increasing effect of amphetamine is much greater on unpunished than on punished responding. Thus, it would appear that rate dependency *per se* is not an adequate explanation of the anxiolytic effect of minor tranquilizers. Some other factor must be invoked to account for the selectivity of their effects on punished responding.

It is now generally accepted that if drugs cause rate-dependent increases in behavior they are acting in a similar way. There may be a general sense in which this is so, but too ready acceptance of this principle impedes the search for differences in drug effects. On many measures benzodiazepines, alcohol, and barbiturates act in the same way, but clearly these drug groups are very different in chemical, pharmacological, neurological, and behavioral terms. Indeed, if their rate-dependency properties are studied in sufficient detail, these are also found to differ. Likewise, both amphetamines and barbiturates have rate-dependent effects on unpunished responding, yet there are both quantitative and qualitative differences.

3. Is the context in which behavior occurs relevant?
Yes, this has been demonstrated in a number of experimental situations, many of which involve the effect of drugs, particularly amphetamines, on punished responding. The study of multiple schedules in which immediate punishment alternates with various other schedule conditions has revealed contrasting effects between the different elements of the complex schedule.

A stimulus does not necessarily have to be present at the time of responding in order to influence a drug effect on that responding. For example, squirrel monkeys were trained on a multiple schedule involving the alternation of 10-min extinction periods with 10 min on a fixed-interval food-reinforced schedule, every thirtieth response being punished with electric shock. The latter component represents immediate punishment and, as expected from numerous earlier studies, d-amphetamine did not increase punished fixed-interval responding. If, however, the context of that responding is changed by replacing the alternating extinction period with shock avoidance, then d-amphetamine was able to enhance markedly the suppressed responding in the immediate punishment segment (McKearney and Barrett, 1975). Thus, in this case neither the event nor the schedule predicted the drug effect. The rate and pattern of responding in the immediate punishment segments of both schedules were indentical, yet the drug effect was opposite. To pursue this, a further modification was studied by Barrett (1977a) in which fixed-interval responding *maintained by shock* presentation alternated with the fixed-interval punishment condition. Under these conditions, amphetamine was again able to increase responding suppressed by immediate punishment, as well as the responding maintained by shock presentation (Fig. 3–7). Thus, the context in which immediate punishment operates clearly modifies the responsiveness of the behavior to drug modification. These are examples of environmental context, but in man *cognitive context* is an important factor.

Although it is possible, for experimental purposes, to isolate and study intero- or exteroceptive discriminative cues, the total environment determining drug action under natural conditions presents a far more complex picture. The experiments of Schachter and Singer (1962) illustrate this very well. Students were asked to take an injection of a harmless substance in a study of its effect on vision. The drug was epinephrine, and some subjects were correctly told that it would produce transient side effects, including hand tremor, increased heart rate, and facial flushing. Others were given inaccurate details of the likely side effects, including foot numbness, itching, and headache. While they were waiting for the drug to take effect, the subjects in both groups were with an individual who had been instructed to indulge in such foolish behavior as playing basketball with scrap paper and flying paper airplanes. Observations of the drugged subjects revealed that the correctly informed group was relatively unaffected by the stooge's behavior, whereas the misinformed subjects exhibited active emotional involvement, joining in raucous behavior with the stooge, far outdoing the excesses of the mysterious stranger. The same physiological background produced by the drug, combined with identical behavior on the part of the stooge, resulted in quite different behavior in the two groups, apparently

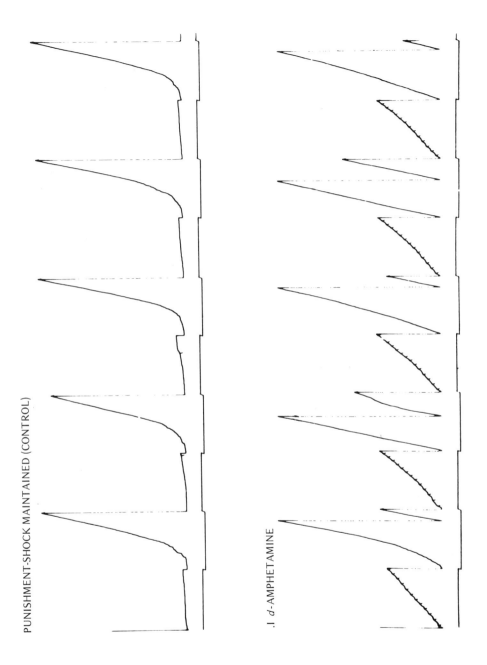

PUNISHMENT-SHOCK MAINTAINED (CONTROL)

.1 *d*-AMPHETAMINE

entirely as a function of what they had been told about the effects of epinephrine. Variations in the normal personality of the subjects must be taken
into account in interpreting drug effects of this kind. However, such observations underline the great importance in human psychopharmacology of
the cognitive set of the subject in relation to drug treatment.

4. Is the behavioral history of the organism of importance?

It is clear that prior experience modifies present behavioral responses. Animals exposed to increasing intensity of electric shock will continue to respond in the presence of intense shock, shock which would eliminate all
behavior in a naive animal. Although immediate punishment suppresses ongoing behavior, the presentation of shock will maintain high rates of responding in animals with experience of shock postponement schedules. Are
the effects of drugs on behavioral baselines similarly influenced by behavioral history? Barrett (1977b) reported that squirrel monkeys with prior
training on shock postponement were trained for one year on a multiple
fixed-interval schedule for alternating food and shock presentation. Identical
patterns of scalloped responding were seen. At this stage the shock presentation element was eliminated and the food element changed by the addition of shock presentation to every thirtieth reinforced response. The animal
was now on a schedule recognized as immediate punishment (Fig. 3–8). As
we have seen, amphetamine does not normally reinstate punished responding. However, in the monkeys with this particular history (shown in panel
A) amphetamine produced a marked stimulation of punished responding.
Naive monkeys with no experience of the shock postponement or shock
presentation schedule did not show increased punished responding after
amphetamine was administered (panel B on right in Fig. 3–8). Thus, the
history with shock stimuli had modified the response to amphetamine.

The effects of drugs on exploratory behavior are also highly dependent on
the behavioral experience of the animal. An example is afforded by Steinberg and her associates (Rushton and Steinberg, 1964) who reported that
the spontaneous motor behavior seen in a Y-maze was increased by am-

---

Fig. 3–7   Top: Control responding by squirrel monkeys on schedule alternating
fixed-interval immediate punishment with fixed interval responding maintained by
the presentation of shock. Bottom: Effect of 0.1 mg/kg d-amphetamine. Responding
in both the immediate punishment and the fixed-interval shock presentation elements of the schedule was increased. (Modified from Barett, 1977a.)

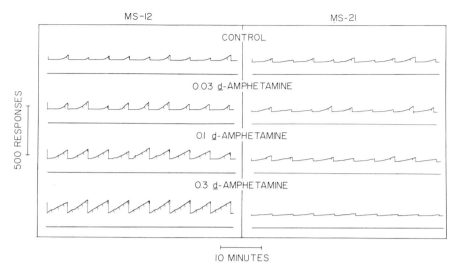

Fig. 3–8 Cumulative response records depicting (A) increases in punished responding with amphetamine after a history of responding under shock-postponement and shock-presentation schedules and (B) the absence of increases in punished responding when no previous exposure was given to schedules of shock. Shock delivery is indicated by a diagonal mark. The recording pens returned to the original position when food was delivered at the end of each fixed interval (Reproduced from Barrett, 1977b).

phetamine if the rats were inexperienced in the situation but that the effect was lost if the rats were experienced.

Turning to experiments that suggest a physiological basis for the importance of experience in modifying drug responses, the classical studies on crowding and amphetamine toxicity may be cited (Moore, 1963). Amphetamine in sufficiently high doses will kill rodents, and the pharmacological measure of these lethal doses is the LD_{50} (the dose killing 50% of the animals within a specified time interval). Amphetamine has a significantly lower LD_{50} in rodents housed in overcrowded conditions than in their normally housed litter mates (15 mg/kg instead of 111 mg/kg). A similar result can be obtained by exposing rodents to shock, stress, noise, or raised temperature.

5. Does experience with a drug modify the response of an organism to that drug?

The reduction in response to repeated administration of a drug is termed tolerance (see Chapter 2). The traditional definition of tolerance requires a reduced response (physiological or behavioral) to the same dose of drug and a concomitant need to increase the dose with chronic treatment. Within this context many terms have crept into use; metabolic, physiological, and behavioral tolerance are referred to, and "dependence" and "tolerance" are often used interchangeably. The relationships between these various correlates of tolerance are not understood. An excellent review by Corfield-Sumner and Stolerman (1978) covers much of the classical literature.

The phenomenon of tolerance has been most widely investigated in relation to morphine and other opiate drugs. Worthy of further comment in this context is the term *learned tolerance*, because its introduction has generated new and interesting questions about tolerance. Clearly, there are marked physiological and metabolic correlates of behavioral tolerance to opiates, and there can be no question that these processes represent a major feature of withdrawal.

However, Siegel and others have emphasized the importance of corollary learning processes which proceed with the development of physiological tolerance. According to these workers, such learning influences the development of the dependent state, the characteristics of the behavioral tolerance observed, and the nature of any subsequent withdrawal symptoms.

In one of his experiments Siegel (1976) demonstrated that tolerance to the analgesic effect of morphine developed when rats were tested in the environment in which they had previously received morphine and been assessed, but not when tested in a different environment. These results suggest an association between environmental cues (CS) and the unconditioned stimuli (UCS) associated with the morphine injection. As a consequence of the regular pairing of these conditioned and unconditioned stimuli, the conditioned stimuli come to elicit unconditioned responses in the absence of the morphine (unconditioned stimulus). It has been frequently reported that the conditioned drug responses are opposite in direction to the unconditioned effects of the drugs. Thus, after morphine is administered in a distinctive environment, those conditioned stimuli would tend to induce hyperalgesia rather than analgesia; the analgesic effect would, thus, be partially reversed and the rats would be showing tolerance to the analgesic effect of the drug when the conditioned stimuli are present.

Wikler (1965) emphasized the importance of a conditioned association between the euphoric state or "high" induced by the intake of addictive drugs and the stimuli associated with the drug-taking act in its broadest sense (ranging from the place where the drug pusher is seen, to the paraphenalia of the syringe and needle). Wikler believes that curing a drug habit must involve extinction of the associated Pavlovian conditioning, as well as withdrawal of the drug itself.

Kesner et al. (1976) provided independent evidence that tolerance to the analgesic effect of morphine represents a form of learning mediated by memory processes and cellular mechanisms similar to those underlying conventional learning. Under certain conditions morphine tolerance can be demonstrated after a single dose of morphine. Kesner and his associates showed in the rat that electroconvulsive shock or subseizure stimulation of frontal cortex soon after the initial administration of morphine disrupted the development of one-trial tolerance on the "flinch jump" test. Such manipulations are known to disrupt the retention of other learned experiences.

IMPORTANCE OF THE VARIOUS DETERMINANTS FOR DISTINGUISHING DRUG CLASSES

There are clearly many determinants of drug action, and all of them should be studied in order to characterize any particular drug fully. The hope is that in this way different classes of psychoactive compounds may be distinguished and the ways in which they influence behavior defined. This has not been achieved, but some examples will be given of how certain drug groups may be characterized by applying the methods of behavioral analysis we have described.

Analgesics

Morphine and barbiturates are prescribed for the relief of intractable pain. Weiss and Laties (1958) have used an ingenious titration method for determining shock threshold to measure the increase in pain threshold after morphine injections (see Chapter 8). Studies of shock-punished behavior, however, make it clear that a change in pain threshold is not sufficient to alleviate pain in all situations, and, indeed, that reinstatement of behavior suppressed by shock is not likely to be mediated by such a mechanism. Although morphine markedly increases pain thresholds, it will not, for example, reinstate behavior suppressed by punishment. In a typical experiment, pigeons were trained in the presence of an orange light for five reinforcements under an FR 30. The light was then changed to white, and, although the FR 30 was still in operation, every tenth response was punished (Kelleher and Morse, 1964). Behavior in the white light was suppressed, and morphine did not reinstate it.

In contrast, barbiturates resulted in an immediate reinstatement of the punished responding, and further evidence that this was not related to an analgesic effect was afforded by the observation that if shock was omitted suddenly in undrugged sessions, behavior was reinstated but less quickly than after barbiturates. Morphine and barbiturates clearly act to relieve the anxiety associated with pain in different ways.

Major vs. minor tranquilizers

Minor tranquilizers (barbiturates in small doses, meprobamate, and benzodiazepines) potently release punished responding, whereas the phenothiazines and other neuroleptics (major tranquilizers) are totally ineffective.

A clear example of this dissociation is found in a study by Morse (1964). Using a multiple VI food/VI punishment schedule (Fig. 3–9), he found that amobarbital increased food-reinforced behavior marginally and punished behavior markedly, whereas chlorpromazine produced a dose-dependent decrease in both behaviors (Fig. 3–10).

Major tranquilizers vs. stimulants

Neither of these groups of drugs attenuate punished responding, but, if they are tested on reinforced patterns of behavior, they are clearly differentiated. Amphetamine increases the response rate on an FI schedule for food and for shock-escape, whereas chlorpromazine decreases both behaviors (Fig. 3–3) (Kelleher and Morse, 1964).

Minor tranquilizers vs. stimulants

Barbiturates in small doses and benzodiazepines have a rate-increasing effect on food-reinforced behavior. The effect is strong in the case of the barbiturates, and, here, they are difficult to distinguish from stimulants. If punished responding is studied, however, they are clearly dissociable; amphetamine is ineffective in restoring punished responding, whereas the barbiturates are highly effective. This example illustrates how drug groups may share a certain property that is primary to one and secondary to the other and how this is only appreciated if they are compared on several behavioral parameters.

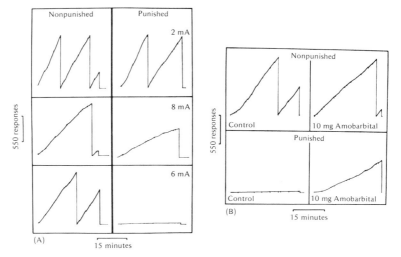

Fig. 3–9   (A) Representative cumulative response records of three pigeons for daily sessions on Mult VI VI + punishment. The nonpunishment and punishment components of the schedule alternated every 4 min. *Left:* nonpunishment periods; *right:* punishment periods. The diagonal marks on the records show food deliveries. Each response during the punishment periods produces a 25-msec electric shock of the current indicated. Suppression during the punishment components varies among the birds. (B) Cumulative response records of one pigeon for a control and drug session on Mult VI VI + punishment. *Left:* control records; *right:* drug records for the following day. The shock current during the punished components was 6 mA, which greatly suppressed the level of responding. After 10 mg amobarbital, the level of nonpunished responding is somewhat decreased (top right), whereas the level of punished responding is greatly increased (bottom right). (Reproduced from Morse, 1964.)

Antidepressants vs. other drug groups

Antidepressants are easily distinguished from stimulants by their failure (except in pigeons and dogs) to increase rates of reinforced behavior. They are also clearly distinguishable from minor tranquilizers because they do not attenuate punished responding. Unfortunately, however, they are extremely difficult to dissociate behaviorally from the major tranquilizers. This is a disconcerting failure of behavioral pharmacology, considering the markedly different therapeutic uses of these drug groups.

The major tranquilizers, like the antidepressants, have rate-increasing effects in pigeons and dogs and do not attenuate punished responding. Only by indirect methods that probably depend on the different neuropharmacological actions of the drugs can these groups be dissociated. Amphetamine-induced locomotor activity, for example, is potentiated by antidepressants of both the tricyclic and MAO inhibitor classes, and this behavior is blocked by major tranquilizers. Similarly, antidepressants, but not chlorpromazine, potentiate the increased rates of responding for intracranial self-stimulation induced by amphetamine.

Indirect methods are perfectly valid in behavioral pharmacology, but it is important to try to develop direct tests to characterize the two major classes of psychoactive drugs that do not reliably increase any behaviors yet studied. Baltzer and Weiskrantz (1970) report an ingenious step in this direction with a potential test for antidepressants involving the Crespi effect (Chapter 1, p. 47).

If an animal that is responding for a regular-sized reinforcement suddenly receives a much larger or smaller one, the rate of ongoing behavior increases or decreases; it is suggested that this reflects "elation" or "depression." Unfortunately, the test has not proved sensitive to antidepressants (Baltzer, Huber, and Weiskrantz, 1979).

Fig. 3–10   (A) The dose–effect curve for amobarbital on punished responding for three pigeons. (B) The dose–effect curve for chlorpromazine on punished responding for three pigeons. (Reproduced from Morse, 1964.)

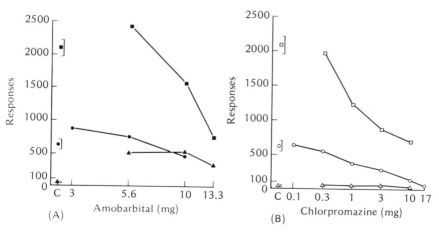

II. Drugs and Behavior

A very wide range of substances have pronounced effects on behavior. Not surprisingly, the drugs that have been used clinically to manipulate the physiological state of the brain in normal subjects, e.g. anesthetics and pain killers, or to alleviate behavioral disorders, e.g. tranquilizers and antidepressants, and those taken by otherwise normal people to induce pleasant psychological changes, e.g. alcohol, nicotine, hallucinogens, have been the most systematically studied. We propose to restrict our discussion to the major groups of drugs that influence selected aspects of behavior, as shown in the accompanying Table.

In each of the subsequent chapters a description of the basic neuropharmacological properties of the drug group precedes a discussion of its effects on behavior and brief comment on some of the animal models developed from such work which may be of relevance to neurology and psychiatry.

There are many different ways of classifying the effects of drugs on behavior: by drug group, by clinical usage, by neuropharmacological properties, by site of action in CNS, or by classes of behavior. All of these have their limitations, but the last has been selected as the most useful in the present text.

The effects of drugs on the various classes of behavior

Chapter	Behavioral state	Drugs with principal effect on state
4	Arousal	Stimulants
		Sedatives
5	Learning and memory	Pituitary hormones
		Protein synthesis inhibitors
		Adrenergic–cholinergic drugs
6	Goal-directed behavior	Adrenergic–cholinergic drugs
		Neuropeptides
7	Mood	Opiates
		Antidepressants
8	Pain	Opiates
9	Anxiety	Minor Tranquilizers
10	Psychosis	Hallucinogens
		Neuroleptics

4. Drugs Affecting Arousal: Amphetamines and Barbiturates

Arousal is probably the most important general variable determining the behavioral responses of animals. Most animals have a diurnal pattern of sleeping and waking, but during the waking phase, when animals respond to the external environment, they may have a wide range of arousal levels. A variety of physiological and psychological variables determines the mean level of arousal at any one time, probably by interacting with the reticular activating system of the brain. Malmo (1959) suggested that there is a U-shaped relationship between the physiological state of arousal and behavioral efficiency. If the arousal level is too low, there is virtually no behavior, and when the optimum level is exceeded, further arousal results in a general disruption of behavior.

Many drugs affect arousal as part of their psychopharmacological profile; the mood-changing opiates, for example, may also stimulate or depress other facets of behavior, whereas antipsychotic drugs, like chlorpromazine, depress all forms of behavior. Some drugs have their main effect on arousal and are used clinically or socially for this reason. The amphetamines and barbiturates will be considered in this context.

AMPHETAMINES AND RELATED COMPOUNDS
Classification

Amphetamine (Fig. 4–1) has several effects on behavior. In particular, it is a stimulant, and it is also an anorexic, i.e. it suppresses appetite for food.

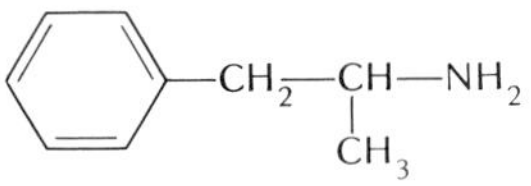

STIMULANTS

Amphetamine

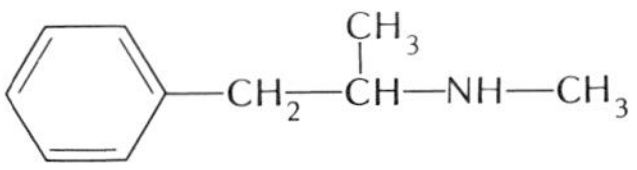

Methamphetamine

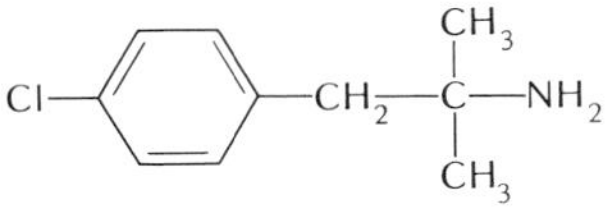

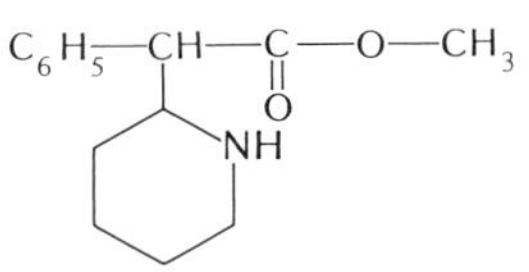

Methylphenidate

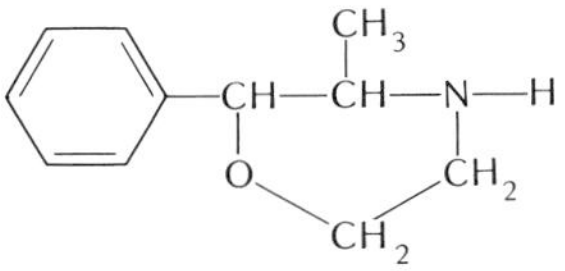

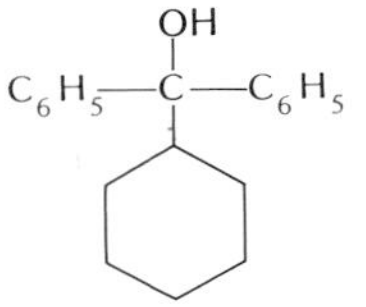

Pipradol

ANOREXICS

Chlorphentermine

Phenmetrazine

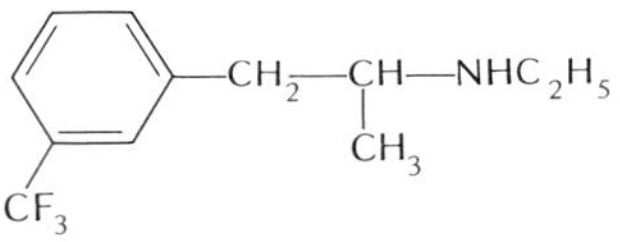

Fenfluramine

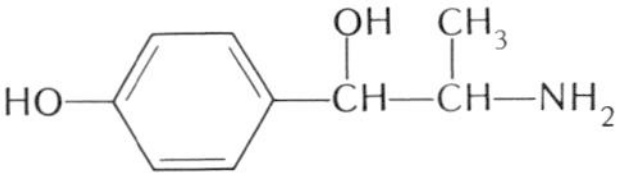

p-Hydroxynorephedrine
(amphetamine metabolite)

Fig. 4–1   Amphetamine and related compounds.

The *d* isomer of amphetamine (DEXEDRINE) is more potent in both respects than the *l* isomer and is the form of the drug commonly used. The related compound *d*-METHAMPHETAMINE ("SPEED") (Fig. 4–1, left) is an even more potent stimulant of behavior, and "rigid" analogues, in which the side chain is cyclized, such as METHYLPHENIDATE (RITALIN) and PIPRADOL, appear to stimulate behavior in a manner very similar to that of amphetamine. Other derivatives, however, are very weak stimulants, while retaining the anorexic effects of amphetamine, e.g. CHLORPHENTERMINE, PHENMETRAZINE (PRE-

LUDIN), and FENFLURAMINE (Fig. 4–1, right). The latter drugs are used clinically as appetite suppressants and have less of the undesirable stimulant and sleep-disrupting properties of amphetamine itself.

Neuropharmacological properties (see Moore, 1978)

The amphetamines are an important group of drugs to neuropharmacologists because their mode of action is fairly clearly defined. Amphetamine is an indirectly acting sympathomimetic amine in peripheral adrenergic systems, that is, it mimics the effects of norepinephrine (NE) by displacing this amine from peripheral adrenergic nerve endings, although amphetamine itself has little or no direct effect on NE receptors. The drug appears to act similarly in the brain, where it has been shown to release both NE and dopamine (DA) from nerves containing these amines. The fact that the powerful central stimulant activity of amphetamine is not shared by other indirectly acting sympathomimetic amines may be explained simply by the ease with which amphetamine penetrates into the brain compared with other amines of this type that are less soluble in lipids (cf. Chapter 2). The notion that amphetamine acts by displacing catecholamines from storage sites in the brain is strongly supported by the finding that pretreatment with drugs that inhibit catecholamine biosynthesis, α-methyl-p-tyrosine, for example, completely prevents amphetamine stimulation of behavior. On the other hand, amphetamine continues to stimulate animals in which brain catecholamines have been depleted by reserpine treatment. This can be explained, however, if it is assumed that amphetamine releases the catecholamines from the small pools of newly synthesized amines that are still present after reserpine treatment. In addition to causing catecholamine release, amphetamine is also a potent inhibitor of the NE- and DA-uptake systems in adrenergic terminals, and this inhibition tends to enhance and prolong the effects of the amines released by the drug by blocking their normal inactivation by these systems.

Although amphetamines appear to cause a release of both NE and DA in brain, their stimulant effects result primarily from the release of DA. The evidence in support of this conclusion is: (1) α- or β-adrenoceptor blocking drugs do not alter the central stimulant actions of amphetamines, (2) Inhibition of NE synthesis, without altering DA synthesis, by inhibitors of the NE synthetic enzyme dopamine-β-hydroxylase fails to block the CNS actions of the amphetamines, (3) Neuroleptic drugs which selectively block CNS receptors for DA (see Chapter 10), such as chlorpromazine, haloperidol, and pimozide, completely prevent the central stimulant effects of amphetamines, and (4) Selective lesions of DA pathways in animals by means of 6-hydroxydopamine administration block amphetamine-induced stimulation, whereas noradrenergic lesions fail to alter the amphetamine response. Thus, Creese and Iversen (1975) reported that injections of 6-hydroxydopamine into rat substantia nigra to destroy the dopaminergic neurons blocked the stimulant actions of d-amphetamine, whereas selective destruction of ascending NE neurons did not. Kelly et al. (1975) showed that 6-hydroxydopamine injections into dopamine-rich areas of brain blocked the stimulant effects of d-amphetamine, even if depletion of NE were prevented by pretreatment of the animals with desipramine, which protects NE neurons from the neurotoxic effects of 6-hydroxydopamine.

When administered in high doses, amphetamines also induce bizarre patterns of repeated behavior in animals, and this "stereotyped" behavior in response to amphetamines also depends principally on dopamine release, particularly in the nigrostriatal system of dopaminergic neurons.

Behavioral pharmacology

One of the most marked behavioral effects of amphetamine is its ability to stimulate various categories of spontaneous motor behavior in all the species that have been studied. A variety of automatic recording devices have been used for quantifying locomotor activity, including running wheels, jiggle cages, photocell devices, circular runways, and electromagnetic movement registering systems (Animex). When interest focused on the effect of arousal-inducing stimuli in the environment on locomotor activity, a variety of situations were devised for varying the nature of such stimulation. These include Y-maze situations with feeding troughs in the arms (Kumar, 1969), boxes with interesting objects placed in them (Carlsson, 1972), operant situations in which a lever press initiates a change in an environmental stimulus, such as a light or, as in the case of Butler's famous monkey experiment, the opening of a window on an interesting vista. A methodological review may be found in Robbins (1977).

Amphetamine has been shown to increase behavior in all these situations. For a number of years, such results have been interpreted simply as evidence of the stimulatory action of the drug. Direct somatomotor facilitation may indeed underlie the running activity seen when a rat is given amphetamine in a familiar environment. Normally an animal is inactive in such an environment, and the drug induces a short-lived burst of running. It has been appreciated recently that, in many of the more complex environments

used for assessing motor behavior, the recorded activity reflects the interaction of responses to several different aspects of the environment. For example, a rat moves about a wire cage resembling its home cage in a certain
way, but it behaves in quite a different way if interesting objects are placed
on the floor of the cage. Ambulation is usually the measure taken, presumably because it is easy to record. But not enough attention has been given
to the consideration that, in different situations, this mean level of activity
reflects the response to several interacting aspects of the environment. Amphetamine increases activity in all situations, but it is important to specify
which aspect of locomotor behavior (e.g. activity related or unrelated to an
investigation of interesting objects) has been changed by the drug.

Berlyne (1955) was one of the first to recognize this point, and he devised
an ingenious apparatus to identify motor responses to different aspects of
the environment. Robbins and Iversen (1973) have used this apparatus to
quantify locomotor behavior in the large area of a box against responses to
interesting objects placed in an alcove at one end of the box. Normal animals
distribute their behavior between these two features of the environment in
a correlated fashion. After amphetamine, a marked increase in locomotor
activity in the large area is seen in conjunction with reduced attention to
the localized stimuli. Similar observations have encouraged the belief that
amphetamine reduces exploration of the environment; it is more likely,
however, that the effect of the drug is not to reduce directly exploration but
that reduction of exploration occurs as a consequence of a direct stimulation
of locomotion in the main cage. The suggestion is that amphetamine increases the probability of certain responses to the disadvantage of others
and that where the opportunity for running exists its probability of occurrence is greatly increased by low doses of amphetamine.

However, conflicting results have been obtained using different measures
of exploratory behavior and, because of these inherent methodological problems, the question of whether or not amphetamine has a direct effect on
exploratory behavior remains unresolved. File and Wardill (1975) used a test
apparatus for rats with three arms and a single floor hole in each; interesting
stimuli were placed under the holes to enhance their novelty. Amphetamine
was found to reduce hole-exploring behavior. Makanjuola et al. (1977)
reached rather different conclusions using an open-field apparatus with six-
teen floor holes, without objects placed under them. They distinguished
"exploratory head dips" as responses to a hole other than the previous one,
and a "stereotyped dip" as one into the same hole as previously. Using this
apparatus, where the probability of exploratory response was high and not

incompatible with stereotyped behavior, they were able to show that amphetamine elicited an increase in *both* exploration and stereotypy, although the time scale and the dose–response profile differed for the two responses. However, there is no independent evidence that a single head dip reflects exploration or that repeated head dips reflect uncontrolled stereotyped responding. It could be that the apparatus encourages head dipping motor activity and that this single response is stimulated progressively by amphetamine. When stimulation was low (soon after the drug was injected and after low doses), repeated head dipping was minimally stimulated and single head dips predominated. At higher levels of stimulation the response was repeated at a higher frequency and appeared stereotyped.

The effects of amphetamine on unconditioned behavior are dose dependent; the maximum locomotor response in photocell cages is elicited by a dose of *d*-amphetamine of 1.5 mg/kg in the rat. If the dose is increased to 5 or 10 mg/kg, locomotor stimulation is no longer seen, and stereotyped behavior emerges. Stereotypy refers to a behavioral state wherein isolated elements of the normal behavioral repertoire, which seem quite inappropriate in the particular environment, are repeated with monotonous regularity. The number of elements of behavior that occur during stereotypy is reduced as the dose of the drug increases. In the rat, for example, stereotyped locomotion, sniffing, neck movements, and rearing are seen in weak stereotypy responses, but when these become intense, gnawing occurs to the exclusion of virtually all other behavior. Schiørring (1971) has also stressed that increasing doses of amphetamine produce a progressively more intense stimulation of fewer and fewer categories of behavior. Amphetamine-induced changes in unconditioned behavior have been studied in a number of vertebrate species (Randrup and Munkvad, 1970). In the cat, side-to-side looking movements with the head (often associated with fearlike responses) and repetitive sniffing movements are seen. As intoxication proceeds during several months of drug treatment a given animal becomes more locked into the stereotypy, returning to the same spot in the cage to sniff, taking up the same posture and sniffing in the same pattern. These studies have been extended to primates. Marmosets tested with *d*- and *l* isomers of amphetamine show a marked reduction in complex acts such as grooming, contact in play and fighting, and manipulating objects. Body activity is increased relatively little but "checking," a rapid side-to-side head movement, is significantly increased. Rhesus monkeys are more interesting because of variations in the responses to amphetamine among individual animals. Certain responses, such as skin-picking and staring, occur in most animals. However, it would appear that the psychological profile and personality of the animal influences the nature of the stereotyped behavior, and, unlike the rat, monkeys are not limited to a highly predictable set of species-specific acts. In monkeys Ellinwood (1971) described biting stereotypies, examining stereotypies, and grooming stereotypies. He noted that an act which is observed to occur at first by chance gradually may emerge as part of a complex stereotyped pattern of behavior. It is interesting that a given animal tends to exhibit the same form of stereotypy each time it is treated with amphetamine. This is reminiscent of the stereotypies described in human amphetamine addicts (Rylander, 1969). Clockmakers dismantle and reassemble clocks, mechanics cars, and housewives may perform repetitious household tasks. The cognitive set and environmental stimuli clearly play a large role in determining the profile of amphetamine-induced behavior in higher primates. Perhaps it is for this reason that complex motor acts become stereotyped in monkeys and man, whereas in rodents continuing stimulation with amphetamine results in a higher and higher frequency of increasingly brief acts, almost all fragments of normal behavior.

In all behavioral tests d-amphetamine is more potent than the optical isomer l-amphetamine. For example, Taylor and Snyder (1971) found the d isomer to be some ten times more potent than the l isomer in stimulating locomotor activity in the rat (see, Fig. 2–3), although there was only a small difference in potency between the two isomers in eliciting stereotyped behavior. Their suggestion that this might imply that release of brain norepinephrine was importantly involved in the locomotor response, whereas dopamine release was more important for the stereotyped behavior response has been largely discounted by subsequent neurochemical and behavioral studies, which strongly suggest that release of brain dopamine is the key factor underlying both of these behavioral responses.

Effects of amphetamine on conditioned behavior

Conditioned response patterns are also affected by amphetamine. The characteristic pattern of responding under fixed-interval schedules of reinforcement is stimulated by amphetamine (Dews, 1955b). The low rate of responding immediately after a reinforcement is particularly sensitive to the rate-increasing effect of the drug. In contrast, the high rates at the end of the interval show less increase and indeed may even be depressed, as are the high rates of responding seen on fixed-ratio schedules.

On the basis of such results, Dews (1958) has proposed a "baseline" theory of the stimulant action of the drug: that low rates of ongoing behavior are stimulated relatively more than high. An analysis of the increase in responding relative to baseline in the sequential segments of the fixed interval supports this proposition.

In reviewing the effects of amphetamine on behavior Dews and Morse (1961) suggested that: "All these findings are compatible with the view that an important determinant of the effects of the amphetamine is the control rate of responding per se, irrespective of species, or type of motivation, or response studied." Although the rate of ongoing behavior is a major determinant of amphetamine action, it is clearly not the only factor. In several different experiments, amphetamine has failed to increase low rates of ongoing behavior and, in other situations, the stimulatory action of the drug is associated with disruption rather than facilitation of performance. Lyon and Randrup (1972) have proposed that response topography should also be considered in relation to the stimulatory action of amphetamine. One of their experiments illustrates the point elegantly. Groups of rats were trained on one of two shock reinforcement schedules. One group was required to make a discrete lever press to turn off a shock and to delay further (and thus avoid) subsequent shocks. The other group was required to hold the lever depressed to escape and avoid shock. The effect of 1 to 5 mg/kg of d-amphetamine was studied on these two behavior patterns. A dose of 1 mg/kg increased lever pressing and lever release as part of the general stimulatory action. As a consequence, avoidance was facilitated on the lever-press schedule and was disrupted on the lever-hold schedule. In contrast, the stereotyped behavior induced by 3 and 5 mg/kg d-amphetamine tended to "immobilize" animals in the vicinity of the lever and disrupted lever-holding behavior less than lever-pressing responses. The authors propose that amphetamine may disrupt or enhance responding depending on the compatibility of the response with elements of behavior stimulated by amphetamine.

A major theoretical advance in this field was made by Lyon and Robbins (1977). In reviewing the earlier observations on rate dependency and response compatibility, and in synthesizing a vast body of experiments on the behavioral effects of amphetamine, they proposed the most parsimonious explanation to date: *that the basic effect of amphetamine is to enhance responding, and that the probability of different behaviors being emitted at the time of drug treatment is the major determinant of the predominant drug-induced behavior.* A number of factors determine response probabilities. In the case of unconditioned behavior, the natural response tendency will predominate, although this may be modified by the design of the environment. This is well illustrated by the range and frequency of different behaviors seen in the various exploratory situations mentioned earlier. In the case of conditioned behavior, reinforcement largely determines the probability of the given responses. With the following provisos, their theory has an impressive generality.

1. *Response incompatibility*—Responses most compatible with the trained response or those biologically innate and easy for the animal to make are likely to be most stimulated.

2. *Time required to complete behavior*—High levels of stimulation invoke physiological constraints in the motor apparatus. A response is generated before the previous one is completed and thus behavior becomes fragmented. Behaviors that normally require a short period for completion retain their identity for the longest time. Neck movements, sniffing, licking, and gnawing all fall within this category. Responses involving sequences of motor acts, like grooming, are not enhanced because there is no longer time for their completion and they are quickly overridden by the brief responses. In both rats and monkeys, grooming and social behavior are the first response elements to disappear during amphetamine treatment.

3. *Baseline response rate*—Highly probable responses occurring at a low rate increase more than equivalent responses occurring at high rate.

4. *Control exerted by environmental stimuli*—If behavior is under the control of strong environmental stimuli, that behavior is very likely to be enhanced by amphetamine and performed in the appropriate stimulus location.

So much for the theoretical basis of the view that a primary action of amphetamine is to stimulate response output by focusing behavior toward certain motor acts. This may be revealed as a form of motor attention which, within its normal limits, would enhance behavioral efficiency. Motor responses are guided by sensory stimuli. There is growing evidence that amphetamine, in addition to its effects on responses, also enhances the control that stimuli exert over those responses and, thus, in a real sense, enhances the associative processes essential to learning and memory. It has been established that amphetamine releases DA in the striatum (Nieoullon et al., 1979). DA release presumably occurs also in the limbic areas and in these sites is essential to the locomotor enhancement seen with moderate doses of amphetamine. This behavioral process has been termed "motivational arousal" (Iversen, 1977) and is considered to be essential in enabling animals to locate, recognize, and respond in the presence of the stimuli most appropriate to their immediate needs.

An event whose presentation sustains behavior is termed a reinforcing

stimulus and is said to be rewarding; both interoceptive and exteroceptive
stimuli can serve that function. Commonly we think of food, water, or sex-
associated stimuli in this context. Animals will respond, or learn to respond,
to obtain such stimuli and amphetamine appears to enhance the way in
which such stimuli gain control over behavior. Animals will also learn to
press a lever and continue to press it at very high rates to obtain electrical
stimulation of certain areas of the brain. This phenomenon is termed INTRA-
CRANIAL-SELF STIMULATION (ICS) and has been the focus of much experimental investigation [reviewed admirably by Milner (1971)]. It is generally
accepted that the brain systems which are most sensitive to ICS are involved
in the process by which sensory stimuli acquire their rewarding or reinforcing property. Reward has thus come to have both procedural and physiological definitions.

The self-stimulation method differs in no formal way from other behavioral techniques based on the use of positive reinforcers. All that is involved
from the point of view of method is the substitution of an electrical stimulus
to the brain instead of a conventional reinforcer like food. It is generally
accepted that ICS reflects activation of pathways in the brain central to the
process of reinforcement. Amphetamine enhances the rate of ICS. It would
seem that in the presence of the drug the reinforcing quantity of a stimulus
is enhanced. This has been demonstrated in a number of ways. For example, the level at which a current has reinforcing power can be assessed
using a titration method to determine ICS threshold. Stein and Ray (1960)
devised a two-lever test situation in which every response to one lever delivered brain stimulation and decreased its intensity by a set amount. A
reward lever was available which reset the current to its initial level. The
current level at which the rat approached the second lever would indicate
the reward threshold, that is, the point at which the gradually decreasing
current lost its reinforcing property. After amphetamine administration, rats
reset the current at a lower point than normal, indicating that the brain
stimulation had become more rewarding. After the administration of DA
receptor blocking drugs, such as pimozide, the reverse was true, and rats
reset the current at a much higher point than normal, suggesting that the
current was not as rewarding as it had been. It has often been suggested
that DA is merely concerned in processes of motor control required to perform ICS rather than with the coding of rewarding stimuli. In support of
this view the commonly reported reduction in rates of responding for ICS
after neuroleptics (DA receptor blocking drugs) are given is said to be due
to motor incapacitation rather than to an attenuation of reward. Two-lever
situations that incorporate measures of rates of responding, as well as cur-

rent preference, answer this question directly. By this means Zarevics and Setler (1979) have shown that amphetamine enhances and pimozide decreases the rewarding value of ICS (Fig. 4.2) independently from their effects on motor output. Recently, ICS has also been studied in terms of rate-intensity functions. This simply means that under a given set of conditions the rate of ICS responding is measured for a range of current intensities. If the brain stimulation then becomes more or less rewarding, the curve relating rate of responding to current intensity shifts to the left or right, respectively. Amphetamine shifts rate-intensity functions to the left, or in other words low intensities of current sustain higher rates of responding than under control conditions; neuroleptics do the opposite.

A number of forebrain sites, particularly in the limbic system, sustain self-stimulation and there is growing evidence that dopaminergic pathways play a central role in the activity of these brain regions. Forebrain sites that sustain the highest and most reliable levels of ICS have dopaminergic innervation: they either provide the trajectory of DA neurons as in the case of the medial forebrain bundle, or lie on such trajectories as in the case of the lateral hypothalamus. Selective interference with brain DA systems by means of α-methyl-p-tyrosine, neuroleptics, or lesions (Cooper et al., 1974; Clavier and Routtenberg, 1976; Rolls et al., 1974) attenuates self-stimulation. Continuing efforts are being made to demonstrate that such manipulations attenuate the rewarding value of ICS and do not merely depress motor output and prevent the performance of the ICS-seeking response (Koob et al., 1978). Similar manipulations of NE pathways do not attenuate ICS. Presumably amphetamine enhances the effect of rewarding brain stimulation by release of DA in these critical pathways. In support of this hypothesis Phillips and Fibiger (1978) demonstrated that amphetamine was no longer able to stimulate ICS responding after biochemical depletion or destruction of forebrain DA pathways. However, it would be misleading to leave this topic without pointing out that some experimenters feel that the importance of NE pathways to reward processes has been underestimated because of the recent emphasis on the role of DA systems. This issue is well argued by Stein et al. (1977) and Routtenberg and Santos-Anderson (1977). At many of the anatomical sites in question it is difficult to selectively lesion NE systems without influencing the DA systems, and the pharmacological methods available for interfering with the synthesis or the synaptic actions of catecholamines [e.g. α-methyl-tyrosine, FLA 63, diethyldithiocarbamate (DDC) or chlorpromazine] influence both NE and DA neurons. For these reasons the issue has not been definitively resolved.

If a neutral stimulus is paired with a reinforcing event, that stimulus ac-

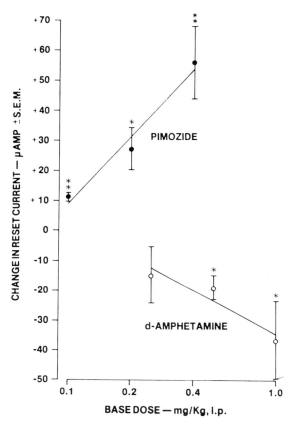

Fig. 4–2 Dose–response curves for the effect of pimozide and d-amphetamine on ICS "threshold" expressed as the change in μA of reset currents. Pimozide produced a significant dose-related increase and amphetamine a decrease in reward "threshold." (* $p < 0.05$; ** $p < 0.01$, two-tailed t-test).
(Reproduced from Zarevics and Setler, 1979)

quires reinforcing properties and becomes a *conditioned reinforcer*. As an extension of Stein's hypothesis that amphetamine enhances the power of reinforcing stimuli, Hill (1970) has proposed that stimulants also, therefore, enhance the control of conditioned reinforcing stimuli over behavior. In the original experiment Hill trained rats to press a lever for sweet milk on a variable interval (2 min) schedule. With each operation of the feeder, its motor emitted a loud hum. Under such conditions the hum acquires a conditioned reinforcing (CR) property and rats trained in its presence extinguish responding when milk is no longer given less quickly than rats trained without the CR. Hill studied extinction with and without the sound in rats treated with pipradol 10 mg/kg or saline. Extinction was significantly slowed by the presence of the CR and to a greater degree in the pipradol-treated rats. Extinction methods for evaluating the power of CR have been questioned (MacIntosh, 1974) because under such training conditions a stimulus may act as a discriminative stimulus *or* as a conditioned reinforcer, and in either case responding in the face of extinction is enhanced. To avoid this problem, Robbins (1978) assessed conditioned reinforcers by their ability to sustain the acquisition of a new operant response; i.e. will rats press an appropriate lever to obtain a stimulus previously associated with food? They did, and pipradol, methylphenidate, and *d*-amphetamine all enhanced the power of CRs to sustain new behavior (Robbins, 1978). Since much behavior is controlled by CRs, it is clear that the hypothesis is of general importance in explaining some of the effects of stimulants on behavior.

If DA release is a correlate of rewarding stimulation and if amphetamine releases DA, then in addition to its ability to enhance the rewarding effect of other stimuli, amphetamine should be rewarding in its own right. This is in fact the case. Rats and monkeys will learn to self-administer amphetamine by pressing a lever to obtain small intravenous injections through an implanted catheter (Woods and Tessel, 1974), and lesions to DA pathways abolish the self-administration of the stimulant cocaine (Roberts et al., 1977).

Amphetamine thus has stimulus properties and, as we have seen in Chapter 1, stimuli control behavior in a number of different ways. For example, if a response is performed in the presence of a stimulus, the latter acquires discriminative properties (S^D). There is growing interest in the discriminative properties of drug states, and it has been shown that animals can use such stimuli to guide behavior (Lal, 1977). This has been shown for amphetamine and for a number of other drug groups including neuroleptics and opiates. In the standard procedure, rats are trained to press the left lever in an operant chamber for food when injected with the drug and the right after a saline injection. Drug and saline test days are given on a random schedule, until the animal reliably approaches and presses the left lever or right lever depending on the injection received. The number of training sessions required varies widely between rats. Once reliable performance to the training dose of the drug is established, drug generalization curves can be obtained. Colpert et al. (1978) found *d*-amphetamine to be five times more potent than cocaine as a discriminative stimulus. Pretreatment with haloperidol did not abolish the discriminative control exerted by the drugs,

suggesting that dopamine does not play an indispensible role in the processes by which a rat learns to respond to the interoreceptive discriminative
cues generated by stimulant drugs, although DA is clearly essential to the
reinforcing property of stimulants.

Insofar as the interoceptive stimuli associated with drug intake can influence similar behavior at a different time, drug-seeking behavior may be
considered "state-dependent." Stretch and Gerber's (1973) study of amphetamine self-administration in the monkey supports this consideration.
Monkeys were trained on progressive ratio schedule (i.e. increasing number
of responses per reinforcement) for infusions of d-amphetamine (Fig. 4–3,
column A). Responding was then extinguished by saline injections (Fig.
4–3, column B). At this stage, amphetamine (1.0, 0.30, or 0.15 mg/kg) was
infused 1 min before the start of a session, and saline injections were continued throughout the sessions. Under these conditions, responses on the FR
schedule re-emerge and reach the level associated with amphetamine reinforcements in the first part of the experiment (Fig. 4–3, columns C, D,
and E).

Many of the effects of amphetamine described above may be explained in
terms of an interaction with DA systems of forebrain. However, it is clear
that amphetamine interacts with other pharmacological substrates of brain
and the task is to differentiate these other sites of action and determine their
contribution to the overall profile of amphetamine effects on behavior. The
best example concerns the anorectic effect of amphetamine, which reduces
food intake in a dose-related manner, an effect that shows rapid tolerance.
Some attempts have been made to account for amphetamine-induced anorexia in terms of response incompatibility. It has been reasoned that it would
be difficult for an animal in a high state of locomotor arousal to focus behavior on feeding. It now seems that there is a better explanation. Amphetamine releases NE as well as DA, and it has been shown that NE release in
the hypothalamus is central to the anorectic effect of amphetamine (see also
Chapter 6).

In addition to its arousing and anorectic effects, amphetamine has other
more recently discovered actions. It seems that in addition to acting as a
reinforcing stimulus, amphetamine can also act as an aversive or punishing
stimulus that reduces the probability of responding. This has been demonstrated using the conditioned taste aversion paradigm. If, after eating, rats
are given an unpleasant sensation they subsequently reject the taste associated with the food. The classic experiments use saccharin as the taste and
intraperitoneal lithium chloride as the unpleasant interoceptive stimulus

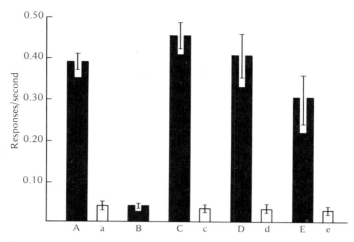

Fig. 4–3   Responses during amphetamine reinforcement, extinction, and amphetamine priming. Columns shown in black (A, B, C, D, and E) refer to the mean (± S.E.) rates of responding during those periods of experimental sessions in which response-contingent infusions of either the drug or saline were available; columns shown in white (a, c, d, and e) refer to mean (± S.E.) rates of responding recorded during time-out (TO). Column A refers to phase 1 (response-contingent infusions of amphetamine); column B to phase 2 (extinction). Columns C, D, and E refer to rates of responding (mean ± S.E.) following amphetamine pretreatment at doses of 1.00 mg/kg (C), 0.30 mg/kg (D), and 0.15 mg/kg (E), respectively. (Reproduced from Stretch and Gerber, 1973.)

(Garcia and Ervin, 1968). Amphetamine in doses upwards of 0.1 mg/kg also induces taste aversion (Cappell and Le Blanc, 1971; Carey and Goodall, 1974).

It may seem paradoxical that amphetamine can act both as a reinforcing and as an aversive stimulus. Confronting this problem directly, Wise et al. (1976) have attempted to demonstrate that amphetamine can act *simultaneously* in an animal as a reinforcing and aversive stimulus. Rats that reliably self-administered amphetamine were tested on the taste aversion paradigm using saccharin solution and a postingestion dose of 1.0 mg/kg amphetamine. Substantial reduction of subsequent saccharin intake was found albeit not as great as in drug-naive animals.

This experiment was difficult to design for two reasons. First, the conditioned taste aversion test should be given early in animal's history of drug self-administration because drug experience reduces the aversive effect of the drug. Ideally, the conditioned taste aversion test should be given on the *first* day the reinforcing effect of the drug is demonstrated. Second, the initial saccharin exposure has to be given before the amphetamine, to satisfy the usual relation between conditioned and unconditioned stimulus for the taste aversion paradigm. Since it is not possible to predict the first day on which the amphetamine will be self-administered, it is impossible to decide the appropriate time for the initial saccharine exposure. Efforts were made to overcome these problems in a second experiment. Rats were first trained to self-administer amphetamine and were then transferred to an equally rewarding stimulant drug, apomorphine. It was assumed that rats would immediately transfer from amphetamine to apomorphine and thus the taste aversion experiment could be performed with confidence on the first day of exposure to apomorphine. This proved to be the case in a number of rats and, again, a reduction in saccharin intake was found in those rats self-administering apomorphine after ingestion of the sweet solution. These are intriguing results, demonstrating that drug injections can be both positively reinforcing and punishing at the same time.

Furthermore, it seems that some stimuli are predisposed to become associated with rewarding events and others with punishment. These constraints on learning are illustrated clearly in taste aversion where in the rat taste stimuli are readily associated with feeling ill, whereas auditory and visual stimuli are found not to be powerful conditioned stimuli in aversion paradigms. If rats drink in the presence of a distinctive light, amphetamine is not able to induce a dramatic reduction of subsequent drinking under the light condition. Such constraints on learning are biologically important; it is more useful to identify poisonous food by taste than by sight or sound.

Reicher and Holman (1977) have shown that rats can learn simultaneously to associate taste stimuli and stimuli from a particular location in the environment with a drug state. Rats were injected with amphetamine and placed immediately or 20 min later on one side of a shuttlebox with access to a flavored solution. On subsequent choice trials without amphetamine, rats chose the side previously associated with the drug state but simultaneously showed aversion to the flavored solution.

How can these widely differing behavioral effects of amphetamine be reconciled? It is now clear that a unitary hypothesis of amphetamine action in terms of pharmacology, site of action in the CNS, and behavior is untenable. A number of studies show that the arousal, anorectic, and aversive effects of the drug are not correlated. Booth et al. (1977) have compared the arousing and aversive effects of a range of stimulant drugs tested at different doses.

They concluded that the potencies of such drugs on the taste aversion task did not correlate with their potencies in eliciting behavioral stimulation. The anorectic and aversive effects of amphetamine do not correlate either. Carey (1978) has compared these effects in separate groups of rats by giving amphetamine before eating to induce anorexia and after eating to induce taste aversion. The development of the two effects had different time scales and showed different patterns of tolerance. 1–2 mg/kg d-amphetamine administered 30 min before eating a preferred high fat food initially almost completely suppressed food intake, but this effect showed rapid tolerance. Given *after* eating there were initially minimal effects on food intake, but with repeated injections almost complete suppression of intake was obtained. It is suggested that the latter effect is due to taste-aversion learning and on this behavioral measure no tolerance was seen to repeated amphetamine administration. At present, it can be concluded that amphetamine acts potently at least on the core DA reinforcement systems of brain and on the hypothalamic regulatory centers. It is possible that some of the more unusual discriminative properties of the drug involve yet other localized neuropharmacological substrates of brain.

Amphetamine psychosis as a model for schizophrenia

Schizophrenia is characterized by bizarre thought disorders, hallucinations, and disturbances of affect leading to withdrawal from meaningful interaction with other people (Wing, 1978). There are several varieties of schizophrenic illness and their etiology is largely unknown, although inheritance is thought to play a significant role. Not surprisingly in these circumstances, it has not proved possible to design a convincing animal model of the clinical condition by manipulation of normal behavioral contingencies. However, two lines of pharmacological evidence have emerged that may lead to useful animal models for schizophrenia research (Snyder, 1972). First, it has been observed that humans addicted to amphetamine show a form of psychotic behavior that closely resembles paranoid schizophrenia; indeed, not infrequently in the clinic, amphetamine addicts have been misdiagnosed as florid paranoid schizophrenics. Second, it has become clear that the neuroleptic drugs which are most successfully used for alleviating the primary symptoms of schizophrenia, act neuropharmacologically as antagonists at CNS dopamine receptors (see Chapter 10).

Amphetamine psychosis in man is characterized by agitation and abnormal cognitive processes, which are often associated with delusions of persecution. Angrist and Gershon (1970) studied the emergence and nature of amphetamine psychosis under hospital conditions. Volunteers, previously addicted to amphetamine, were given large doses of amphetamine over a 24-hr period. Dramatic psychosis emerged consistently on this drug regimen. Thought disorder was conspicuously lacking, although it was possible that the increased level of arousal evoked by the drug masked this sympton. Typically, amphetamine psychosis is associated with delusions, hallucinations in all modalities, and the stereotyped repetition of meaningless patterns of behavior.

If the claim of psychological and neuropharmacological similarity between amphetamine psychosis and paranoid schizophrenia is valid, certain further predictions can be made. Mild schizophrenia should be exacerbated by amphetamine administration, and other drugs that increase brain concentrations of free DA should also induce psychosis. These predictions have been borne out by experimental work in man. Davis (1974) reported that relapse, with the reappearance of hallucinations and delusions, could be induced in recovered schizophrenics and that the *d*- and *l* isomers of amphetamine were equipotent in this respect. It is important to note that amphetamine intensifies preexisting schizophrenic symptoms; it does not precipitate additional symptoms. Patients are able to recognize that their illness worsens under the influence of the drug. In contrast, when they are treated with LSD, schizophrenics can identify the ensuing psychosis as different from their preexisting mental disturbance (Janowsky et al., 1973).

L-dopa, which increases the availability of DA in the brain, might also be expected to induce psychosis. Indeed, psychotic side effects are not uncommon in parkinsonian patients who receive treatment with large doses of L-dopa, and when L-dopa was given to schizophrenic patients an exacerbation of psychosis was observed (Angrist et al., 1973).

Cocaine is another stimulant that induces a form of psychosis similar to schizophrenia in man and shares many of the neuropharmacological properties of amphetamine (Siegel, 1978).

As mentioned earlier, large *acute* doses of amphetamine produce marked behavioral changes in all animal species studied. In the rat and monkey (Randrup and Munkvad, 1970; Ellinwood, 1971) abnormal stereotyped behavior is prominent. Ellinwood et al. (1972) reported observations of catatonic postures elicited in the cat by amphetamine. They described dyssynchrony as "a given body ensemble taking on autonomous movement which did not seem to have purpose or relatedness to other body segments." For example, repetitious repositioning or raising movements of the hind legs on many occasions had little or no relation to the sniffing patterns that involved the head and neck. The active front end and the inactive hind end resulted in a hunchback posture. The cat often appeared to have forgotten where a leg was positioned and left it in an awkward position. Other disjunctive postures included uncomfortable sitting and lying positions, very much like those noted in human catatonics. The importance of postural attitudinal sets for the normal organization of behavior has been stressed.

Amphetamine does not induce stereotypy after selective destruction of the nigro striatal DA pathway, although the increase in locomotor arousal seen after low doses of the drug remains. By contrast, the mesolimbic-cortical dopaminergic pathway is involved in locomotor responses to amphetamine but not in stereotypy. It is likely that in man the stereotypy and agitation are associated with these two sectors of the DA system; it is more difficult, however, to predict the neurological foci for the thought disorder, hallucinations, and affective changes induced by amphetamine.

Are there any other models of schizophrenia in animals which mimic a greater range of the cardinal symptoms of the clinical condition? Amphetamine psychosis and schizophrenia are chronic conditions which cannot be duplicated by acute drug treatment. A means of achieving slow sustained release of amphetamine in animals has been devised (Huberman et al., 1977). The drug is dissolved in a silicone liquid base within a plastic pellet which is implanted subcutaneously. The drug is released slowly and escapes from the plastic pellet through a diffusion hole. Sustained levels of brain amphetamine are found in the rat for up to 10 days after implantation of a pellet containing 48 mg amphetamine. Interesting behavioral results have been obtained in implanted rats habituated in a social colony (Ellison et al., 1978). On days 1 and 2 the predictable increases in general activity and stereotypy were seen in the drugged animals. But as the drug state continued fascinating behaviors emerged in this complex social environment. On day 3 drugged animals withdrew into the burrows where they remained for about 24 hr. On re-emerging they initiated a great deal of abnormal social interaction, often approaching and initiating aggressive encounters with other rats. Surprisingly, these behaviors are seen with sustained brain levels of amphetamine no higher than those seen 30 min after an i.p. injection of 2 mg/kg of amphetamine. Recently, the drug pellet implantation of amphetamine has been used in rhesus monkeys. After the stereotypy phase, bizarre startle, orientation, and fleeing behaviors were frequently observed. As these occurred in the absence of identifiable stimuli they may constitute a form of hallucinatory behavior. Tactile hallucinations also seemed to occur, as intense bouts of skin inspection and picking were observed, reminiscent of the "bug" hallucination in human amphetamine and cocaine addicts. It would seem that models involving social interaction provide interesting new avenues of enquiry.

Animal models for assessing drug actions on brain dopamine and their relevance to Parkinson's disease

Parkinson's disease is a neurological condition associated with muscular rigidity, a paucity of voluntary movements (akinesia), and tremor. It is progressive and seriously debilitating. It has long been known to be associated with neuropathological changes in the basal ganglia. Several different forms and etiologies of the disease have been recognized. In cases where tremor is the dominant symptom, patients have often been treated by the surgical production of lesions in certain thalamic nuclei associated with motor control and thought to be involved in the maintenance of the abnormal tremor. The rigidity and akinesia symptoms that predominate in other groups of patients have been treated with drugs, and anticholinergics were known to alleviate the symptoms long before the neuropharmacological rationale of this therapy was appreciated. When the distribution of amine transmitters in the brain was described, it became apparent that the basal ganglia had a rich dopaminergic innervation, and biochemical analysis of postmortem parkinsonian brain tissue revealed abnormally low levels of DA and tyrosine hydroxylase in the caudate nucleus and other regions of the neostriatum. This biochemical defect, together with evidence of cell loss from the substantia nigra, the site of origin of the dopaminergic nigrostriatal system, confirmed the neurochemical basis of at least the rigidity and akinesia symptoms in Parkinson's disease.

These findings resulted in the development of a new pharmacological treatment for parkinsonism. It was argued that, since the disease was associated with a deficiency of DA in the brain, biochemical manipulations that temporarily replenished DA stores should improve the extrapyramidal motor symptoms. But DA itself could not be given, since it would not pass the blood–brain barrier. It was found, however, that L-dopa, an amino-acid precursor of DA, did enter the brain to increase brain DA in experimental animals. L-Dopa therapy for parkinsonism was introduced and proved highly successful. This represents the first example of the rational development of a drug treatment for a CNS disorder based on a neurochemical understanding of the nature of the disease. As far as the rigidity and akinesia symptoms are concerned, L-dopa has revolutionized the prognosis for many parkinsonian patients. The improvement in motor performance is rapid, once L-dopa treatment is started, and bedridden patients can often resume normal activities.

The neurochemical coordination of basal ganglia structures has been further explored in animal preparations. It appears that the synthesis of DA in the nigrostriatal pathway is controlled partly by a feedback loop from the striatum to the substantia nigra, and ACh is thought to be the transmitter at the regulating synapses. In addition, there is a strong cholinergic input to the striatum itself, and the fact that anticholinergic drugs are used successfully to treat parkinsonism suggests that there is a cholinergic/dopaminergic balance involved in the normal control of motor function.

Animal model systems have been devised to study antiparkinsonian drugs. The apparently simple neurological and neurochemical basis of Parkinson's disease encouraged attempts to produce a similar defect in animals by the placement of lesions in the nigrostriatal system. Such lesions in rats, cats, and monkeys, however, disrupt normal motor behavior but do not closely mimic the clinical syndrome. This is perhaps not surprising. Parkinson's disease develops in patients over a period of many years, and such a gradual eroding of neural substrates may well induce subtle adaptive changes in nervous functions that cannot be mimicked by a sudden experimental assault on the same structure. Larochelle et al. (1971) have pursued this problem in both cats and monkeys. Although discrete substantia nigra lesions in the monkey did not produce parkinsonian symptoms, more extensive extrapyramidal damage involving the substantia nigra and the neural circuit between the red nucleus and the cerebellum induced tremor. Damage to the latter circuit plus treatment with the MAO inhibitor, harmaline, produced the same effect. In monkeys with the combination lesions, L-dopa treatment markedly improved the motor disturbances.

Bilateral substantia nigra lesions, therefore, do not produce an animal model of Parkinson's disease. Ungerstedt (1971), however, has developed a unilateral substantia nigra lesion preparation that has proved useful in evaluating drugs that influence the dopaminergic functioning of the basal ganglia.

The unilateral lesion is made by injecting 6-OHDA through a cannula placed in the substantia nigra to selectively destroy amine-containing neurons, in this case, the nigrostriatal DA pathway; widespread nonspecific damage to nearby systems is thus avoided. After the immediate postoperative effects on motor behavior subside, the rats show circling motor activity if the dopaminergic system is stimulated pharmacologically. The rats are placed in a circular dome to provide an easy way of constraining circling, and a recording mechanism attached to the back of the rat automatically cumulates rotations. In this so-called "ROTOMETER," drugs that release amines (e.g. amphetamine, cocaine) produce turning toward the side of the lesion, whereas DA agonists (e.g. apomorphine, L-dopa) produce turning in the opposite direction (Fig. 4–4). It is suggested that the nigrostriatal degeneration results in the loss of presynaptic DA and postsynaptic supersensitivity on the side of the lesion. Therefore, drugs that release amines have less influence on this side of the basal ganglia, whereas receptor stimulators have more. Amine receptor blocking agents like the phenothiazines and butyrophenones prevent drug-induced rotation. In intact rats, consistent turning behavior can also be induced by unilateral injection of DA or apomorphine directly into the striatum (Ungerstedt et al., 1969). Glick has gone further and suggested that in normal rats there is a natural imbalance between DA levels in the two striata. This imbalance accounts for the spatial preferences shown by rats in behavioral situations, such as a T-maze or a two-lever Skinner box (Zimmerberg et al., 1978).

BARBITURATES
Classification and neuropharmacological properties (see Nicoll, 1978)

There are many different barbituric acid derivatives with sedative properties. They range from drugs with slow metabolism and long duration of action, such as PHENOBARBITAL, to drugs with ultrashort actions, such as THIOPENTAL which are widely used as anesthetics (Fig. 4–5). Before the advent of the minor tranquilizers, drugs like phenobarbital were widely used as antianxiety agents and were given in small doses to reduce emotional tension and produce mild skeletal muscle relaxation (see Chapter 9). The barbiturates, however, readily lead to addicition and tolerance when used chronically. The risk of accidental poisoning or suicide is also much greater than with the newer antianxiety drugs, and thus barbiturates have fallen out of favor for psychopharmacological use.

Within the brain, barbiturates produce a number of effects, in particular a general slowing of oxidative metabolism and a depression of synaptic transmission. These effects do not seem to be confined to any particular neuronal system, and it is possible that the actions of these drugs are related to an overall depressant effect on brain metabolism and activity, related to their anesthetic properties. On the other hand, there is evidence that the barbiturates may act more specifically, for example, by enhancing the inhibitory synaptic actions of GABA (Nicoll, 1978).

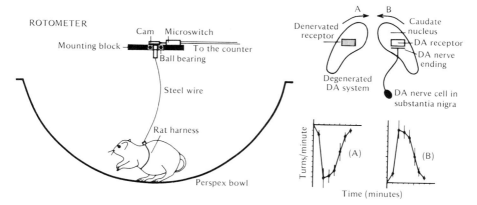

Fig. 4–4 *Left:* A schematic drawing of the rotometer. The movements of the rat are transferred by the steel wire to the microswitch arrangement. *Upper right:* the principal outline of the experimental situation shown in a horizontal projection of the nigrostriatal DA system. When stimulation of the denervated receptor dominates, the animals rotates in direction A. When stimulation of the innervated receptor dominates, the animal rotates in direction B. *Lower right:* the rotational behavior is presented as turns per minute vs. time. The curves are given negative *y*-values when stimulation of the denervated receptor dominates and positive *y*-values when stimulation of the innervated receptor dominates. Each point represents the mean (± S.E.M.) of a certain number of animals. (Reproduced from Ungerstedt, 1971.)

Behavioral pharmacology

In large doses barbiturates suppress ongoing behavior and induce sleep. But in small doses they increase rather than decrease behavioral output. Dews (1955a) reported that pentobarbital increased response rates in pigeons working on a multiple FI/FR schedule of reinforcement. The FI performance was more sensitive than FR responding to the rate-increasing effect of barbiturates. The facilitation seen with small doses may be associated with improved discriminative behavior in certain circumstances. This may be a result of the drug's ability to modulate sensory input, by acting on the reticular activating system, and, thus, maintaining a level of arousal optimal for behavioral efficiency.

The apparently paradoxical ability of depressants and stimulants at some doses to facilitate and at others to impair behavior is conveniently illustrated by an inverted U-shaped relationship between behavioral efficiency and arousal. A particular level of arousal is optimal for any particular behavior. Barbiturates in small doses increase specific arousal by eliminating irrele-

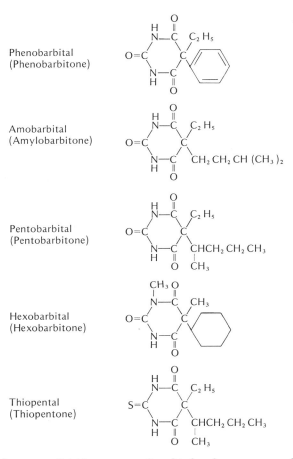

Phenobarbital
(Phenobarbitone)

Amobarbital
(Amylobarbitone)

Pentobarbital
(Pentobarbitone)

Hexobarbital
(Hexobarbitone)

Thiopental
(Thiopentone)

Fig. 4–5   Barbiturates. British synonyms listed in brackets, compounds arranged in order of decreasing duration of effect.

vant stimuli; but they eventually depress arousal. Amphetamine progressively increases arousal, until eventually the level is so high as to be incompatible with efficient behavior. It is, therefore, possible for either depressants or stimulants to enhance behavioral efficiency by inducing the optimum level of arousal. An interesting example of this effect of barbiturates is their reported ability to improve impaired *delayed response* performance in monkeys subjected to lesions of the frontal lobe (Wade, 1947). It has been suggested that these lesions disrupt the normal inhibitory control exerted by the frontal cortex over the hindbrain reticular activating system. The result-ant disinhibition of sensory arousal mechanisms produces a highly distract-able animal that is unable to perform well on certain delay tasks. Barbitu-rates are thought to overcome this difficulty by attenuating sensory input. Weiskrantz et al. (1965) reported that the minor tranquilizer meprobamate improves delayed response behavior in monkeys with frontal lobe lesions to the same degree as pentobarbital. But when a particular element of behav-ior is performed efficiently, the prediction is that further increases in the dose of either class of compound will eventually disrupt behavior; depres-sants because of anesthesia and stimulants because of overarousal.

The similarity of the facilitation seen with both amphetamine and the barbiturates is further emphasized by the finding that the rate-increasing effects of both drugs are related to the level of ongoing behavior. Indeed, Dews (1964) was the first to formulate the baseline phenomenon on the basis of studies of the effect of amobarbital on FI behavior in the pigeon. If successive segments of the fixed interval are examined, barbiturates and amphetamine increase low rates of responding in the initial segments and decrease high rates of responding in the terminal segments.

The stimulatory property of these drugs explains their use for inducing "high" states in man, and both barbiturates and amphetamines are drugs of abuse. It is suggested that the arousal-inducing function of both groups is mediated at the level of the reticular-activating system. There is electro-physiological support for this in the case of the barbiturates, and the fact that amphetamine excites many neurons in the reticular-activating system, when iontophenetically applied, encouraged Bradley (1968) to make the same claim for amphetamine.

When these drugs are given in combination, potentiation of the rate-in-creasing effects are seen. Rushton and Steinberg (1964) reported that naive rats in a Y-maze showed greater stimulation after a combination of ampheta-mine (0.75 mg/kg) and amobarbital (15 mg/kg) than after either drug alone. Since rats experienced in the situation did not show such effects, the authors suggested that these drugs result in stimulation by reducing fear, which would presumably be at a much higher level in naive rats. An alternative explanation could be that the low level of spontaneous behavior in naive rats, unlike the higher levels in experienced animals, is increased by am-phetamine and low doses of barbiturates. Rutledge and Kelleher (1965) fa-vor such an interpretation, having shown similar potentiation of the rate-increasing effects by amphetamine and barbiturates in pigeons pecking on a multiple FI/FR schedule of reinforcement. In neither of these schedule conditions, could fear be proposed as an intervening variable, and yet the drugs given singly or in combination increased low rates of responding in the early part of the FI and did not affect the high levels of responding characteristic of the FR schedule.

Marked tolerance is seen on repeated dosage with barbiturates, i.e. progressively larger doses are needed to elicit the same effects. The neuropharmacological basis of this effect is obscure, but an interaction between hypnotics and brain NE has been discussed. In support of this hypothesis are observations that depletion of brain NE prevents the development of behavioral tolerance to phenobartital ethanol in mice (Tabakoff et al., 1978), although evidence of physical dependence is still found. Mice were treated intraventricularly with 6-OHDA and then fed phenobarbital in the diet. On removal of the drug, withdrawal symptoms indicated the existence of physical dependence. Functional tolerance was assessed 44 hr after withdrawal by studying the sleep time and body temperature change when phenobarbital was re-administered.

The second matter of concern in the literature is the effects of barbiturates and alcohol on cognitive performance. Here the results are mixed. A number of earlier studies showed that even with depressant doses of barbiturates, responses to simple discriminative stimuli in the environment remain unimpaired, despite general motor depression and ataxia.

Pigeons on an FI/FR schedule, with red and blue lights used as the stimuli associated with the two schedules, will, under a large dose of barbiturate, appear grossly uncoordinated and ataxic in the Skinner box. Nevertheless, when the colored light indicating that FR performance is demanded appears on the key, they will struggle to the key and respond quickly with the required number of pecks.

This is the case only when relatively simple levels of stimulus control are operating. Dews showed, for example, that when red and blue S^D and S^Δ alternated during a fixed-interval schedule, pentobarbital (3 mg/kg) left discrimination performance intact. If, however, there was a different S^D and S^Δ stimulus during each segment of the FI, and discrimination accordingly became more difficult, the same dose of pentobarbital disrupted discriminative control, and considerable responding during the S^Δ was seen (Fig. 3–4).

Furthermore, monkeys on a difficult size discrimination task and pigeons on a conditional brightness discrimination task (Blough, 1957) show decreased accuracy of discrimination after pentobarbital. This cannot be attributed to a depressant effect of the drug because, in the latter experiment, increased response rates were associated with the impaired accuracy of discrimination. The temporal discrimination required for successful performance on DRL schedules is also severely disrupted by pentobarbital. Not all CNS depressants have this effect; ethanol, for example, although it generally depresses responding, leaves temporal discrimination unaffected (Sidman, 1956).

Delay discrimination tasks reveal another feature of depressants—although the registration of information may be impaired by the drug, its subsequent retrieval may be enhanced. During the delay, irrelevant stimuli are normally responded to, and interference occurs. The longer the delay, the greater the interference and, consequently, the poorer the retention. Depressants in small doses depress the arousal mechanism, which not only impairs registration but also reduces the level of interference. Jarvik (1964) found this to be the case in monkeys trained on a 1- or 8-sec delayed response task. The accuracy was reduced by pentobarbital, but the normal deterioration in performance as the delay lengthened was eradicated. Summerfield (1964) described impaired registration and improved retention in man using the gaseous anesthetic nitrous oxide as the depressant.

Unfortunately in those earlier studies the behavioral measures used, the responses recorded, and the analysis of the results make it impossible for experimenters to distinguish between the various hypotheses to account for the observed changes in performance. More recent studies have used highly controlled behavioral paradigms and mathematical models for distinguishing the contribution of various aspects of performance to improved or impaired behavior. Amylobarbital-induced disruption of discrimination behavior in the pigeon has been analyzed with signal detection methods to differentiate changes in sensory function and response bias (Hulme et al., 1979). As in the case of the benzodiazepines (see Chapter 9), the disruption is associated with disinhibition of responding rather than sensory loss. The task is to discover if drugs, such as the barbiturates and benzodiazepines, have more specific effects on information processing which cannot be accounted for in terms of general response disinhibition. The indications are that indeed there are additional and more specific effects on cognitive performance.

Such findings are exemplified in a study by Sahgal and Iversen (1979) employing the Konorski paradigm. On this task the animal monitors pairs of stimuli; if A follows A, or B follows B, one response is required, but a different response must be made to dissimilar pairs. The discriminability of A and B can be varied at either the sample or the matching phase; the delay between the presentation of the stimuli can also be varied. By manipulating these variables, levels of performance after a drug or a lesion can be equated, and the rate of decay of information during the memory phase can be assessed, independently of difficulties in the encoding or retrieval of information. Such analysis reveals that in the pigeon amylobarbital and ethanol impede the encoding of visual information in addition to any effect such drugs may have on response probability. (The other group of anxiolytic drugs, the benzodiazepines, have the same effect on this task.)

A third and major effect of the barbiturates is that they possess anxiolytic actions similar to those seen with other minor tranquilizers, notably the benzodiazepines. This subject will be dealt with separately, in Chapter 9.

To summarize, barbiturates influence arousal levels as well as specific aspects of cognition, and act as potent anxiolytics. Their site or sites of action in the CNS and their neuropharmacological properties at these sites remain obscure. It seems unlikely that a single specific or nonspecific aspect of their action will account for the range of behavioral effects they can precipitate. However, this matter remains to be resolved.

5. Effects of Drugs and Hormones on Learning and Memory

INTRODUCTION

The plasticity of the brain that allows its functions to change adaptively in response to experience is one of the highest functions of the CNS and also one of the least clearly understood at this time. The cellular and biochemical changes associated with learning and memory are largely unknown. Most neurobiologists believe that these phenomena are associated in some way with changes in the connectivity of neurons in the brain, but there is very little clear-cut evidence in mammals that such changes occur in any particular learning situation. Striking progress, however, has been made in studying the electrophysiological correlates of learning in simpler animals, such as Aplysia, a marine mollusc with a simple but well-defined nervous system and behavioral repertoire (Kandel, 1978).

There have been many attempts by biochemists to explain the processes of learning and memory in simple chemical terms—suggestions, for example, that memory may be associated with the synthesis of specific informational macromolecules in the brain (see Dunn 1976, 1980 for reviews). Such naive hypotheses, however, seem to bear little relation to the real nervous system. A number of claims that "memories" could be transferred from the brains of trained animals to those of untrained animals by means of extracts containing such specific chemical substances as ribonucleic acids, proteins, or peptides have also failed to stand up to the crucial test of reproducibility when examined in other laboratories. The unsatisfactory state of our knowledge in this area does not mean that drug effects on the processes of learning and memory cannot be studied; indeed, a large literature exists on such effects and their pursuit remains an active focus of research interest. Such studies may eventually provide pharmacological tools for enhancing normal memory or reversing its inadequacies induced by disease or aging.

In mammals arousal and the processes fundamental to learning and memory have traditionally been linked in theoretical terms. It is likely that increased levels of CNS arousal, whether induced by specific or nonspecific interaction of drugs with CNS, will facilitate processes essential to the storage and retrieval of information. Certainly stimulant and convulsant drugs such as strychnine, metrazol, and amphetamine (see Chapter 4) facilitate learning and memory. This is also the case for low doses of barbiturates, which, it has been pointed out (Chapter 4), enhance behavioral output. However, the possibility exists that some drugs may act much more specifically to influence learning and memory. In the following sections we consider examples of such drugs; some, like the protein synthesis inhibitors, have been studied for a number of years; others, including the neuropeptides, represent an exciting new class.

EFFECTS OF PITUITARY PEPTIDES

Particular interest has focused during the past few years on the reports of de Wied and co-workers that the pituitary peptides ACTH, α-MSH, vasopressin, and oxytocin have effects on the acquisition, storage, and retrieval of information (de Wied, 1974, 1978). The discovery that a number of pituitary hormones (including these four) are found in brain, where their existence appears to be independent of the pituitary, has reinforced the view that their effects on information processing are independent of their neuroendocrine effects (Krieger and Liotta, 1979).

ACTH

The studies of de Wied and his colleagues began with the observation that hypophysectomized rats, which lack the normal source of ACTH, showed an impaired acquisition of avoidance conditioning and an unusually rapid extinction of such behavior once it had been established. Administration of small doses of ACTH to such rats restored normal acquisition and extinction behavior (summarized in de Wied, 1974). The obvious interpretation of this finding was that ACTH was effective because of its ability to stimulate corticosteroid release from the adrenals. However, a number of fragments of the ACTH molecule were found to possess the same behavioral effect as the full molecule; these include the melanocyte-stimulating hormone (α-MSH) and $ACTH_{4-10}$. As these fragments are devoid of any effect on the adrenals, their behavioral actions cannot be attributed to stimulation of circulating cortiocosteroids. This discovery was extremely important, and provided the first evidence that pituitary hormones might exert direct effects on the brain, unrelated to their peripheral endocrine actions. The amino acid sequence $ACTH_{4-10}$ appears to represent the minimum needed for behavioral activity, and since this sequence occurs also within the related pituitary peptide β-LIPOTROPIN it is perhaps not surprising that this molecule shares the same behavioral activity, and is in fact considerably more potent than $ACTH_{4-10}$ (see Fig. 7–4).

Despite its ability to reverse the behavioral deficit on avoidance tasks after hypophysectomy, ACTH has no significant effects on the acquisition of shock avoidance behavior in normal rats. However, it was found that ACTH and the fragments $ACTH_{4-10}$, $ACTH_{1-10}$, and α-MSH markedly retard extinction of such learning. In one of the tasks used by de Wied and colleagues, rats learn to climb a pole to avoid electric shock. The shock is then disconnected and extinction is assessed in terms of how many trials the rat required to realize that the floor is no longer electrified. The effect of ACTH in delaying extinction is shown in Fig. 5–1. Similar results have been obtained in a number of shock avoidance learning tasks and also, although less reliably, on appetitive learning tasks.

The experimenters have viewed these results in terms of a specific effect of ACTH to strengthen the memory of the original learned pole jumping response. However, extinction is a complex behavioral phenomenon (see Mackintosh, 1974 pp. 405–418) which has been accounted for in a number of different ways. For example, it seems reasonable to assume that an associative process by which the animal learns that the floor is no longer electrified, occurs during extinction. ACTH could slow down this learning process. It turns out to be very difficult to design specific behavioral tests to distinguish such hypotheses but this is the challenge which must be taken up in an effort to define more precisely the influence of ACTH and related peptides on the processes of learning and memory.

Taste aversion induced with lithium in rats is a different and interesting form of learning. Smotherman and Levine reported (1978) that ACTH delays the extinction of this learned response. It has also been found that

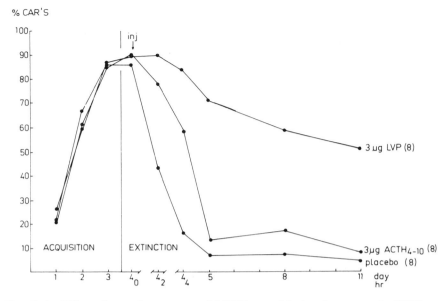

Fig. 5–1   Effect of a single injection of $ACTH_{4-10}$ and lysine-8-vasopressin (LVP) on the extinction of a conditioned shock avoidance (pole jumping) response. The effect of LVP in delaying extinction is greater and more long lasting than that seen with $ACTH_{4-10}$. (Kindly supplied by Dr. Tj. B. van Wimersma-Greidanus.)

ACTH is able to alleviate the amnesia produced in rats by carbon dioxide inhalation, electroconvulsive shock, or intracerebral administration of the protein synthesis inhibitor puromycin.

It is possible that these and other effects of ACTH can be explained in terms of an effect on the registration or memory of fear responses. For example, male rats groom excessively in novel environments, a reflection, it is suggested, of the experienced novelty which is fear-inducing. Hypophysectomy or intraventricular infusion of antiserum to ACTH reduces such novelty-induced grooming (Dunn et al., 1979). On the other hand, increasing brain ACTH levels by intraventricular or intranigral infusion of the peptide induces intense grooming behavior. These results could be interpreted in terms of ACTH enhancement of fear. File (1979) has also recently suggested that ACTH is *anxiogenic*, as she found that ACTH decreases the amount of social interaction between male rats to the same degree that experience of a novel, frightening environment does. By contrast, anxiolytic drugs (minor tranquilizers) increase such social interaction (File and Hyde, 1978).

In a rather different situation, Roche and Leshner (1979) found that administration of ACTH to male mice enhances the memory of being submissive in a fight. Defeated mice were given a single subcutaneous injection of ACTH and tested for submissiveness 24 hr, 48 hr, and 7 days after the initial encounter. The effect of ACTH lasted for 48 hr.

A different behavioral paradigm was used by Martin (1978). Mallard ducklings show imprinting behavior during the first days of life. The strength of approach behavior to the imprinting model is inversely related to plasma corticosterone levels, and injections of corticosterone reduce approach behavior. In contrast, $ACTH_{1-10}$ (which lacks any endocrine effect on the adrenals) enhances rather than reduces imprinting behavior. Corticosterone binding sites have been found in the optic tectum of the bird, and the author suggested that "the amount of glucocorticoid or ACTH-like peptide present in this area may modulate the input to higher brain centers and thus influence the behavioural excitability or arousal of the young bird after exposure to the imprinting object" (which incidentally becomes an object of fear, inducing withdrawal after the sensitive period for imprinting is past).

Whether these ACTH effects on the response to fear-inducing events can be encompassed within a mnemonic hypothesis remains to be determined. It should also seriously be considered that the behavioral effects of ACTH may reflect changes in a more general process related to the arousal induced by motivationally significant stimuli.

Attempts have been made to identify the site of action of ACTH and related peptides in brain. Lesions to the nucleus parafascicularis in the thalamus block the effect of $ACTH_{4-10}$ in delaying extinction. Lesions to the anterior hippocampus are similarly effective. Local injections of ACTH in the medial posterior thalamus produce a delay in extinction. It would thus appear that the midbrain limbic circuitry is essential for the effects of ACTH.

It has been suggested that ACTH and other peptides influence CNS functions by modulating the effects of neurotransmitters in the brain. There is a literature suggesting a relationship between ACTH, corticosterone, and norepinephrine (NE) in the expression of avoidance responding. Ögren and Fuxe (1977) found severe impairment of shock avoidance behavior after a combined lesion of the adrenals and the locus coeruleus (the origin of the dorsal NE pathway innervating the hippocampus and cortex). Treatment with corticosteroids reversed this deficit, which was not observed after either lesion alone. However, a number of behavioral tasks have been described which are impaired by lesions to the dorsal NE bundle. These are all situations in which the animal must learn not to respond to nonrewarded stimuli. These include extinction of previously rewarded responses, partial reinforcement paradigms, S^D/S^Δ discrimination tasks. Mason and Iversen (1979) have suggested that successful performance on such tasks represents an important form of attentional behavior. The hippocampus appears to be a site of possible importance for the integration of the responses to ACTH, corticosterone, and NE. In an elegant series of iontophoretic and electrophysiological studies of hippocampal pyramidal neurons, Segal and Bloom (1976) have suggested that NE in hippocampus plays an important role in processes related to attention. It is also known that the hippocampus contains a high density of corticosteroid receptors. Finally, Segal (1976) has found that ACTH can antagonize the response of hippocampal pyramidal neurons to NE.

Vasopressin

This peptide hormone of the posterior pituitary has also been investigated by de Wied's group on the same experimental memory paradigms (van Ree et al., 1978). Like ACTH, vasopressin delays the extinction of shock avoidance behavior. The Brattleboro strain of rat, which lacks the ability to synthesize vasopressin due to a mutation, has provided a useful model for studying the role of vasopressin in behavioral control. In these animals, which exhibit diabetes insipidus and are deficient in acquiring shuttlebox avoidance responses, the learned response extinguishes more rapidly than in normal animals.

In normal rats a single subcutaneous injection of lysine$_8$-vasopressin (LVP) or arginine$_8$-vasopressin (AVP), the natural antidiuretic hormone in the rat, has an inhibitory effect on the extinction of pole-jump avoidance which lasts for several weeks (Fig. 5–1). Desglycinamide-lysine$_8$-vasopressin (DG-LVP), which has only weak antidiuretic and vasopressor properties, has a similar behavioral effect, suggesting that, as with ACTH, the behavioral and endocrine actions can be dissociated. As with ACTH, the posterior thalamus (including parafascicular nuclei) was found to be a positive injection site. Bilateral lesions to this area abolished the normal effect of subcutaneous ACTH in delaying extinction and resulted in the requirement of higher doses of LVP for the same effect. An interaction with forebrain NE systems is again suggested by the observation that the effect of AVP in facilitating one-trial passive avoidance was blocked by a lesion to the dorsal NE system made in the locus coeruleus (Kovacs et al., 1979).

The effects of ACTH and vasopressin on the retention of avoidance behavior differ in duration. ACTH effects can be detected for up to 2 days, whereas vasopressin effects are longer lasting (>7 days) see (Fig. 5–1). It has been suggested (de Wied and Gispen, 1977) that ACTH acts by intensifying fear-like responses to the shock experience, whereas vasopressin has an effect on the processes underlying the storage of learned experiences. However, it is difficult to devise behavioral tests to distinguish such hypotheses regarding the bases of behavioral deficits. It is particularly so in this case, because the tests that have proved most sensitive to the effects of ACTH, vasopressin, and related peptides involve the use of shock-motivated behavior.

PROTEIN SYNTHESIS INHIBITORS AND MEMORY

There have been many studies of the effects of antibiotic drugs that inhibit nucleic acid or protein synthesis on learning and memory (see Dunn, 1976, 1980). The most consistent results have been obtained with compounds that inhibit protein synthesis, such as PUROMYCIN, CYCLOHEXIMIDE (and its more potent analogue ACETOXYCYCLOHEXIMIDE), and ANISOMYCIN. It is clear that these compounds can produce amnesia in animals, although doses sufficiently high to cause nearly complete (> 90%) inhibition of cerebral protein synthesis for prolonged periods are required. Since such treatments are highly toxic, it is impossible to use the drugs repeatedly for long periods of time, and it is important to distinguish specific effects that such drugs may have on learning and memory from nonspecific effects caused simply by their toxic action. Nevertheless, in properly controlled studies this distinction can be made, for example by demonstrating that the antibiotics do not impair the acquisition of a learned task, although they subsequently impair its retention. For example, Barondes and Cohen (1968) showed that acetoxycycloheximide, when given to mice at doses large enough to cause nearly complete inhibition of cerebral protein synthesis, does not prevent the animals from learning a simple positional or light/dark discrimination in a T-maze. Retention of this learning also remains normal for up to 3 hr after initial acquisition, although retention at 6 hr, 1 day, or 7 days after learning is markedly impaired (Fig. 5–2). These and similar results suggest that whereas learning itself does not depend on ongoing protein synthesis, the process of consolidation of long-term memory may be crucially dependent

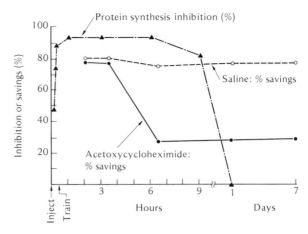

Fig. 5–2   Effect of acetoxycycloheximide on protein synthesis in the brain and on memory. Mice were injected subcutaneously with 240 μg acetoxycycloheximide 30 min before training to escape shock by choosing the lighted limb of a T-maze to a criterion of five out of six consecutive correct responses. Different groups were tested for retention (percent savings) at each of the indicated times. (From Barondes and Cohen, 1968.)

on cerebral protein synthesis. Inhibitors of protein synthesis, like electro-convulsive shock treatment, can also lead to retrograde amnesia if given during this consolidation period, which seems to start during the acquisition itself and continues for some hours thereafter. Thus, in mice or goldfish trained on simple discrimination tasks, electroconvulsive shock, cyclohex-imide, or puromycin can prevent long-term memory formation if given im-mediately after the training period but not if administration is further de-layed.

Despite their interesting effects on memory, however, the antibiotics have proved to be of only limited usefulness in providing insights into the biochemical or pharmacological basis of memory. It is not even clear that their behavioral actions are caused by an inhibition of protein synthesis in the brain. Puromycin, for example, causes abnormal seizure-like electrical activity in hippocampus, and puromycin-induced amnesia can be antago-nized by the anticonvulsant drug diphenylhydantoin. Its amnesic actions might thus be due to a convulsant effect similar to that produced by electro-convulsive shock treatments. Another hypothesis is that the amnesic effects of the antibiotics are a secondary consequence of their ability to impair cerebral neurotransmitter metabolism, in particular to inhibit catecholamine biosynthesis, but this remains controversial (Dunn, 1980). It has even been suggested (Nakajima, 1975) that the amnesic actions of the antibiotics might be attributed to effects on peripheral rather than on central targets. Nakajima proposed that the drugs might act to block steroid hormone synthesis in the adrenal glands, and showed that administration of corticosteroids such as hydrocortisone or corticosterone could reverse the amnesic effects of cycloheximide in mice.

It is clear that a number of stimulant drugs such as amphetamine can reduce the amnesic effects of the antibiotics. Flood et al. (1978), for example, found that anisomycin-induced amnesia of a passive avoidance response in mice could be reversed if the stimulants caffeine or nicotine were administered 30 min after training. The depressant drugs sodium phenobarbitone or chloral hydrate, in contrast, had an additive amnesic effect when combined with anisomycin. These observations emphasize the importance of adequate arousal for memory storage and suggest the possibility that the antibiotics may impair memory by altering the arousal state.

Even if the amnesic actions of the antibiotics do depend on inhibition of cerebral protein synthesis, we are no nearer to understanding the functional significance of such an action, since it is not clear which particular brain protein(s) are crucially involved. Indeed, inhibition of neuropeptide synthesis in the brain by the same inhibitors may be more important than protein synthesis inhibition. In summary, the hope that antibiotics might prove to be "magic bullets" that would provide insight into the fundamental mechanisms of memory has not been fulfilled.

DRUGS ACTING ON ADRENERGIC AND CHOLINERGIC MECHANISMS

There is considerable evidence that ascending neurotransmitter systems are involved in learning and memory and mediate the effects of a number of drugs which influence learning and memory (Hunter et al., 1978). Kety (1972) originally proposed that the widespread release of norepinephrine in the forebrain could serve as a synaptic facilitator of information storage. Studies of learning and memory in animals after selective lesions of NE pathways by means of 6-hydroxydopamine suggest that NE is indeed involved in certain forms of attentional behavior fundamental to learning, although it does not appear to be essential for all forms of learning (Mason and Iversen, 1979). It is clear, however, that in the absence of forebrain NE, many forms of associative learning are perfectly normal. Less extensively studied in this context are dopamine and serotonin, although claims have been made that dopamine release in the striatum is a prerequisite for adequate associative learning. On the other hand, there is an extensive literature on cholingergic mechanisms in relation to learning and memory. In a wide range of species and tasks, the anticholinergics (i.e. drugs that block cholinergic receptors), such as atropine and scopolamine, have been shown to impair learning (Berger and Stein, 1969). The tasks studied include active and passive avoidance, conditioned suppression using shock, habituation to a novel stimulus, and performance on matching to sample of colors. Some theorists (Carlton, 1963) have suggested that the cholinergic system is most important for tasks that involve some kind of behavioral inhibition, i.e. responding under one condition and not under another, as in a go, no-go discrimination task. The generality of this thesis remains to be explored in situations in which responding is eliminated with differential reinforcement, extinction, and punishment.

The behavioral actions of scopolamine and atropine are clearly due to an effect on CNS, since their quaternary nitrogen derivatives, which do not pass the blood–brain barrier, are inactive. Carlton (1963) found that atropine methyl nitrate did not affect avoidance behavior in the rat, and Jarvik and collaborators reported that scopolamine methyl bromide did not impair accuracy of matching to sample in the monkey, although the response rate was depressed on this task. If anticholinergics impair learning, substances that enhance cholinergic activity at the synapse would be expected to enhance acquisition, and, indeed, this is the case. Anticholinesterases, which inhibit the ACh degrading enzyme and thus result in more transmitter being available in the synaptic cleft, are reported to facilitate acquisition of bar-pressing alteration and brightness-detection tasks in rats (Warburton, 1972). On both these tasks, anticholinergics impair learning.

Warburton concluded that cholinergic manipulation affected the sensory decisions of the animals rather than their response strategy. Jarvik's observation of impaired accuracy in matching to sample in the absence of response impairment supported this conclusion. Enhanced cholinergic activity appears to improve sensory filtering processes, thereby strengthening the tendency to ignore irrelevant stimuli and improving discrimination. The ascending reticular formation projections to the sensory cortex are likely to be the neural substrate for this cholinergic mechanism. A related cholinergic circuit passing through the hippocampus is also involved in this form of behavioral control.

Not surprisingly, memory is also affected by cholinergic manipulation. Anticholinergics used as preanesthetic medication have long been observed to produce amnesia in man. Oliverio (1968) found that scopolamine impaired acquisition and retention of avoidance behavior in the mouse. In an intriguing series of experiments, Deutch (1971) investigated the effect of cholinergic manipulations at various times after the learning experience. During the initial period after training (1–3 days) cholinesterase inhibitors had no effect on retention, but from 5 to 14 days after training cholinesterase inhibitors produced a progressively greater disruption of the previously learned response. The drug effects, however, were temporary; this suggests an action on retrieval mechanisms, leaving the original memory intact. Finally, at about 28 days after memory formation, when normal animals show evidence of forgetting, cholinesterase inhibition caused a facilitation in retention. The effects of the anticholinergic drug scopolamine were opposite to those produced by the cholinesterase inhibitors. Similar complex triphasic patterns resulting from cholinergic manipulations have been reported by others (for review see Zornetzer, 1978).

There is no area in behavioral pharmacology more fraught with experimental traps than the study of pharmacologically induced changes in learning and memory. Only the most carefully designed experiments avoid the pitfalls (Weiss and Heller, 1969). Even then the final answer is complicated in the case of cholinergic drugs. In addition to effects on acquisition and retention, the cholinergic drugs alter the habituation response of the animal to the testing environment. Even more important, the physiological changes induced peripherally by, for example, injections of the anticholinergics can serve as interoceptive discriminative cues, and ideal conditions for state-dependent learning effects are thus created (Overton, 1966).

DRUG TREATMENT OF DEMENTIA?

The most obvious and urgent clinical application of improved knowledge of drug effects on learning and memory would be in devising effective drug treatments for human *dementia*. Senile dementia, a general term used to describe impaired cognitive function in the elderly, is an increasingly common condition in the Western world as life expectancy has increased. In 1978 some 11% of the U.S. population were older than 65 years. Fifty years from now, in 2030, between 17 and 20% of the U.S. population will be older than 65 years and the absolute number of persons in this age group will be more than 50 million, of whom as many as one in ten will suffer from senile dementia. Although there are many different factors that may lead to senile dementia, including cerebral vascular disease, alcoholism, brain tumors, and injuries, it has become clear that the single largest category, accounting for more than 50% of all cases, is *Alzheimer's senile dementia*. This is a condition of unknown origin which is characterized by a shrinkage and loss of cells from cerebral cortex, and by the occurrence of characteristic pathological changes in cortical tissue. Numerous amyloid-containing plaques and neurofibrillary changes in damaged neurons are evident in such tissue on microscopic postmortem examination. Although this and other dementias are still poorly understood in biological terms, recent biochemical findings in postmortem brain tissue from patients dying with Alzheimer's senile dementia have offered a potentially important clue. Several groups have reported that there is an apparently selective loss of cholinergic neurons, especially from cortical areas, in this form of dementia. This loss is reflected by reduced levels of the cholinergic enzymes acetylcholinesterase and choline acetyltransferase, and the extent of these changes parallels the severity of the cognitive impairment and of the neuropathological changes (Perry et al., 1978; Katzman et al., 1978).

If the cholinergic deficit in Alzheimer's senile dementia does indeed prove to be a specific neurotransmitter abnormality, similar in character to the loss of dopamine from basal ganglia in Parkinson's disease, then it may prove possible, at least temporarily, to alleviate the distressing symptoms of this form of dementia by cholinergic replacement therapy. This hypothesis would also be consistent with animal and human data as outlined above, which suggest that blockage of cerebral cholinergic function leads to impaired learning and memory, whereas increased cholinergic function may facilitate such processes.

6. Goal Directed Behavior

There have been many studies of the pharmacological control of appetitive behavior and of the underlying CNS neurotransmitter mechanisms. For detailed reviews see Hoebel (1978), Setler (1978) and Meyerson and Eliasson (1978). The few examples here are those for which we have begun to understand the underlying neurotransmitter mechanisms involved in modulating behavior, and where pharmacological agents may be useful in controlling that appetitive behavior.

FEEDING BEHAVIOR

The norepinephrine (NE) innervation of the hypothalamus appears to play a central role in the initiation and suppression of feeding behavior (reviewed in Iversen and Iversen, 1975). Studies of this control mechanism have advanced by the use of local injections of neurotransmitter substances and drugs into brain. For a number of years, the literature on this topic was confusing, with some workers claiming that NE initiates feeding and others that it induces satiety and reduces food intake (Iversen and Iversen, 1975). Over the past few years, however, more detailed attention to the sites of injection and the judicious use of specific α- and β-adrenoceptor agonists and antagonists have helped to clarify the picture. NE initiates feeding in satiated and hungry rats when injected in the medial paraventricular nucleus and periventricular area of the hypothalamus. It is considerably more potent than dopamine and this stimulatory effect is mediated by α-adrenoceptors. NE can also suppress feeding in hungry rats when injected into the perifornical region and β-adrenoceptors appear to be involved in this response. Dopamine has also been implicated in this mechanism by the finding of a strong suppression of feeding after peripheral injections of the DA agonists L-dopa and apomorphine.

In earlier studies it was reported that the perifornical region of the lateral hypothalamus was the site where injections of amphetamine produced their most dramatic anorectic effects (cf. Chapter 4). Thus, amphetamine-induced release of endogenous NE and DA, or application of exogenous catecholamines to this site reduces food intake (Leibowitz and Rossakis, 1979).

Lesion experiments have been performed to evaluate the role of NE, DA, and 5-HT on the effects of amphetamine and other related anorectic agents (Garattini et al., 1978). NE depletion following bilateral electrolytic lesions to the ventral noradrenergic bundle reduces the anorectic effect of amphetamine, whereas depletion of striatal DA following 6-hydroxydopamine lesions is without effect. Interestingly, these manipulations do not attenuate the anorexia induced by fenfluramine, whereas lesions of the 5-HT system of the medial raphe nuclei do. This result suggests that 5-HT systems may also play a role in food intake behavior and offers an alternative pharmacological approach to the control of obesity.

There is reason to believe that the release of both NE and DA may contribute to amphetamine-induced anorexia in a dose-dependent manner. The anorexia associated with low doses of amphetamine in the rat (<0.5 mg/kg) appears to be predominantly a NE-mediated phenomenon because: 1. The effect is not blocked by selective DA antagonists such as pimozide, α-flupenthixol, and spiperone. 2. Low doses of amphetamine exert a more potent inhibition of the reuptake of NE than of DA (Garattini et al., 1978). 3. Lesions to NE pathways in the brain antagonize the anorexia caused by low doses of amphetamine (Ahlskog, 1974; Carey, 1976).

At higher doses of amphetamine DA mechanisms appear to contribute to the anorexia because: 1. The effect is blocked by specific DA antagonists at doses of these neuroleptics which do not themselves reduce spontaneous food intake (Burridge and Blundell, 1979). 2. Particularly interesting are the recent findings of Burridge and Blundell (1979) that atypical neuroleptics, like clozapine and thioridazine, however, fail to antagonize the anorexia caused by any dose of amphetamine. These drugs are DA antagonists that also possess potent anticholinergic properties (antimuscarinic) and this apparently counteracts the functional consequence of their DA receptor blocking actions, making them ineffective in blocking some behaviors mediated by DA mechanisms (see also Chapter 10).

DA pathways outside the hypothalamus also seem to contribute to the control of feeding behavior. Ungerstedt (1971) showed that bilateral lesions to the origins of the DA pathways in the rat substantia nigra resulted in a total loss of feeding and drinking behavior and rapid death. The effect of the lesion on feeding, however, may well be secondary to the profound lack of motor arousal produced by the lesion. Interestingly, Blundell (personal communication) has shown that although amphetamine reduces overall food intake in the rat, careful scrutiny of the actual feeding behavior reveals simultaneous stimulation of the motor acts involved in feeding. This is a good example of two simultaneous but pharmacologically and neurologically distinct actions of a single drug on behavior.

DRINKING BEHAVIOR

When food and water are freely available and climatic conditions are stable, thirst is probably never experienced. Drinking is largely anticipatory of future needs for water and seems to be governed by an innate circadian rhythm. (Fitzsimons, 1976)

Nevertheless, animals can be induced to drink by intracellular or extracellular dehydration. There are two principal organs that control water intake: the brain determines drinking behavior and the kidney controls loss of water. The ultimate effect of any drug on water balance and drinking will depend on its pattern of influence on these two complementary control mechanisms. The β-adrenoceptor agonist *isoproterenol* induces copious drinking, but despite the water load urine flow is delayed because of the antidiuretic action of the drug. On the other hand, the diuretic substance *frusemide* induces urine flow, and drinking does not occur until there is a substantial negative fluid balance. Thus isoproterenol is a true dipsogen, inducing thirst and primary drinking, probably through activation of the renin–angiotensin system, whereas frusemide would appear not to be.

It is known that sensitive areas exist in the hypothalamus which respond to cellular dehydration (i.e. osmotic changes) and thereby initiate drinking and simultaneously activate the secretion of vasopressin from the pituitary to control fluid loss by the kidney. A second control mechanism has long been known to exist in the renin–angiotensin system of the kidney. Extracellular dehydration induced by hemorrhage, for example, activates this control system. The enzyme RENIN is released from the kidney, and promotes the formation of the potent vasoconstrictor peptide ANGIOTENSIN II in blood, which then contributes to the restoration of body fluid balance. Apart from the peripheral actions of this peptide, angiotensin can act directly on certain areas of the brain to promote drinking behavior. Thus, extracellular, like intracellular, dehydration controls both the kidney and drinking behavior to reinstate fluid balance. The subfornical organ (SFO) and the organum vasculosum, on the wall of the third ventricle, are the sites most sensitive to angiotensin II. The threshold dose in the subfornical organ is only 0.1 to 1.0 pg and the effect has been demonstrated in reptiles, birds, and mammals (Fitzsimons, 1975, 1976). The biosynthetic pathway for angiotensin II involves the enzyme renin, the tetradecapeptide RENIN SUBSTRATE, and the immediate precursor ANGIOTENSIN I. All of these components are present normally in brain, and act, like angiotensin II, as dipsogens when injected intracerebrally. Lesions of the subfornical organ or infusion of the angiotensin receptor blocker SARALASIN block the drinking response to angiotensin II. Although the exact cellular mechanisms involved are not understood, the activation of drinking behavior by intracerebral administration of angiotensin II is one of the most intriguing and dramatic examples of selective behavioral activation by a small peptide.

Which CNS transmitter systems are involved in the basic control mechanisms relating to drinking remains unclear. Carbachol injected directly into the hypothalamus induces a marked drinking response. Angiotensin II-induced drinking, however, does not seem to involve a cholinergic mechanism since atropine abolishes carbachol-induced drinking but leaves the response to angiotensin II unaffected. Angiotensin II-induced drinking is reduced after 6-hydroxydopamine lesions and can be blocked by the DA antagonist haloperidol, suggesting an involvement of CNS DA mechanisms.

Other peptides have been investigated for their dipsogenic effects. Intracranial injections of substance P and the related peptide eledoisin elicit drinking in the pigeon, and in this species eledoisin is almost as potent a dipsogen as angiotensin II. However, in the rat substance P does not act in this way, and instead is an antagonist of angiotensin II-induced drinking.

SEXUAL BEHAVIOR

Two aspects of sexual behavior have received most attention (1) the copulatory act and (2) sexual motivation, i.e. the strength of the urge to gain contact with a sexually active partner. In the female rat copulation is assessed by observing the lordosis response, the position assumed by the female to aid penetration by the male, and in the male by mounting and ejaculatory responses.

In studying the effects of manipulations of brain transmitter levels and drugs on reproductive behavior it is essential to control the hormonal status of the subject. Typically ovariectomized females are used which have been stabilized by administration of estrogen and progesterone. A number of brain transmitter substrates have been implicated in female copulatory behavior, but the most consistent finding is that forebrain 5-HT pathways exert an inhibitory effect. Thus, depletion of 5-HT by treatment with p-chlorophenylalanine increases lordotic behavior. Increased dopaminergic activity is also inhibitory, and amphetamine decreases lordosis as it induces stereotypy, suggesting that these two effects of amphetamine are mediated by different neural substrates. Stimulation of muscarinic receptors with pilocarpine decreases copulation in the rat and hamster, an effect that seems to involve 5-HT systems, as it can be prevented by pretreatment with p-chlorophenylalanine.

In the male opposite effects of 5-HT and dopamine on the activation of copulatory behavior seem to exist. A selective increase of DA facilitates mounting behavior, whereas the opposite effect is obtained by increasing 5-HT. Intraventricular injections of β-endorphin (1–3μg) in the male rat reduce mounting behavior, an effect that can be reversed with naloxone. This effect may have a clinical parallel, since long-term users of narcotic analgesics often complain of frigidity and impotence. The stable enkephalin analogue D-Ala$_2$-Met$_5$-enkephalinamide also inhibits male sexual activity in the rat, and treatment of sexually inactive males with the opiate antagonist naloxone can induce copulation (Gessa et al., 1979).

Another remarkably specific behavioral response to a peptide is the effect of luteinizing hormone-releasing hormone (LHRH) on sexual behavior. LHRH is a peptide released from hypothalamus, which controls the secretion of luteinizing hormone and follicle stimulating hormone from anterior pituitary; it may also be released within various brain areas. LHRH markedly facilitates lordosis behavior in the estrogen-primed ovariectomized rat when administered systemically or by local injection of very small amounts (1 ng or less) into the preoptic area (Moss, 1978). The effect is of long latency and duration, with the first effects observed 2 hr after LHRH injection and a peak response after 5 hr. The phenomenon appears to involve a direct action of LHRH on CNS, and cannot be mimicked by administration of luteinizing hormone or follicle stimulating hormone, or by other hypothalamic peptides such as TRH.

7. Drugs Affecting Mood: Antidepressants and Opiates

Drugs whose principal effects are on mood, or affect, have important clinical applications in the treatment of depression. The opiates are also included in this chapter, since their mood-elevating effects can be discussed separately from their actions as pain-relieving drugs (Chapter 8).

ANTIDEPRESSANTS
Classification and neuropharmacological properties

Clinically, depression is characterized by a lowering of mood and is often classified as "endogenous" or "reactive." Endogenous depression often recurs in a regular phasic manner and is not obviously correlated with environmental events; depression of mood alternates with periods of normality in the so-called unipolar depressions. In many other cases, abnormal heightening of mood (mania) alternates with the periods of depression in the so-called bipolar or manic-depressive psychoses. The reactive depressions, by contrast, consist of mood abnormalities elicited by stressful environmental events. Depressive psychoses, although they resemble to some degree the mood changes of schizophrenia, are not characterized by the thought disorders, hallucinations, and lack of contact with the real world that mark schizophrenia.

As with many other classes of psychoactive drugs, the antidepressant and antimanic drugs were discovered by accident. During treatment of patients for tuberculosis with the compound IPRONIAZID, it was noticed that this drug had a significant mood-elevating effect. This discovery was followed by the observation that iproniazid is a powerful inhibitor of the enzyme mono-amine oxidase (MAO), and this led to the development of a whole family of antidepressant drugs that are MAO inhibitors. A second important series of drugs was discovered when numerous structural analogues of chlorproma-zine were synthesized and tested. Replacement of the sulfur atom in the phenothiazine ring of the drug promazine with a methylene bridge gave the compound IMIPRAMINE, which has no neuroleptic properties but was in-stead found to have an important mood-elevating action. This change from the flat tricyclic phenothiazine structure to a "skewed" three-ring system based on the iminodibenzyl nucleus led to the evolution of another large family of compounds known as the tricyclic antidepressnats (Fig. 7–1).

A variety of MAO inhibitors and tricyclics are currently in use as antide-pressant drugs. Many of the MAO inhibitors are hydrazine compounds that evolved from iproniazid but are considerably more potent than the parent compound, e.g. PHENIPRAZINE (Catron). Others are nonhydrazines, such as PARGYLINE (Eutonyl) and TRANYLCYPROMINE (Parnate) (see Fig. 2–16). The tricyclics include imipramine (still widely used), its desmethyl derivative DESIPRAMINE, the 3-chloro analogue CLOMIPRAMINE, and another impor-tant series of compounds derived from AMITRIPTYLINE-NORTRIPTYLINE and PROTRIPTYLINE (Fig. 7–1). Imipramine and amitriptyline are metabolized *in vivo* by the liver to give the demethylated derivates desipramine and nortriptyline (Fig. 7–1), and these are both pharmacologically as active or even more active than the parent compounds. This is thus a good example of drug metabolism giving rise to active products, a process that may be related to the delayed and prolonged actions of the parent drugs.

Some drugs have specific effects on mania, which is in many ways the opposite of depression, with abnormally elevated mood, often accompanied by excitement, hallucination, and violence. Thus, the neuroleptic drugs, or major tranquilizers (see Chapter 10) have specific antimanic actions, and a remarkable discovery has been that long-term treatment of patients with simple inorganic salts of LITHIUM has a beneficial effect: it prevents the recurrence of manic episodes (Schok, 1963). Lithium may also protect against the recurrence of depression in manic-depressive patients.

Neuropharmacological properties
The MAO inhibitors, as their name implies, are powerful inhibitors of monoamine oxidase (MAO) in the brain and in other tissues. All of the com-

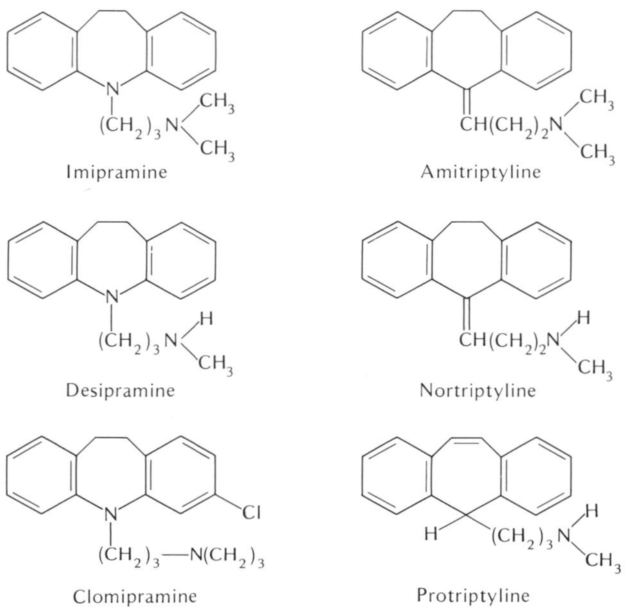

Imipramine

Amitriptyline

Desipramine

Nortriptyline

Clomipramine

Protriptyline

Fig. 7–1   Tricyclic antidepressant drugs.

pounds in clinical use as antidepressants produce an irreversible inhibition of this enzyme when administered *in vivo*, and their effects are thus very long lasting. Indeed, recovery of MAO activity in brain and peripheral tissues after treatment with such compounds as pargyline occurs only as new enzyme molecules are synthesized to replace the irreversibly inhibited enzyme. As mentioned in Chapter 2 (p. 95), MAO is involved in the metabolic breakdown of both the catecholamines and 5-HT. After treatment with an MAO inhibitor, there is a rise in the concentration of NE, DA, and especially 5-HT in animal brains, and it is generally assumed that the drugs act to make more of these transmitter amines available for release at adrenergic and triptaminergic synapses in the brain. There have been, however, no direct demonstrations that this is the case, in either the CNS or the peripheral adrenergic neurons. A rise in the storage level of transmitter need not necessarily mean that more transmitter will be released in response to nerve activity—nevertheless, this remains the most plausible explanation of the mode of action of MAO inhibitors.

The idea that MAO inhibitors act by making more catecholamine or 5-HT available at aminergic synapses also fits neatly with the postulated mode of action of the tricyclic antidepressant drugs. These compounds do not inhibit MAO, but they are all potent inhibitors of catecholamine- and 5-HT-uptake mechanisms. Imipramine, amitriptyline, and especially their desmethyl analogues are among the most potent inhibitors of the NE uptake system in noradrenergic neurons known (see Chapter 2, p. 96). They are effective in *in vitro* experiments at concentrations as low as 10^{-8}M (the equivalent of only a few picograms of drug per milliliter). The same drugs, however, are also very potent inhibitors of the 5-HT uptake system associated with 5-HT-containing neurons in the CNS. There is a somewhat different structure–activity relationship for inhibition of 5-HT and NE uptake by the tricyclics (Table 7–1), desipramine being the most potent inhibitor of NE uptake and clomipramine the most potent inhibitor of 5-HT uptake. Nevertheless, since the clinically used drugs are moderately potent inhibitors of both systems, it is impossible to say whether the action on one or the other amine system is the more important. The tricyclic antidepressants are, however, very much less active as inhibitors of DA uptake in dopaminergic neurons, so this seems to be ruled out as a site of action. At synapses using NE or 5-HT as transmitters, the tricyclic antidepressant drugs would be expected to enhance and potentiate the effects of the released transmitter by preventing the normally rapid removal of released amine by tissue uptake mechanisms. In peripheral adrenergic systems, this is exactly the effect observed; drugs such as imipramine or desipramine markedly potentiate the responses of smooth muscle tissues to sympathetic nerve stimulation or to applied NE.

It seems likely, therefore, that antidepressant drugs owe their action to a potentiation of NE and/or 5-HT at synapses in the CNS. This hypothesis is supported also by the behavioral effects of these drugs, particularly their ability to antagonize or counteract behavioral depression induced by reserpine or tetrabenazine, which act in the opposite manner to reduce the availability of catecholamines and 5-HT in the brain. It should be remembered, however, that we do not know whether the effect on NE or on 5-HT is the most important in explaining the mood-elevating effects of these drugs. Indeed it is quite possible that such effects are related to neither compound. For example, it has been suggested that the antidepressant activity of the tricyclic drugs is related to their rather potent actions as antagonists of histamine receptors in brain (Kanof and Greengard, 1978). The relative importance of amine uptake inhibition should become clearer as the results of clinical trials with newly developed more selective drugs become available. Thus the compounds MAPROTILINE, NISOXETINE, and NOMIFENSINE are potent inhibitors of catecholamine uptake with little effect on 5-HT uptake,

Table 7–1. Inhibition of amine uptake by tricyclics

Amine	IC$_{50}$* (μM)		
	5-HT	NE	DA
Clomipramine	0.04	0.30	—
Imipramine	0.50	0.20	8.70
Desipramine	2.50	0.03	50.00

*IC$_{50}$ values (drug concentration needed to cause 50% inhibition of amine uptake) were determined in rat brain synaptosome preparations.

and ZIMELIDINE, FLUOXETINE, and CITALOPRAM are selective 5-HT uptake blockers (see Iversen and Mackay, 1979).

The inhibition of MAO in the liver and intestine by MAO inhibitors gives rise to undesirable side effects which limit the clinical usefulness of these drugs. The enzyme is very abundant in these peripheral tissues, where it normally plays an important role in destroying and rendering harmless such pharmacologically active amines as tyramine; these amines are present in substantial amounts in many foods of plant origin and are absorbed in quite large quantities from the diet. Because this detoxification mechanism is abolished after MAO inhibition, ingestion of foods rich in these amines, such as certain cheeses and wines, can have undesirable and even fatal consequences in patients being treated with such drugs. A sudden absorption of a large dose of tyramine can lead to serious cardiovascular disturbances, since this amine stimulates the entire cardiovascular system by promoting a release of NE, which it displaces from sympathetic nerve terminals. For this reason, patients treated with MAO inhibitors must observe strict dietary precautions; the potential toxicity of the MAO inhibitors has led to their gradual replacement in clinical use by the tricyclic antidepressant drugs, which do not produce these undesirable side effects.

The inorganic salts of lithium have a variety of effects on excitable tissue. Lithium ions can replace sodium in the generation of the nerve action potential, but, unlike sodium, lithium is not rapidly pumped out of cells by the active pump mechanism; it tends, therefore, to accumulate, rendering the tissue less readily excitable. The precise mode of action of the antimanic actions of lithium salts, however, it not known. The antimanic actions of neuroleptic drugs, such as chlorpromazine are thought to be related to the ability of such drugs to antagonize CNS receptors for DA (see Chapter 10).

Behavioral pharmacology of antidepressants
Tricyclic compounds
The behavioral effects of the tricyclic antidepressants are extremely difficult
to characterize and dissociate from those of the neuroleptic phenothiazines.
This should perhaps not be surprising in view of their chemical similarity
and their shared efficacy in modulating affect and mood. When relatively
large doses are given, both have a sedative effect on spontaneous motor
behavior, although motor depression after imipramine is not associated with
catatonia. Imipramine produces dose-dependent decrements in responding
on FR schedules for food reinforcement. FI responding is also depressed,
and the scalloped pattern of responding is reduced to a low regular pattern
throughout the interval. Responding maintained by shock-escape or shock
avoidance is affected in a similar manner (Cook and Kelleher, 1962).

There are reports, as with chlorpromazine, that in conditioned avoidance
situations, where both avoidance and escape can be evaluated, imipramine
will abolish the avoidance response, leaving the escape response intact.
A change in the power of environmental stimuli to control behavior is
cited as an explanation for this and related results. This is supported by the
finding that avoidance under certain conditions is not impaired by either
chlorpromazine or imipramine. Cook and Kelleher describe a concurrent
schedule for the squirrel monkey in which shock is avoided on a nondiscri-
minated Sidman schedule, and every 100th response is reinforced with
food. The low avoidance rate after each reinforcement is not affected by
imipramine, although the high rate of responding just before each reinforcement is depressed.

The same authors also investigated imipramine on their two-key paradigm, where presses on one key produced reinforcement and presses on the
other discriminative stimuli (S^D or $S\Delta$), indicating whether or not reinforcement was available on the other key. In the pigeon, imipramine, like chlorpromazine, increased responding to the "discrimination" key, and it was
concluded that "imipramine and chlorpromazine have some common pharmacological properties."

It has also been stated, as with chlorpromazine, that negatively reinforced
behavior is more sensitive to the disruptive effects of imipramine than is
positively reinforced behavior. But these interpretations must be accepted
with caution and should be examined in the way Dews and Morse (1961)
evaluated the reports of a similar effect for chlorpromazine. The soundest
approach to this problem is to *equate* the baseline behaviors controlled by
shock and food. This has been achieved by Kelleher and Morse (1964) in the
squirrel monkey, using either FI shock-escape or FI food reinforcement

schedules. In this case, imipramine produces an identical dose-dependent depression of both behavioral baselines. Different monkeys were trained on the two schedules, and it remains to be shown on an alternating FI escape FI food schedule that the same results would be found. If imipramine has any selective effect on negatively reinforced behavior, it has yet to be clearly defined.

In the search for behavioral methods of characterizing antidepressants, various indirect methods have been investigated. First, tricylic antidepressants have been found to potentiate the behavioral effects of amphetamine. Stein, for example, reported such a potentiation of amphetamine-induced increases in the rate of intracranial self-stimulation in rats with implanted stimulating electrodes. Several authors have demonstrated a potentiation of amphetamine-induced locomotor activity in the rat. This effect has now been shown to be due to the fact that the tricyclic antidepressants impede the enzymatic degradation of amphetamine. The effect is species-specific and is not found, for example, in the mouse. Second, and again unlike chlorpromazine, the tricyclics antagonize the depressant effects of reserpine and tetrabenazine in some species. McKearney (1968b) has shown that, in the rat, imipramine does *not* antagonize the depressant effects of tetrabenazine on operant responding. Antagonism is seen in the pigeon, but, as McKearney points out, this is a species in which imipramine alone has marked rate-increasing effects.

MAO inhibitors

Behavioral studies of the MAO inhibitors have been closely correlated with neuropharmacological studies of these compounds. The inhibition of MAO results in an accumulation of amine transmitters in the brain, and behavioral correlates of these neuropharmacological changes have been sought. Since MAO inhibition affects the synaptic availability of DA, NE, and 5-HT, it has been difficult to correlate any behavioral change with any particular amine. A slow increase in spontaneous activity has been reported, which corresponds in its time course to the increase in amine levels after certain MAO inhibitors. Because of their chemical structural similarity to amphetamine, some MAO inhibitors have additional stimulant properties and can induce a faster increase in spontaneous locomotor activity.

Intracranial self-stimulation (ICS) is one behavioral measure that has yielded positive effects with antidepressants. As discussed, the tricyclics potentiate amphetamine-induced ICS by increasing brain amphetamine levels. The MAO inhibitors, however, increase ICS behavior directly, which may well relate to their own effect on amine systems. Poschel and Ninteman

(1963) reported that 100 mg/kg iproniazid increases ICS markedly after the second dose. Tranylcypromine at doses that do not affect locomotor activity prevents the normal abolishment of ICS responding by tetrabenazine.

MAO inhibitors will also reverse tetrabenazine-induced depression of shock-avoidance behavior in the rat. On this parameter they again differ from the tricyclics (Fig. 7–2).

Stein and Wise (1969) suggested that ICS reflects activity in reward systems in the hypothalamus/limbic areas, and it has also been suggested that depression could reflect sluggishness in such systems, which can be reversed with drugs that increase the synaptic availability of amines. If this is the case, it is surprising that tricyclics, which also increase synaptic amines by blocking uptake, have no such effect on ICS behavior when given alone.

Animal models of depression

It is one of the enigmas and frustrations of behavioral pharmacology that a behavioral model of depression in animals has not yet been developed. Attempts to devise a behavioral model mimicking the conditions associated with human depression have continued, with the aim of finding a simple, predictive behavior for detecting drugs of potential clinical value. Psychological theories of depression have focused attention on maternal deprivation and negative reinforcement as behavioral variables likely to yield models of depression (Aikisal and McKinney, 1975). Progress has been mixed. The infant monkey, when separated from its mother for long periods, exhibits behavior termed *anaclitic depression*, which includes many of the symptoms seen dramatically in institutionalized children. Of the drugs used in earlier studies, antidepressants were not able to normalize the social behavior of these infants. The major tranquilizer chlorpromazine was found to be beneficial, probably because of its quietening effect. Less activity and distress was seen, but there was no improvement in social behavior. In a recent study (Hrdina et al., 1979), infant rhesus monkeys were separated from their mother for 2 or 3 weeks at 6–8 months of age. A number of behavioral categories were recorded during baseline, separation, and reunion. Daily desipramine (5 mg/kg) significantly reduced distress and self-directed behaviors and reinstated play activities.

Pursuing the theme of negative reinforcement and stress, Seligman (1975) used procedures in dogs and rats involving the repeated presentation of aversive stimuli, in conditions where escape or avoidance is not possible. These paradigms result in a conditioned immobility which has been likened to the helplessness seen in reactive depression; the effects of drugs on this

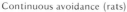

Continuous avoidance (rats)

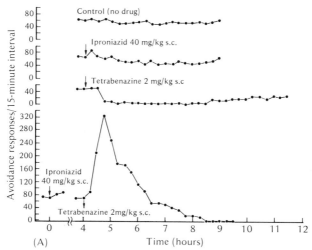

Continuous avoidance (rats)

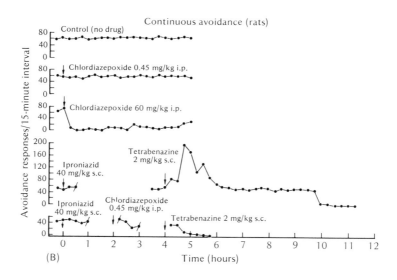

behavioral model have not been studied yet. In a similar vein, Porsott et al. (1978) devised a swimming tube test. Naive rats are placed in a vertical plexiglass cylinder for test periods of 15 min. Typically the rats are highly active during the first few minutes seeking escape from the tube. Activity then subsides and the rats become immobile, holding the head just above the water level. In subsequent test sessions rats quickly become immobile and remain so for about 75% of the session. A wide range of antidepressants significantly reduce this immobility when given systemically. This effect is not due to direct motor stimulation, as locomotor behavior'in the open field is not increased by these drugs. The test seems to be capable of distinguishing several drug groups which are known to influence mobility. Amphetamine, for example, is active in the swimming test but also increases open-field activity. The minor tranquilizers fail to effect immobility even at doses producing ataxia and the major tranquilizers, like reserpine and chlorpromazine, increase immobility and also decrease open-field behavior. Antidepressants are recognized normally on a battery of pharmacological tests in animals involving potentiation of catecholamine effects: most clinically useful drugs potentiate amphetamine effects, antagonize reserpine-induced ptosis and hypothermia, and block NE and 5-HT uptake. A number of compounds have been synthesized, however, which do not fulfill these criteria, and yet have been found to be clinically effective in depression. Such compounds include IPRINDOLE, a tricyclic indole; MIANSERIN, a tetracyclic compound; VILOXAZINE, a β-blocked derivative; and NOMIFENSINE, all of which antagonize immobility in the rat swim test. Indirect approaches to the problem of finding a simple and reliable test for antidepressants, however, have

---

Fig. 7–2   (A) Effects of iproniazid, tetrabenazine, and the combination on rate of lever pressing of rats in the continuous avoidance procedure. *First record:* avoidance response rate during a 5-hr control session; *second record:* iproniazid alone had no significant effect on behavior; *third record:* tetrabenazine alone produced a nearly complete loss of responding; *fourth record:* in rats pretreated with iproniazid, tetrabenazine produced marked stimulation shown by the increased rate of lever pressing. (B) Effect of chlordiazepoxide on the stimulation induced by iproniazid and tetrabenazine. *First record:* Control behavior; *second record:* a small dose of chlordiazepoxide had no effect on normal avoidance behavior; *third record:* it was necessary to increase the dose of chlordiazepoxide to 60 mg/kg to markedly suppress normal avoidance behavior; *fourth record:* stimulation produced by iproniazid and tetrabenazine; *fifth record:* administration of a small dose of chlordiazepoxide 2 hr prior to tetrabenazine, in rats pretreated with iproniazid, completely blocked the stimulation. (Reproduced from Zbinden and Randall, 1967.)

yielded interesting, if puzzling, results. A surgical model has been intensively researched by Cairncross et al. (1979). Removal of the olfactory bulbs in the rat results in a number of neurochemical changes in brain including a reduction of forebrain NE, and results in learning deficits on appetitively and aversively motivated tasks, including stepdown passive avoidance, oneway avoidance, and conditioned taste aversion. These deficits are correlated with marked increases in blood corticosteroid levels. Treatment with antidepressants normalizes the steroid level and reverses the behavioral deficits.

Neurochemical theories of depression

Research on the biological basis of affective disorders has focused for many years on the "monoamine hypothesis," which proposes that the underlying disorder is due to a functional decrease in NE or 5-HT activity at synapses in the brain. A corollary is that the therapeutic effects of antidepressant drugs can be explained by their ability to increase the activity of NE and/or 5-HT at these synapses. The hypothesis has been reviewed in detail elsewhere (Van Praag, 1978; Schildkraut, 1978; Sachar and Baron, 1979), but some of the highlights of the supporting evidence are as follows:
1. Reserpine, which depletes brain NE and 5-HT, precipitated some sort of depressive syndrome in as many as 15% of the people who were treated with this drug in the 1950's, when it was used in hypertension therapy.
2. Tricyclic antidepressants block the reuptake of released NE and/or 5-HT, which suggests that they act to enhance the actions of these transmitters in the brain. Similarly, the MAO inhibitors prevent the metabolic breakdown of NE and 5-HT, thereby enhancing their effects.
3. Amphetamine, which releases catecholamines in the brain, elevates mood in normals and in some depressed patients.
4. Some studies report that the 5-HT precursor, tryptophan, potentiates the therapeutic effects of MAO inhibitors, and 5-HTP has also been reported to have antidepressant actions.

   Although this evidence provides strong support for the monoamine hypothesis, many problems remain. It is difficult, for example, to account for the slow onset of clinical improvement in patients treated with tricyclic antidepressants who may require 1–3 weeks of drug treatment before they show a beneficial effect, whereas the blockade of NE and 5-HT uptake occurs rapidly. Furthermore, tricyclic antidepressants and MAO inhibitors affect both NE and 5-HT mechanisms and it is not clear which of these may be more important. In this context, clinical results with the newer drugs which have more selective effects on the uptake of NE or 5-HT should be revealing. One school of thought favors the catecholamine mechanism. In support of this view, it can be argued that an inability to respond to reinforcement appears to be a core feature of depression. In animal experiments, ICS (intracranial self-stimulation) has proved to be a valuable model for studying the pharmacological properties of reinforcement processes, and some authors (Stein et al., 1977 for review) have argued strongly that release of brain norepinephrine is the key feature explaining the basis of ICS behavior. On the other hand (see pp. 159 above), the validity of this assumption has been questioned by others, who have suggested that brain dopamine systems may be equally important in explaining self-stimulation behavior (Routtenberg and Santos-Anderson, 1978).

An attractive hypothesis is that "depression" may have a number of different biochemical explanations, and in particular there may be some subgroups that can be categorized as "low norepinephrine" and others as "low 5-HT." Biochemical studies on depressed patients offer some support for this idea. Although it is difficult to assess brain NE or 5-HT function in living patients, some indirect approaches are available. Thus, measurements of the concentration of the 5-HT metabolite 5-HIAA (see Fig. 2–18) in cerebrospinal fluid, and measurements of the rate of increase in cerebrospinal fluid 5-HIAA after blockade of its normal efflux from the brain with PROBENICID gives an index of 5-HT activity. Several studies have reported abnormally low levels of 5-HIAA in cerebrospinal fluid samples from depressed patients, and a subgroup of patients can be distinguished. Measurements of the NE metabolite MHPG (see Fig. 2–15) in urine or cerebrospinal fluid also provide an index of CNS noradrenergic function. Animal studies suggest that as much as half of the urinary MHPG derives from NE metabolism in the brain. There have been several reports of a reduced urinary excretion of MHPG in depressed patients, and a subgroup appears to be abnormally low. Again, the trial of selective amine uptake inhibitors should help to resolve this question. For example, drugs such as MAPROTILINE and NISOXETINE which are "pure" NE uptake inhibitors would be predicted to be effective only in patients in the "low NE" category, whereas "pure" 5-HT uptake inhibitors such as FLUOXETINE and CITALOPRAM should benefit patients in the low 5-HT group.

The precise nature of the biochemical abnormalities underlying depression, and the areas of brain involved remain unknown. Although the monoamine hypothesis remains attractive in general terms, much more specific information is needed. For example, depression is often accompanied by disorders in neuroendocrine function. An extensive literature has shown that excessive secretion of steroids (cortisol) secondary to excessive ACTH secretion often occurs in severe depression. It is possible that a deficiency of NE and/or 5-HT at the hypothalamic level could be responsible for such endocrine disturbances (Sacher and Baron, 1979).

OPIATES AND ENDORPHINS

Classification and neuropharmacological properties (for review see Snyder and Childers, 1979)

The group of drugs known as the *opiates* or sometimes as the *narcotics* comprises the various naturally occurring alkaloids of the opium poppy, of which MORPHINE is the principal example, and various synthetic drugs with similar actions; these include HEROIN, LEVORPHANOL, MEPERIDINE, PENTAZOCINE, and ETORPHINE (Fig. 7–3). The unique psychopharmacological and pain-relieving (ANALGESIC) actions of morphine have been known to man for several thousand years. In contrast, the discovery that the brain normally contains its own endogenous morphine-like chemicals, the ENDORPHINS, is a very recent one. The endorphins are a group of peptides, of which the principal members are LEU-ENKEPHALIN and MET-ENKEPHALIN:

Leu-Enkephalin = TyrGlyGlyPheLeu
Met-Enkephalin = TyrGlyGlyPheMet

These two small peptides differ only in the carboxy-terminal amino acid, leucine or methionine. They are the principal endorphins in brain and spinal cord, where they are found in specific groups of neurons (see Fig. 2–24). Enkephalin-containing nerve terminals are particularly abundant in sensory nuclei in spinal cord and brainstem, where they are thought to act to modify transmission in pain pathways. The enkephalins are also abundant in many other regions of brain, including globus pallidus and various regions of the limbic system. The larger peptide β-ENDORPHIN is found in small amounts in brain (Fig. 2–24) and in much larger amounts in the pituitary gland. β-Endorphin incorporates the structure of metenkephalin at its amino-terminal end. In biosynthesis, β-endorphin is made from a series of larger peptides from which the pituitary hormone ACTH also derives (Fig. 7–4), and it seems likely that cells in the pituitary or neurons in brain which contain β-endorphin also contain ACTH, or an ACTH-like peptide. This is particularly intriguing because of the behavioral effects of ACTH-like peptides described above (p. 178). The neurons in brain that contain β-endorphin, however, appear to be quite distinct from the more numerous and widespread systems of neurons containing enkephalins.

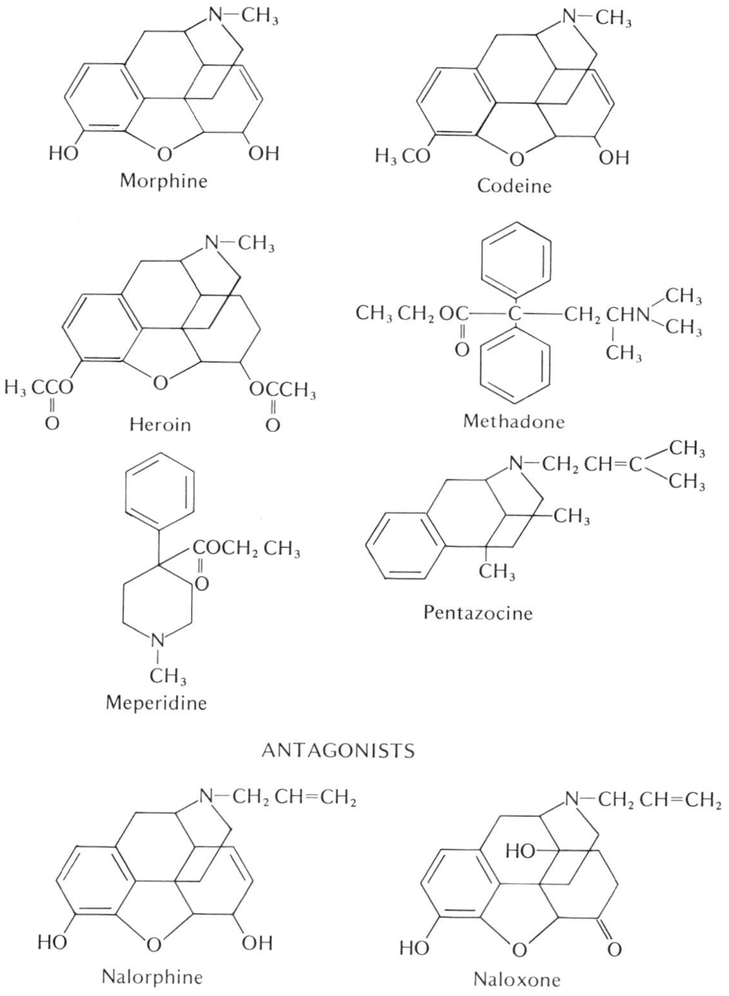

Fig. 7–3 Structures of some morphine-like drugs and antagonists.

Opiates and endorphins act on "opiate" receptors, which were first detected in CNS by radioligand binding studies using radioactively labelled opiate drugs as ligands (Snyder and Childers, 1979). Opiate receptors occur in particularly high densities in regions of brain which contain enkephalins. The enkephalins and β-endorphin compete with radiolabelled opiate drugs for binding to such receptors. Endorphins also mimic the actions of opiates on various pharmacological test systems involving actions on peripheral tis-

PRECURSOR RELATIONSHIPS OF
CORTICOTROPINS AND PITUITARY
ENDORPHINS

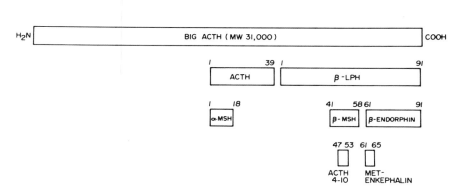

Fig. 7–4.   In the pituitary gland, and probably in brain, a single large precursor molecule (BIG ACTH) contains within its amino acid sequence the entire ACTH and β-lipotropin hormone (β-LPH) molecules. In turn, the ACTH sequence contains within it that of α-melanotropin (α-MSH); and the β-LPH sequence contains β-MSH and β-endorphin. Furthermore, the sequence of amino acids 4–10 in ACTH is repeated within the β-LPH sequence. Although the amino acid sequence of met-enkephalin is contained in the first five residues of β-endorphin, free met-enkephalin has not been detected in significant quantities in the pituitary gland. Moreover, there is no evidence that β-endorphin is the precursor of met-enkephalin synthesis in the brain. (From Snyder and Childers, 1979.)

sues. Thus, the opiates and endorphins inhibit the electrically evoked contractions of guinea pig gut or mouse vas deferens *in vitro*. In such tests the availability of specific antagonists for opiate receptors has proved critically important. Some compounds structurally related to opiates possess antagonist rather than agonist effects; these include NALOXONE, NALORPHINE, and DIPRENORPHINE, and naloxone has become the most commonly used antagonist drug.

The endorphins, and especially leu- and met-enkephalin, are degraded rapidly by metabolizing enzymes (peptidases) in brain and in blood and other peripheral tissues. Therefore, the enkephalins are not suitable for use as centrally acting drugs. They are not absorbed after oral administration and penetrate into CNS only poorly. However, synthetic analogues of enkephalins have been developed in metabolically stable forms; some can even be absorbed after oral administration and retain full morphine-like properties. Thus, it is likely that enkephalin-derived drugs will soon be available for clinical testing.

The opiates have complex neuropharmacological actions. They are extremely useful drugs clinically for the alleviation of severe pain (see Chapter 8). Their analgesic action, however, is also associated with complex psychological effects, of which their ability to induce a state of euphoria is the main reason for their importance as drugs of abuse. The particular state of well-being induced by the opiates in addicts defies description; after intravenous administration, these drugs lead to immediate physical sensations that are extremely pleasurable. The marked tendency of repeated drug administration to lead to tolerance and physical dependence, however, makes them dangerous drugs of addiction.

Tolerance and dependence

The opiates are the drugs *par excellence* for illustrating the phenomena of tolerance and dependence. Tolerance is readily induced in man or animals by repeated drug administration (see Fig. 2–4). After some weeks of drug administration, the animal or human addict may require twenty to forty times the dose of drug initially used to obtain a given effect. Animals can be trained to self-administer opiate drugs, and the dose of drug administered in this way shows a progressive increase as tolerance develops. Tolerance cannot be explained simply in terms of an increased rate of drug metabolism after chronic use, although this may play some role in the overall process. The development of "cellular tolerance" of unknown mechanism seems to be far more important (see Chapter 2, p. 62). Cross-tolerance is seen among all the opiate agonists described above.

Physical dependence invariably accompanies the development of tolerance to the opiates. Thus, addicts or chronically treated animals may appear superficially normal, but a withdrawal syndrome is easily precipitated by stopping drug treatment or, more immediately, by the administration of an opiate antagonist drug such as NALOXONE. The withdrawal syndrome is a complex process with many different components; in man, these include restlessness, craving for the drug, perspiration, chills, fever, vomiting, panting, insomnia, and hyperactivity of the sympathetic system (dilated pupils, piloerection, and hypertension). The withdrawal syndrome can be reversed immediately by administration of morphine or any other opiate agonist drug. The rapid effects of opiate agonists and antagonists in reversing or precipitating withdrawal symptoms strongly suggest that after tolerance has developed a continued occupation of receptor sites by an opiate agonist drug is needed to prevent the onset of withdrawal.

The idea that enkephalin-derived drugs might prove to be nonaddictive seems unlikely to prove correct. Repeated administration of these peptides to animals, by direct intracerebral injection or infusion, leads to tolerance and also to signs of dependence in such animals when challenged with naloxone.

Many theories of the cellular basis for tolerance and dependence have been proposed. It seems likely that some long-term changes take place in the synthesis of macromolecules involved in the action of the drugs. Studies with radiolabelled receptor-binding drugs have so far failed to reveal any long-term change in the number of opiate receptor sites in brain tissue from tolerant animals; moreover, there are no changes in the enkephalin levels in such animals either.

Behavioral pharmacology

The mood-changing properties of morphine and heroin form only part of a complex profile of psychological and physiological effects induced by these drugs.

In common with other CNS sedatives and hypnotics, small doses of morphine stimulate behavior, whereas large doses are depressant. For example, small doses stimulate locomotor activity in rodents, and Goldstein and Sheehan (1969) used this simple behavioral response as an elegant model system for quantifying tolerance to morphine and its analogues. A single dose of 20 mg/kg of levorphanol induces a "running fit" in mice, and, if this dose is repeated every 8 hr, tolerance develops rapidly (Fig. 2–4). The running fit meets the essential criteria for a typical effect of the opioid narcotics. It shows the same high degree of specificity, levorphanol being active whereas its stereoisomer dextrorphan is inactive: the slopes of the dose–response curves are the same for the running fit and analgesia, and both are antagonized by nalorphine.

Attention has turned more recently to the stimulatory effects of morphine in the rat. In this species morphine is usually considered to produce a profound form of catalepsy. However, if the animals are observed for longer periods and a range of doses is studied, a different picture emerges. At low doses morphine induces locomotor activity in rats, and at a slightly higher dose a characteristic form of stereotyped behavior is seen. Finally, after large systemic doses, a cataleptic state is seen, the duration of which varies with dose. However, when the animal emerges from this depressed state, marked locomotor stimulation is seen. The stimulatory effect of morphine on unconditioned behavior can be distinguished from that caused by amphetamine. Whereas the latter drug depresses social interaction and increases only responses of short duration, morphine increases social responses, including rearing and grooming and a wide range of other species-specific responses. Schirring and Hecht (1979) contrasted the "selective" stimulation of amphetamine with the "polyactivation" seen after morphine.

If animals are injected repeatedly with the same dose of morphine, tolerance develops and at this stage, withdrawal of the drug or injection of opiate antagonists results in severe withdrawal symptoms. In the rat these include diarrhea, squealing, writhing, "wet-dog" shakes, ptosis, teeth chattering, and weight loss. Although dependence and withdrawal are associated with all the natural, synthetic, and endogenous opiate-like compounds yet described, it is still not known which opiate receptors in the CNS are centrally involved in the expression of withdrawal behavior.

It is possible to demonstrate a degree of abstinence after a single dose of morphine. Pilcher and Stolerman (1976) devised a novel application of the taste aversion paradigm to determine the minimum dose of morphine in rats from which abstinence could be precipitated. Rats were given access to water for 1 hr daily. When adaptation to this drinking regime was established, saccharin (0.1%) was substituted on every third day and immediately after the drinking session the rats were injected with naloxone. For 10 days prior to the first presentation of saccharin and for the remainder of the experiment, morphine (10 mg/kg) or saline was given twice a day. In the saline treated controls repeated pairings of naloxone with saccharin failed to reduce subsequent saccharin intake. But after a single pairing in the morphine-treated rats, a significant reduction in saccharin intake was found, which became greater with subsequent saccharin-naloxone pairings. In later experiments doses of morphine as low as 1 mg/kg were sufficient to produce naloxone-induced aversion. Single doses of morphine were able to produce detectable aversion 1.5 h after the first injection, emphasizing that morphine dependence can occur very rapidly.

Turning to conditioned behavior, Verhave et al. (1959) studied rats trained in a shock avoidance task. The conditioned-avoidance response was lost with a dose of 4 mg/kg, but escape was less affected. In dogs, however, Domino et al. (1958) did not find a loss of shock avoidance except at doses that produce motor deficits and, at this level, escape behavior was more affected than avoidance. McMillan and Morse (1967) studied the depressant effect of morphine on food-reinforced responding in pigeons, and these effects, like the excitatory effects, show tolerance after daily injections (Fig. 7–5). When

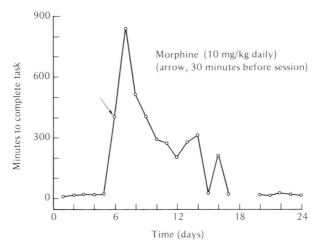

Fig. 7–5   The development of tolerance to the effects of 10 mg/kg of morphine daily on schedule-controlled performance in the pigeon. *Abscissa:* daily sessions; *ordinate:* time to complete the four schedule components composing the daily session. The first five points show the control performance. From the 6th session (arrow), 10 mg/kg of morphine were given 30 min before the session. The time to complete the session increased greatly and then gradually returned to control values. The pigeon was injected but not tested on days 18 and 19. (Reproduced from McMillan and Morse, 1967.)

tolerance has developed, the same dose will frequently stimulate response rates rather than depress them (Fig. 7–6). Stimulatory effects of morphine have been seen in man, where convulsions eventually occur.

With the discovery of opiate receptors and endogenous opioid peptides in brain, interest has focused on localizing the sites of action for the various behavioral effects of morphine. In the forebrain, high concentrations of opiate receptors and enkephalins exist in anatomical proximity to the ascending DA pathways. It has now been shown that morphine and endorphins injected at the site of this interaction result in profound behavioral effects. The mesolimbocortical (MLC) DA system is involved in locomotor arousal and the nigrostriatal (NS) system with sensorimotor integration and motor sequencing (Iversen, 1977). Morphine, enkephalin, and β-endorphin injected into the region of the DA cell bodies of the MLC system induce a marked stimulation of locomotor behavior (Joyce and Iversen, 1979). In the DA terminal areas of the MLC system morphine and enkephalin also induce locomotion. In the most systematic study of this effect Costall et al. (1978)

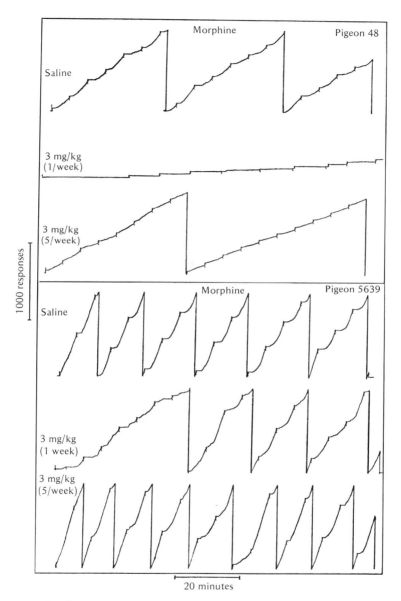

Fig. 7–6   The development of tolerance to the effects of 3 mg/kg of morphine on schedule-controlled performance in the pigeon. Cumulative response records under multiple FR 30 FI 5, pigeons 48 and 5639. The records show the effect of saline, 3 mg/kg of morphine during the first 1/week series, and 3 mg/kg of morphine during the daily morphine series. (Reproduced from McMillan and Morse, 1967.)

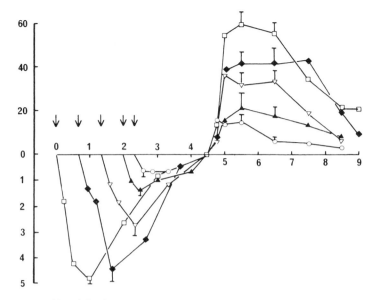

Fig. 7–7.   Profile of the biphasic motor behavior induced by 1 (○), 3.125 (▲), 12.5 (▽), 50 (◆), or 100 (□) μg of morphine injected bilaterally into the nucleus accumbens. The ordinate shows activity in a positive direction (which was assessed as the number of interruptions of a photocell light beam occurring within a 10-min period) and shows catalepsy in a negative direction (scored according to Costall's system). Abscissa: time (hours). Each point is the mean response from 5 to 8 rats. Standard errors of the maximum values are shown. Arrows indicate the relative times of injection for each dosage group following superimposition of graphical data. (Reproduced from Costall et al., 1978.)

described a dose-dependent biphasic locomotor response to morphine injected into the nucleus accumbens (Fig. 7–7). At all the doses studied morphine injected bilaterally into the nucleus accumbens produces catalepsy initially, followed by locomotion. The size and duration of these two effects are dose-dependent (Fig. 7–7).

Morphine-induced catalepsy appears to be associated with the MLC rather than the striatum. Dill and Costa (1977) failed to induce this behavior after injecting 22.5 μg of enkephalin into the striatum, whereas in the nucleus accumbens this dose produces marked catalepsy. β-Endorphin has a similar action and Segal et al. (1977) have compared the behavioral features of this opiate-induced catalepsy with that seen after neuroleptic treatment, and found them to differ. Local injections of morphine and enkephalin into the origins of the nigrostriatal DA system induce the steretyped behavior associated with activation of that system. After unilateral injection into the substantia nigra, turning behavior is seen. The various effects of morphine and opioid peptides are reversed by naloxone, by lesions to the DA pathways, or by neuroleptics, suggesting a functional relationship between opiate receptors and DA neurons in the mediation of motor behaviors.

If, as is generally accepted, the dopamine systems mediate the processes essential to reward and if opiates interact with DA neurons, it may not be surprising to find that animals will respond to obtain morphine injections. This is true of other reinforcers like food, water, escape from aversive stimuli, and electrical stimulation of certain areas of brain. However, the high rates of responding seen in animals seeking rewarding drugs are in a certain sense paradoxical, since the initial presentation of these drugs is almost certainly aversive.

Earlier, the evidence that amphetamine acts as an aversive stimulus in some circumstances was discussed, and yet amphetamine infusion is clearly rewarding in self-administration paradigms. The same is true of morphine. The first injection of morphine is reported to be aversive in man, and morphine can punish saccharin drinking in conditioned taste aversion paradigms. Animals may have *to learn* which stimuli are rewarding. Perhaps there are not such things as "innate" reinforcers. There is evidence that animals have to learn about food reinforcement. This is certainly the case for brain stimulation reward. More recently, mild tail pinch has been identified as a reinforcer and in this case rats clearly have to learn about the nature of this motivating stimulus (Koob et al, 1976). It is a small step to suggest that stimuli which themselves directly facilitate learning and memory have a high probability of acquiring independent reinforcement properties. Mondadori and Waser (1979) developed these important theoretical issues relating learning and memory to reinforcement. Such reinforcers as food or electrical brain stimulation improve retention of different tasks if given post-trial. These authors showed that morphine (40–100 mg/kg) facilitates learning of one-trial passive avoidance in drug-naive mice. Undoubtedly such doses of morphine would be shown to be aversive under other conditions.

In agreement with these findings of facilitation, Rigter (1978) reported that in rats systemic treatment with the pentapeptides met- and leu-enkephalin reduce the amnesia for one-trial avoidance responding induced by carbon dioxide inhalation. The dose required to produce this effect was 30 μg or less, whereas 100 μg or more injected intracerebrally is required to induce analgesia (Belluzi et al. 1976).

Experimental studies of morphine self-administration

It is interesting to speculate why some psychoactive drugs are highly addictive, whereas others are not. Both antidepressants and opiates produce elevation of mood, but only the latter are addictive.

It has been found generally that animals will self-administer those drugs which are known to be highly addictive in man. This is fortuitous for the study of the processes fundamental to addiction. Our knowledge of the processes essential to drug addiction is not great but it is sufficient to imply that all these drugs are not addictive for precisely the same reasons. However, if we consider the three major addictive drug groups—stimulants, depressants, (ethanol and barbiturates), and opiates—they have three shared properties. First, they are all reinforcers; second, animals are able to recognize and discriminate the complex of interoceptive responses induced by the different drug groups; third, and probably as a consequence of the first and second effects, conditioning effects can readily be demonstrated between the drugged state and the environment in which the drugged state is experienced.

Rats will self-administer morphine orally or via implanted catheters. As with traditional reinforcers, animals will learn a new response to obtain the drug. Furthermore, morphine can be presented on schedules and the resulting patterns of drug-seeking responses are identical to those seen for food, water, or shock-avoidance.

Studies demonstrating that animals are able to discriminate the "states" following treatment with a number of psychoactive drugs have also been well reviewed (Colpaert and Rosecrams, 1978). It has long been known that drugs can act as discriminative stimuli and awareness of state dependency (or lack of awareness) has dogged behavioral pharmacology for many years. It is essential to take into account state dependency if one is studying the effect of a drug on subsequent behavior. This proved of great importance in studying the effects of drugs on learning and memory (see Hunter et al., 1977). In the case of addictive drugs, their discriminative properties may relate directly to their reinforcing power.

The phenomenon of conditioning associated with the presentation of rewarding drugs or the withdrawal of those drugs is receiving more experimental attention since Wikler (1965) recognized that the control of addiction presented behavioral as well as pharmacological problems. Wikler suggested that in opiate dependence stimuli reliably and regularly associated with withdrawal could eventually elicit withdrawal even in people no longer taking drugs. The theory has been extended to include a similar condition-

ing process occurring between the environment and the "high" associated
with drug. Thus stimuli reliably associated with the "high" acquire some
reinforcing value in the absence of the drug. Attempts have been made to
measure these conditioning effects in human addicts and O'Brien (1976)
cited an example of conditioned withdrawal:

The patient was a 28 year old man with a 10 year history of narcotic addiction. He
was married and the father of two children. He reported that, while addicted, he
was arrested and incarcerated for 6 months. He reported experiencing severe withdrawal during the first 4 or 5 days in custody, but later, he began to feel well. He
gained weight, felt like a new man, and decided that he was finished with drugs. He
thought about his children and looked forward to returning to his former job. On the
way home after release from prison, he began thinking of drugs and feeling nau-
seated. As the subway approached his stop, he began sweating, tearing from his eyes
and gagging. This was an area where he he had frequently experienced narcotic
withdrawal symptoms while trying to acquire drugs. As he got off the subway, he
vomited onto the tracks. He soon bought drugs, and was relieved. The following day
he again experienced craving and withdrawal symptoms in his neighbourhood, and
he again relieved them by injecting heroin. The cycle repeated itself over the next
few days and soon he became readdicted.

He also reported on a 2-year study of eight heroin addicts, drug-free at the
time of the study. All subjects reported periodic episodes of discomfort (including tightening in throat, yawning, rhinorrhea, back or abdominal pain,
and nausea), termed "sickness." At other times feelings termed "craving"
were experienced. Three subjects were not able to relate these feelings to
specific environmental stimuli. Five subjects were able to relate sickness
and craving to distinct stimuli and to rate these stimuli in order of potency.
In a later study of 100 patients on methadone, a high proportion (58–62%)
were able to rate stimuli associated with sickness and craving and there was
a 0.88 correlation, suggesting that the same stimuli produced both feelings.

In rats and monkeys maintained on opiates, evidence of these forms of
conditioning can be obtained. Goldberg and Schuster (1967) made monkeys
dependent on morphine. The animals were trained to work for food on a
schedule of reinforcement, and, when nalorphine was administered, withdrawal occurred and responding for food was depressed. Then a buzzer was
sounded during the withdrawal induced by nalorphine, and, after such conditioning, presentation of the buzzer alone induced withdrawal symptoms
and depression of bar pressing, even though morphine was still being given.

In following up these studies, Schuster and Woods (1968) found that sensory stimuli associated with opiate administration itself could also be conditioned. The monkeys worked on a 6-hr multiple schedule, which started
with a 2-hr time-out when no food or drug was available; during 1 hr, in the

presence of a green light, food reinforcement was available, and this was followed by 1 hr of white light, with infusion of morphine every 2.5 min in the presence of a red light. The 5th hour was the food schedule and the 6th hour a time-out.

After 60 days of drug infusion, the animals were put into morphine extinction. On alternate days, during the 4th hour, the red light without morphine was presented, or the red light was presented, and saline infusion was given. Under the latter condition, an increase in responding was seen in the presence of the red light plus the physical manipulations associated with placebo injection (Fig. 7–8). Since the red light alone did not have this effect, it is suggested that the stimuli associated with the injection had acquired conditioned reinforcing properties because of their earlier association with morphine infusion. These are most important observations for understanding the behavioral basis of morphine addiction. The implication of the results with humans and with animals is that one cannot successfully withdraw opiate from an addict unless the conditioned stimuli are also extinguished. In the absence of the drug, the sight of the familiar pusher elicits either craving or withdrawal symptoms, both of which encourage the addict to seek the primary reinforcer, the drug. To look at the problem from a different viewpoint, the stimuli conditioned to a drug state could be used to manipulate the process of withdrawal. The presentation of stimuli conditioned to be "high," if presented during withdrawal, should weaken the intensity of the unconditioned responses seen in withdrawal. This has been demonstrated by Drawbaugh and Lal (1974). Rats were made morphine-dependent by injections in the presence of a bell. A 24-hr withdrawal induced a hypothermic response, which was reversed if the bell was presented. Withdrawal from morphine also disrupts conditioned responses; for example, patterns of responding maintained by schedules of reinforcement in the rat are disrupted by large doses of morphine, but rapid tolerance to this disruption is seen if the morphine injections are continued, and indeed escalated. In the dependent state normal patterns of responding are seen, which on withdrawal are grossly distorted. If morphine injections are given regularly in the presence of a stimulus (auditory tone), the presentation of the tone during withdrawal prevents the disruption of conditioned responding seen typically in rats conditioned and withdrawn in the absence of the tone (Tye and Iversen, 1975). In both of these studies naloxone-induced withdrawal symptoms were not modified by the presentation of the conditioned stimulus. The fact that naloxone blocks the psychological responses evoked by conditioned stimuli in the same way that it blocks the uncondi-

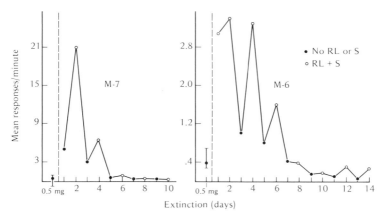

Fig. 7–8. Responses of two monkeys during morphine extinction sessions. On each graph the far left point is the final 5-day average of response rate for morphine reinforcement. To the right of the dashed line, points show extinction data—solid points, absence of response consequence (i.e. no morphine or conditioned stimuli); open circles, response consequence of saline plus red light. Absolute response rates differ in the two animals, but in both the presence of conditioned stimuli increases extinction responding. (Reproduced from Schuster and Woods, 1968.)

tioned morphine effects has both theoretical and practical implications. Of theoretical importance is the suggestion that the conditional stimulus may evoke activity in the brain pathways specifically sensitive to the agonistic actions of morphine and to morphine dependence. The practical importance of this finding is related to the use of narcotic antagonists in the therapy of narcotic addiction. The current rationale behind the use of narcotic antagonists in the treatment of heroin addicts is that these drugs extinguish heroin consumption because they block the "high" sought from the agonist effects of the drug. Since narcotic antagonists appear to block the effects of conditioned stimuli associated with drug intake, as well as the response to the drug itself, they may be valuable in extinguishing a morphine habit associated with the conditional placebo effects of morphine-seeking behavior. These effects have been considered to be major factors in "cured" morphine addicts who go back to morphine use.

   In conclusion, the interoceptive stimuli associated with addictive drugs are rewarding, discriminative, and readily associated with neutral stimuli in the environment. Advancement of knowledge on this important topic awaits an understanding of the CNS processes underlying these three properties of the drugs of abuse.

8. The Pain-Relieving Actions of Morphine and Related Opiates

Despite the addictive liability of morphine and its congeners, and the undesirable autonomic side effects of these drugs, they are still the most effective pain-relieving agents (ANALGESICS) known, and these drugs play an important role in the clinical management of severe and chronic pain. Although an intensive search has been conducted for many years to discover safer analgesic drugs with the pain-relieving properties of morphine, but without its addictive and psychotropic properties, this effort has met with only limited success. Although many synthetic analogues of morphine have been discovered—for example, levorphanol, meperidine, pethidine, and methadone—none of them differs basically from morphine in addiction potential. The most promising discovery has been that some drugs such as PENTAZOCINE (see Fig. 7–3) and BUPRENORPHINE are potent analgesics with reduced addiction potential, and they appear to act as partial agonists or as mixed agonists/antagonists at opiate receptor sites. The discovery of the endorphins has led to hectic activity in the design and testing of synthetic analogues of the naturally occurring enkephalins as potential new analgesic drugs, but it is too early to assess whether these agents will differ qualitatively from the existing opiate alkaloids and synthetic congeners.

In this chapter we will review the contribution of animal experiments to studies of pain mechanisms and the actions of analgesic drugs.

ANIMAL MODELS FOR ASSESSING ANALGESIC DRUGS

Pain is an intensely subjective experience and as such cannot be measured in animal experiments. However, animal tests can measure the threshold of responsiveness to painful stimuli, and such methods have been of major importance in screening and evaluating analgesic drugs. The hot plate test and the tail-flick withdrawal test have been widely used. In the former the rodent is placed on a hot plate set at a fixed temperature (e.g. 55 ± 1°C). The latency to lick a paw or jump from the plate is a measure of the responsiveness to thermal pain. In the tail-flick test, the tail is placed in an appropriate restraining groove under a radiant heat source. Again the latency to respond is recorded. Flinch-jump tests have also been described with application of electric shock to the feet. Here, regardless of the response, the intensity of the shock is systematically raised and lowered to determine the threshold of responsiveness rather than the speed of response to a fixed stimulus. Titration methods have also been used in rats and monkeys. For example, Yaksh et al. (1977) confined rats in an operant chamber with their tail projecting through a hole in the back wall. Electrodes were taped to the tail and the apparatus was programmed so that a 5-sec shock to the tail was delivered every 3 sec. The shock intensity increased in 26 equal steps from 0 to 6 mA. If the rat pressed the lever during the 5-sec shock, it was turned off immediately and its intensity was reduced by one step during the next shock period. Thus the response of the animal determined the intensity of shock presented.

The analgesic actions of morphine, nalorphine, and the benzomorphan compounds have been demonstrated by Weiss and Laties (1964b) using an elegant titration method to determine the maximum electric shock level monkeys would tolerate. Monkeys sat in a restraining chair and were shocked through shoes on the feet. The apparatus was programmed so that the animal received a shock of increasing intensity (<5 mA) every 2 sec. A lever press between shocks prevented this increase. Thus, by pressing regularly the animal could "hold" the shock at a low level of intensity. Six-hr sessions were given. After a 2-hr control run, morphine or a related compound was injected, and the shock threshold plotted for a further 4 hr. The shock was controlled by a recording attenuator, an apparatus that systematically changes the intensity of a stimulus and plots out its value on a continuous paper record. Both morphine and the synthetic benzomorphan analgesic (WIN 20,740) (Fig. 8–1) increased the level of shock monkeys would tolerate; 4 mg/kg of morphine raised the shock level to nearly its maximum (Fig. 8–2).

DO OPIATES REDUCE THE INTENSITY OR THE UNPLEASANTNESS OF PAIN SENSATIONS?

During the past twenty years concepts of how opiates act to relieve pain

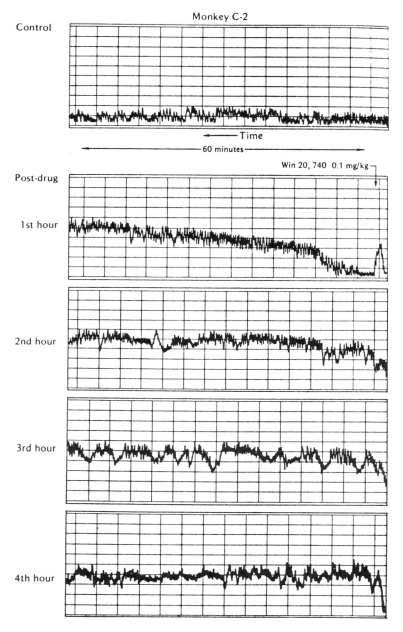

Fig. 8–1   Recording attenuator record of the response of one monkey to 0.1 mg/kg of WIN 20,740. Each segment represents 1 hr; the control segment is the last hour of the 2-hr predrug sample. Time reads from right to left; maximum shock is represented by the top of the record. Each 1-hr segment begins with the shock level reset to zero. (Reproduced from Weiss and Laties, 1964b.)

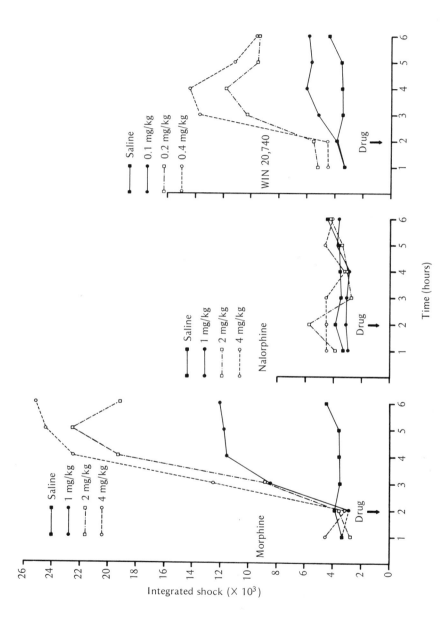

Saline
1 mg/kg
2 mg/kg
4 mg/kg

Morphine

Saline
1 mg/kg
2 mg/kg
4 mg/kg

Nalorphine

Saline
0.1 mg/kg
0.2 mg/kg
0.4 mg/kg

WIN 20,740

Integrated shock (X 10³)

Drug

Time (hours)

have been considerably influenced by the work of Beecher (1959). He distinguished between *pain sensations* that relate to the intensity of noxious stimuli and a variety of *pain reactions* that reflect complex emotional and cognitive responses elicited by such stimuli. The latter are influenced by personality, past experience, and experiential context. Beecher proposed that opiates produce clinical analgesia primarily by altering the unpleasantness of pain reactions rather than by altering the intensity of pain sensations. In other words, the patient may still feel the pain but it no longer hurts. This view attracted considerable attention, and suggested that the effects of opiates on mood and their possible antianxiety effects might be intimately related to their actions in relieving pain. When morphine was studied on one of the classical behavioral tests for assessing antianxiety drugs in animals, however, the results did not support the contention that there is such a relationship between analgesia and mood. In the Geller procedure, rats are reinforced and simultaneously punished with electric shock for lever pressing. Minor tranquilizers (benzodiazepines and barbiturates) produce a marked release from the suppressive effects of punishment, but morphine in doses of 4 mg/kg is quite ineffective, despite the fact that this dose must be clearly analgesic (Geller et al., 1963). Kelleher and Morse (1964) also failed to reinstate punished responding with morphine in the pigeon (Fig. 8–3). However, they found that when the punishing electric shock was actually switched off (and presumably pain was totally eliminated), responding was reinstated much less quickly (Fig. 8–4) than after benzodiazepine or barbiturate administration (see Fig. 9–3). This suggests that although the procedure involves a painful stimulus, responding is being controlled by some additional factor which can be modified with anxiolytic drugs but not with morphine. This lack of effect of morphine on punished behavior

---

Fig. 8–3 Effect of morphine on behavior suppressed by punishment. The first four frames show performance of pigeon 235 on the fixed-ratio procedure in which nonpunishment and punishment components alternated. Shocks were scheduled in punishment components except where indicated. *First record:* control performance; *second record* (start): performance on the same procedure following the intramuscular injection of morphine (1 mg/kg); at the large arrow, scheduled shocks were omitted; *third and fourth records:* the effects of larger doses of morphine—20 min in which no responses occurred have been omitted from the 10 mg/kg record; *fifth record:* the effect of morphine on the performance of pigeon 234. Scheduled shocks were omitted at the beginning of the record and then reinstated at the larger arrow. Note that morphine did not prevent the almost immediate return of suppression by punishment with electric shocks. (Reproduced from Kelleher and Morse, 1964.)

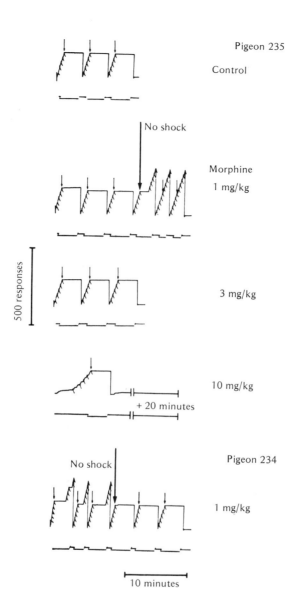

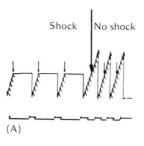

(A)

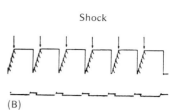

(B)

500 responses

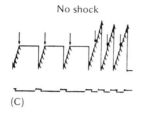

(C)

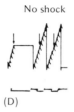

(D)

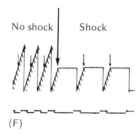

(E)

(F)

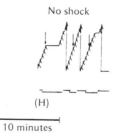

(G)

(H)

10 minutes

seemed well established until McMillan (1973a) found that under certain conditions morphine would reinstate punished responding in the pigeon. This result was obtained using a multiple FI/FI punishment schedule, with every response during the punishment component being followed by a 2.5 – 5.2 mA shock of 50-msec duration. Morphine in 0.3 and 1.0 mg/kg amounts restored responding during the punishment component to the same degree as did the benzodiazepines. The failure to obtain this result in earlier experiments is difficult to explain. There are, however, differences in species, schedule, and shock parameter between the three studies. In the Geller procedure, rats were used and every response was both rewarded and punished during the punishment component, but the shock level was low, 0.75 mA. Kelleher and Morse (1964) used high shock levels but punished only the first ten responses of each rewarded FR 30 in the punishment component of their schedule. McMillan (1973a) also punished every response made during a rewarded 5 min FI with a high shock. This punishment-releasing effect of morphine is clearly an important finding, and the discrepancy between this study and the previous results is worth further investigation, especially in view of the fact that McMillan (1973b) reported that on a FR 30, FI 5 min schedule, with every response in both components punished, morphine failed to reverse suppression.

The results of animal experiments, thus, do not make it clear that opiates possess anxiolytic properties. A report by Gracely et al. (1979) also seriously questioned the view, put forward by Beecher (1959), that opiate analgesics act principally by reducing the unpleasantness rather than the sensation of pain. In this study 40 dental patients were asked to rate the magnitude of painful electrical stimulation of the tooth pulp before and after the intrave-

---

Fig. 8–4   The effects of omitting and reinstating scheduled electric shocks on behavior suppressed by punishment. In nonpunishment components, a 30-response, fixed-ratio schedule of food reinforcement was in effect in the presence of an orange stimulus; nonpunishment components terminated after five reinforcements as indicated by the small arrows. In punishment components, a 30-response, fixed-ratio schedule was in effect in the presence of a white stimulus; each of the first ten responses of each ratio produced a brief electric shock. Punishment components terminated after five reinforcements or 3 min, as indicated by the resetting of the pen to the bottom of the record. The frames show successive daily sessions except between B and C, where one session is omitted, and between F and G, where two sessions are omitted. The periods during which scheduled shocks were omitted are indicated. Note the records (frames C, D, and H), showing suppression of responding at the beginning of sessions in which scheduled shocks were omitted (spontaneous retrogression). (Reproduced from Kelleher and Morse, 1964.)

nous administration of either the short-acting opiate analgesic drug, fentanyl, or saline placebo. The responses were registered by choices of verbal descriptions from lists of either sensory intensity (weak, mild, intense) or unpleasantness (annoying, unpleasant, distressing). Fentanyl clearly reduced the sensory intensity of the painful stimulation without affecting its unpleasantness, indicating, in contrast to the previously held view, that opiate-induced analgesia may involve a significant attenuation of pain sensation.

SITES OF ACTIONS OF OPIATES IN CNS

In their classical intracranial electrical stimulation studies, Olds and Milner described an extensive range of sites, focused in the periaqueductal grey (PAG) of the brainstem and midbrain, where stimulation is highly aversive. This "punishment" system stood in complementary relationship to the "pleasure" system extending from the forebrain through diencephalon and mesencephalon to tegmental areas close to the aversive sites. Mayer et al. (1971) made the important observation that electrical stimulation of PAG induces profound analgesia without a general loss of sensori-motor function. In mapping sites in monkey brain at which local microinjections of morphine were effective in inducing analgesia, assessed by a shock titration procedure, Pert and Yaksh also found the PAG to be a key site for opiate-induced analgesia (reviewed by Yaksh and Rudy, 1978). Opiates were also found to cause analgesia in the rat when injected into the PAG. Biochemical experiments have shown that this region of brainstem contains unusually high local concentrations of opiate receptors and enkephalins, and the analgesic effects of both locally injected morphine or electrical stimulation of PAG are blocked by naloxone—suggesting that they are mediated by an action on opiate receptors (Akil et al., 1976). In the case of electrical stimulation, the mechanism may involve a local release of enkephalins in the PAG region. Electrical stimulation of the central grey also produces relief in patients suffering from intractable pain, and this effect is naloxone reversible (Hosobuchi et al., 1977).

What is the basis of PAG-induced analgesia? Does activation of opiate receptors in this region modify the transmission of sensory pain information to the forebrain by an influence on ascending systems or is pain input blocked at the spinal cord level by activation of descending pathways from PAG to spinal cord? It seems that both mechanisms operate. It has been shown that descending NE and 5-HT fibers from the raphe nuclei modulate the transmission of pain stimuli in the dorsal horn of the spinal cord, and these systems are activated by PAG stimulation. Lesions to the raphe magnus (Chance et al., 1978) or pharmacological depletion of brain catecholamines or 5-HT (York and Maynert, 1978) attenuate the analgesic effect of morphine.

In addition, opiate receptors and enkephalins are found in locally high concentrations in the dorsal horn of spinal cord, in the region of termination of the small sensory fibers that transmit painful information from the periphery. Melzak and Wall (1965) put forward the important idea that gating mechanisms exist at the spinal cord level to modulate the transmission of painful stimul to supraspinal regions. It is now clear that opiates may induce analgesia directly at spinal cord level, as shown by Yaksh and Rudy (1977) who were able to elicit analgesia in the rat following direct application of morphine to spinal cord through a catheter inserted into the subarachnoid space. Jessell and Iversen (1977) proposed a possible substrate for the pain gating mechanism in spinal cord. They suggested that opiates (or naturally occurring enkephalins) may act on sensory nerve terminals in dorsal horn to suppress the release of the pain transmitter (possibly a peptide, substance P). The opiates are thus able to elicit analgesia by actions both at spinal cord and brainstem levels, and these sites appear to complement each other synergistically, so that application of morphine to both PAG and spinal cord simultaneously is far more effective in causing analgesia than stimulation of either site alone.

There remains the question of the role of opiates and enkephalins in the forebrain in relation to pain and anxiety. It has been reported that bilateral injection of morphine into the corticomedial amygdala in rats elevates pain thresholds, assessed by means of a modified "flinch-jump" test (Rodgers, 1977). Without objective tests of analgesia it is impossible to determine if the analgesia elicited by opiates at forebrain sites is qualitatively similar to that elicited at PAG or spinal cord sites. Manipulations of brain levels of 5-HT and catecholamines modify opiate-induced analgesia after amygdala injections, as they do for analgesia induced at more caudal sites.

A dynamic balance exists between pain and pleasure. It may be significant that some of the sites where electrical stimulation induces analgesia will also sustain self-stimulation. It may be that analgesia represents heightened pleasure and relief from anxiety. It is tempting to speculate that opiate receptors and enkephalins in the forebrain are involved in modifying the affective, rather than the sensory response to painful stimuli. This, however, is not a simple hypothesis to pursue in experimental animals. Objective, quantitative tests are needed to evaluate the sensory and affective responses to painful stimuli, and at present they are lacking.

FUNCTIONS OF THE ENDOGENOUS ENDORPHINS

Many experiments have confirmed that the endogenous opioids leu- and met-enkephalin and β-endorphin can also induce analgesia. Intraventricular injections of leu- or met-enkephalin or microinjections directly into the PAG induce analgesia, albeit short-lived, in the rat. Synthetic analogues of leu- and met-enkephalin, or β-endorphin, which are less rapidly degraded by metabolism in brain, are very effective in causing long-lasting analgesia after intracerebral administrations. These results suggest that the endorphins in brain may represent an endogenous mechanism for attenuating painful or distressing stimuli. It has been suggested that such a mechanism would be of great survival value to injured animals or to those in biologically threatening situations.

We think it likely that all mammals possess a set of powerful and endogenous centrifugal mechanisms of pain control within the brain stem. Lower animals may have little access to these systems except under the most dire circumstances, such as during strong appetitive, aggressive, or self-protective drive states, and especially during the goal-directed behaviours associated with these states. In man, however, it may be that there are better developed pathways of access (perhaps of telencephalic origin) to these brain stem systems. Thus our cognitive capacities to think, to believe, and to hope enable us, probably all of us under the appropriate conditions, to find and employ our pain inhibitory resources. The important challenge in the years to come for behavioural scientists involved in pain research will be to explore and ultimately bring under control those precise circumstances and techniques that will reliably enable people to make use of these resources when needed. (Liebeskind and Paul, 1977)

There are a number of predictions of such a hypothesis:

1. Acute stress should promote analgesia.
2. These effects should be naloxone reversible.
3. Acute stress or pain should result in the release of endogenous opioids.
4. Blockade of the effects of endogenous opioid peptides with naloxone should result in behavioral changes.

There is clear experimental support for *1–3* (see Rossier et al. 1977). The evidence for *4*, however, remains equivocal both in experimental animals and in man (Grevert and Goldstein, 1978). Intriguing results have been obtained by Herman and Panksepp (1978) and Panksepp et al. (1978), who found that separation of infant guinea pigs from their mother produced distress calling which was reversed by systemic morphine and enhanced by naloxone. The problem may be to find the appropriate baseline of stress-induced behavior with which to study endorphin mechanisms.

9. Drugs with Anti-Anxiety Properties: The Minor Tranquilizers

CLASSIFICATION AND NEUROPHARMACOLOGICAL PROPERTIES

The minor tranquilizers are used for treating neurotic as opposed to psychotic symptoms. Neuroses are varied but are generally characterized by anxiety and tension. A variety of pharmacological agents have been used over the years—alcohol being perhaps the most common.

BARBITURATES in small doses have been used extensively for their antianxiety effects. Their use for this purpose is not favored at present, because of the problems of tolerance and dependence and the possible hazards of accidental overdose or suicide associated with the regular prescribing of such drugs to anxious and depressed patients. Nevertheless, as we shall see, barbiturates share the specific attributes of the more potent minor tranquilizers, MEPROBAMATE and the more recently discovered BENZODIAZEPINES.

When meprobamate was first described, its behavioral effects appeared to be similar to but less dramatic than those of chlorpromazine. The term "minor tranquilizer" came into use to differentiate such drugs from the "major" neuroleptic tranquilizers. In their 1963 review, Cook and Kelleher stated that meprobamate and chlordiazepoxide (Librium) "are prescribed for mild behavior disorders." Now that the major and minor tranquilizers have been studied in a wide range of behavioral stiuations, it is apparent that the differences between them are qualitative rather than quantitative. It is for this reason that we prefer to use the terms "antipsychotics" or "neuroleptics" and "minor tranquilizers" in this book rather than the traditional major/minor tranquilizer terminology.

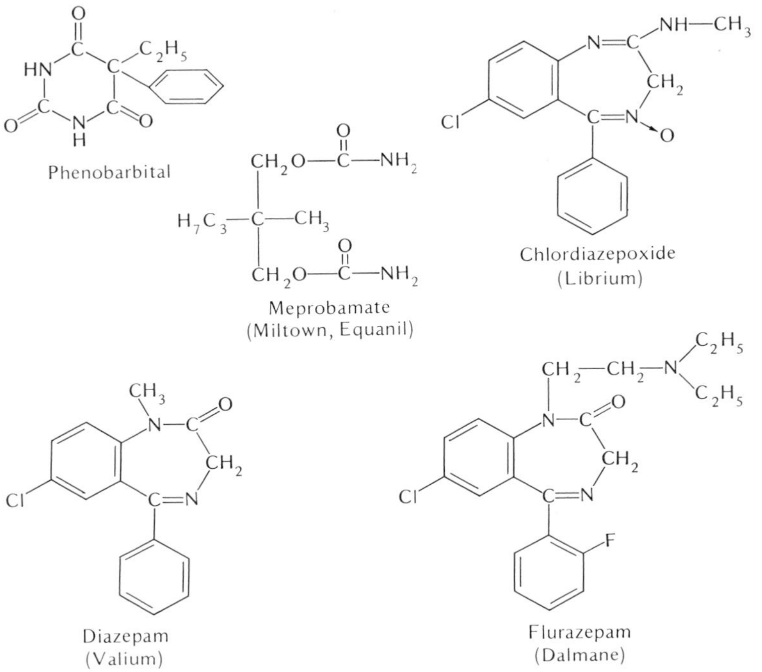

Fig 9–1   The minor tranquilizers.

The benzodiazepines, exemplified by CHLORDIAZEPOXIDE (LIBRIUM) and DIAZEPAM (VALIUM) (Fig. 9–1), have found great favor because they combine specific calming and antianxiety effects with very low toxicity, so that there is little danger of the accidental or intentional overdose that so frequently occurs with the barbiturates. A large number of related benzodiazepine derivatives have been synthesized and tested, and several of these compounds have proved clinically useful, for example, FLURAZEPAM (DALMANE) (Fig. 9–1) and NITRAZEPAM (MOGODON). The latter compounds are more powerful hypnotics than chlordiazepoxide or diazepam and are used to induce sleep rather than to tranquilize.

The precise neuropharmacological actions of the minor tranquilizers are still unclear. It has been suggested that the ability of barbiturates and benzodiazepines to reduce the rate of turnover of brain 5-HT may be critical in explaining their behavioral effects (Stein et al., 1973). However, more attention has focused recently on the alternative possibility that the primary action of barbiturates and benzodiazepines may be to enhance the effects of the inhibitory transmitter GABA in CNS. An important development has been the description of specific benzodiazepine receptors in brain by use of radioligand binding techniques, using radioactive DIAZEPAM or the more potent analogue FLUNITRAZEPAM as ligands. In this way it has been shown that brain tissue contains high affinity binding sites for benzodiazepines; these sites do not recognize GABA or other known transmitters, but benzodiazepines inhibit the binding of ^{3}H-diazepam in a rank order of potency similar to their behavioral effects in animals *in vivo* (Fig. 9-2). The benzodiazepine receptor, however, remains a mysterious entity. Although some interactions between GABA and GABA-mimetic drugs and benzodiazepines can be demonstrated biochemically, these are indirect in nature. Thus, benzodiazepines do not directly interact with GABA receptors, using ^{3}H-GABA as a ligand for such sites, and GABA-like drugs do not directly affect benzodiazepine sites. Furthermore, the distribution of GABA and benzodiazepine receptors in brain is not parallel; the highest densities of benzodiazepine sites occur in cerebral cortex, while the GABA receptors are most abundant in cerebellum. An intriguing possibility is that the brain may normally contain some hitherto unknown chemical which may act as the endogenous ligand for the benzodiazepine receptors—in the same way that the endorphins act on opiate receptors. Meanwhile, the suggestion that benzodiazepines and barbiturates may act by enhancing the effects of GABA remains a plausible working hypothesis.

BEHAVIORAL PHARMACOLOGY
Meprobamate

The tranquilizing effect of meprobamate was originally detected when it was observed that it could "tame" monkeys. In doses of 250-400 mg/kg, the drug makes normally truculent monkeys easy to handle, and they do not respond aggressively to man. Although tranquilized, the animals remain responsive to the environment; this taming effect contrasts with the equally potent effect of chlorpromazine in this respect, which leaves the animal withdrawn from the environment. Experimentally induced aggression is also attenuated by meprobamate. Surgical lesions of the septum result in marked aggression in certain species, such as the rat, and meprobamate in doses of 240 mg/kg abolishes this aggression. Chlorpromazine will also sedate such animals, but they become vicious if aroused. If isolated in individual cages for 2 to 3 weeks, mice show attack behavior when they are

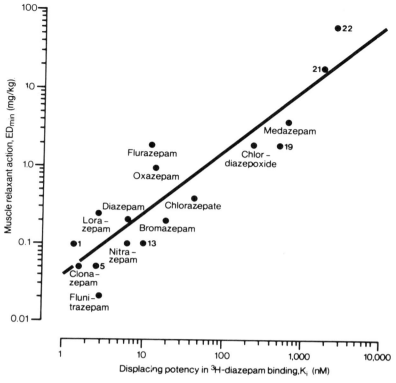

Fig 9–2   Correlation between *in vivo* pharmacological activity of a series of benzodiazepines [cat muscle relaxant test, minimum effective dose (ED_{min}) in mg/kg orally]
with potencies of same drugs in displacing ^{3}H-diazepam binding to membrane receptors in homogenates of rat cerebral cortex; potencies measured as K_i values in na-
nomolar; equivalent to drug concentration needed to half-saturate receptor sites *in
vitro*. Correlation coefficient $r = 0.905$ ($P<0.0001$). The numbers refer to the following Hoffmann La Roche test compounds: 1 = Ro 5–3027; 5 = Ro 5–3590; 13 = Ro
5–2904; 19 = Ro 5–3636; 21 = Ro 5–5807; 22 = Ro 5–4933. (From Möhler and
Okada, 1977.)

again placed in social situations, and meprobamate will reduce such fighting. Electric foot shock will induce fighting in pairs of rats, and meprobamate is effective in this situation as well.

   In studies of this kind, meprobamate has often been compared with chlorpromazine, barbiturates, and benzodiazepines. When such comparisons are
made, meprobamate is invariably found to be the least potent. There is

some controversy about the specificity of the behavioral effects induced by these various drug groups. All of the drugs are sedatives, but, at least in the case of meprobamate, the anxiety-reducing effects are correlated with the ability to induce muscle relaxation.

Barbiturates also induce muscle relaxation; unlike the barbiturates, meprobamate has an antianxiety effect at doses that do not impair motor or intellectual performance. Chlordiazepoxide is claimed to be unique in its selective taming effect, but there is no general agreement on this point.

Cook and Kelleher (1963) reviewed the effect of meprobamate on a wide range of behaviors controlled by schedules of positive reinforcement and found it to have generally rate-increasing effects. The low rates of responding engendered by a DRL schedule are markedly reversed by meprobamate. Inter-response times are shortened, and reinforcements are thus lost. Other low rates of responding, e.g. FI 5 min and VI 1.5 min schedules were also increased. Rates of bar pressing for intracranial stimulation (ICS) are also increased by meprobamate.

These rate-increasing effects of meprobamate can be demonstrated in monkeys, as Cook and Kelleher (1962) showed, using a multiple FI 10 min and FR 30 schedule with interposed time-outs. Responding was also markedly increased by 50–199 mg/kg meprobamate without any overall loss of discrimination. These authors observed that meprobamate and chlordiazepoxide, which was included in the study, increase behavioral output without overt signs of stimulation and, in this sense at least, can be distinguished from amphetamine, which produces similar behavioral effects on these parameters.

Finally we come to the behavioral effects of meprobamate that are unique to the minor tranquilizers—their ability to reinstate behavior suppressed by punishment. The Estes-Skinner procedure again yields equivocal results, but on the Geller procedure with immediate punishment, the effects are clear. Meprobamate (120–135 mg/kg) increases the number of shocks a rat will tolerate, even when intense shock levels are used (Geller and Siefter, 1960).

Barbiturates used as minor tranquilizers

We shall not dwell on this topic because barbiturates as tranquilizers have been largely supplanted by more specific drugs and also because the effects of barbiturates have been described at greater length in another section (Chapter 4).

In brief, the behavioral effects elicited by small doses of barbiturates are very similar to those of meprobamate. They do not share the powerful taming effect of chlordiazepoxide, and yet they show equally powerful releasing effect on behavior suppressed by immediate punishment. This has been demonstrated with the Geller-Seifter procedure (1960), an FR/FR punishment schedule (Fig. 9–3) (Kelleher and Morse, 1964), and a multiple VI/VI punishment schedule (Morse, 1964) (Fig. 3–9). The latter is especially interesting because the stimulation of reinforced and punished behavior was demonstrated simultaneously. Their powerful effect on punishment together with their general facilitutory effect may explain why the barbiturates were previously used so successfully as minor tranquilizers. Indeed, in many studies, barbiturates proved to have a more powerful punishment releasing effect than the benzodiazepines, which are promoted as specific antianxiety drugs. The dissociation of the effect of amphetamines from that of barbiturates on punishment suggests that brainstem arousal mechanisms do not underlie this effect. Nor do the depressant effects of barbiturates account for their effects in releasing behavior suppressed by punishment, since 10 mg/kg of pentobarbital, which reinstates punishment-suppressed behavior, also stimulates reinforced behavior. Morse and Kelleher (1964) with their multiple FR/FR punishment schedule (Fig. 9–3) have shown that pentobarbital will sustain higher rates of responding in the shock component than actual removal of the shock itself. Indeed, on the basis of this effect, which is believed to reflect the antianxiety effect of minor tranquilizers, it could be claimed that small doses of barbiturates are as effective as small doses of the benzodiazepines.

Benzodiazepines (chlordiazepoxide, diazepam, oxazepam)

The benzodiazepines have not been as intensively studied as meprobamate or the barbiturates. Nevertheless, there are reports of the effects of chlordiazepoxide on aggression, spontaneous motor activity, positively reinforced behavior, and immediate punishment that indicate that the benzodiazepines show the same profile of behavioral effects as meprobamate.

Furthermore, with respect to the specific behavioral effects that characterize minor tranquilizers, taming and reinstatement of punished responding, chlordiazepoxide is claimed to be more potent and selective than either meprobamate or the barbiturates.

Geller, Kulak, and Seifter (1962) first described the potent antipunishment effect of chlordiazepoxide. Their behavioral procedure was based on

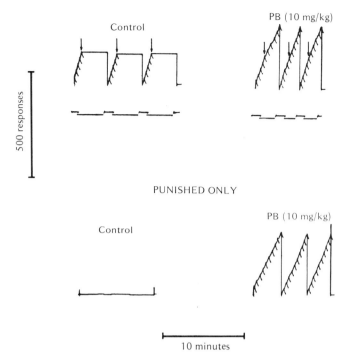

Fig. 9–3 Effects of pentobarbital (PB) on key pecking suppressed by punishment. Each frame shows a complete control session followed by a complete drug session. The drug was given intramuscularly 15 min before the beginning of the drug sessions. *Upper:* in nonpunishment components (event record displaced upward), a 30-response, fixed-ratio schedule of food presentation was in effect in the presence of an orange light. The termination of each nonpunishment component is indicated by a small arrow. In punishment components (event record displaced downward), a 30-response, fixed-ratio schedule was in effect in the presence of a white light; each of the first ten responses of each ratio produced a 35-msec electric shock of 6 mA, 60 cycles ac, delivered through gold wire electrodes implanted around the pubis bones of the bird. The termination of each punishment component is indicated by the resetting of the pen to the bottom of the record. *Lower:* the punishment procedure was in effect throughout each session in the presence of a white light. Note that under both procedures pentobarbital attenuates the suppression of responding by punishment. (Reproduced from Kelleher and Morse, 1964.)

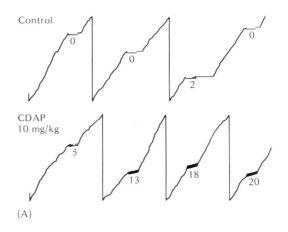

Control

CDAP
10 mg/kg

(A)

HIGH SHOCK

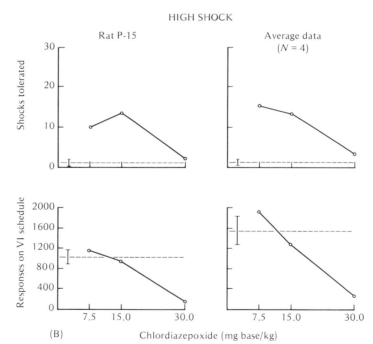

Rat P-15

Average data
(N = 4)

Shocks tolerated

Responses on VI schedule

(B)   Chlordiazepoxide (mg base/kg)

238

the work of Estes (1944). A rat was trained to lever press for a milk reward on a VI 2-min schedule. When the lever pressing had stabilized, a tone was introduced every 15 min for 3 min, and this signaled a change from VI to continuous reinforcement. After further stabilization, every response during the tone periods produced not only reinforcement but also a shock to the feet. In this conflict situation, the immediate punishment virtually abolished responding during the tone (Fig. 9–4A). Chlordiazepoxide in doses up to 15 mg/kg reinstated responding during the shock periods without changing the responding during the "safe" VI periods (Fig. 9–4B). This may be contrasted with earlier findings with meprobamate and pheno- and pentobarbital. These compounds also increase punished responding, but there are invariably associated changes in the rate of nonpunished VI responding.

The classical Geller-Seifter paradigm is a laborious one and does not lend itself to the testing of large numbers of rats or wide dose–response curves when anxiolytic compounds are studied. Pollard and Howard (1979) sought to modify the procedure to obtain reliable control responding during short test sessions. They described a 15-min alternating schedule, presenting 12 min of a food-reinforced VI 1-min schedule followed by 3 min of food VI plus punishment. The shock is presented on an escalating scale; each response during conflict increases the intensity of the shock by 0.05 mA. All known anxiolytic agents including meprobromate and pentobarbital result in a dose-dependent release of responding during conflict.

This selectivity of the effect of chlordiazepoxide in behavioral situations involving shock was also noted by Cook and Kelleher (1962) using a concurrent avoidance fixed-ratio procedure with the squirrel monkey. The monkey was shocked every 30 sec if it did not respond to the lever. Every response postponed the shock for 30 sec, but at the same time every 100th response

---

Fig. 9–4 (A) Cumulative response records showing the effects of chlordiazepoxide (CDAP) upon a punishment discrimination maintained with a high shock. The pen offsets indicate tone periods; upward pips of the pen represent responses that were simultaneously rewarded with food and punished with shock. The numbers of such responses appears under the shock period. (B) Effects of CDAP upon a punishment discrimination maintained with a high shock. *Left:* charts show the number of shocks tolerated during tones and intertrial VI rates for an individual rat under each drug condition. The drug points are averages for three injections. *Right:* chart show the same data averaged for four rats. Dotted lines, control values (individual data $N = 36$, grouped data $N = 144$). I---, two mean standard deviations. These means were computed by averaging the mean standard deviations of four rats, each based on 36 control observations. (Reproduced from Geller et al., 1962.)

(FR 100) resulted in delivery of a food pellet. Behavior on this schedule is maintained by two conditions of reinforcement; shock avoidance (negative reinforcement) and food reward (positive reinforcement). Chlordiazepoxide has a unique effect on performance, disrupting the avoidance component and increasing the shocks taken without affecting the overall response rate on the fixed-ratio schedule of reinforcement. By contrast, meprobamate and phenobarbital eliminate the high response rates characteristic of the fixed-ratio component but only increase shocks taken at doses that produce signs of neurotoxicity. Rats give the same response to benzodiazepines on continuous avoidance schedules, showing a significant increase in the number of shocks taken at doses well below the tranquilizing dose.

Zbinden and Randall (1967) pointed out that chlordiazepoxide and oxazepam (0.05 mg/kg) can abolish the ability of iproniazid to accentuate the stimulatory effect of tetrabenazine on continuous avoidance behavior. This is an important test because, although the benzodiazepines do have pronounced effects on Sidman and the discrete-trial avoidance tests, these effects are similar to the effects of the major tranquilizers. Heise and Boff (1962) proposed that the Sidman avoidance results can be used to differentiate these drug groups if a ratio measure of the minimum effective dose (MED), which causes escape failure, to the minimum dose, which just increases the number of shocks, is calculated. The benzodiazepines, with which increased shock tolerance is seen at a much lower dose than escape failure, give a high ratio, whereas for chlorpromazine these doses are very similar. This comparison also emphasizes the specificity of benzodiazepines in aversive situations because the other minor tranquilizers (meprobamate and barbiturates) closely resemble the neuroleptics when the MED ratio values are considered (Table 9–1).

There are some species difference in the responses to benzodiazepines. Cats, for example, show pronounced muscle relaxation at very low doses. Scheckel (1965) used delayed matching of colors as an anxiety-inducing behavioral procedure with rhesus monkeys. The matching delay is increased in an orderly way each time the animal correctly matches colors at the existing delay between cue sample and choices. Very small doses of chlordiazepoxide (0.3 mg/kg) significantly increase the delay that can be tolerated (Fig. 9–5).

The apparently specific behavioral effects of certain psychoactive drugs have been explained in terms of the so-called "baseline" phenomenon discussed in Chapter 3. Chlorpromazine, for example, which is thought to interact more strongly with behavior controlled by shock than by positive re-

Table 9–1. Minimum effective doses and dose range ratio in the continuous avoidance procedure

Compound	Rats				Squirrel monkeys			
	Route of admin.	Shock rate increase (MED, mg/kg)	Escape failure (MED, mg/kg)	Dose range ratio	Route of admin.	Shock rate increase (MED, mg/kg)	Escape failure (MED, mg/kg)	Dose range ratio
Chlordiazepoxide	p.o.	5.2	60.0	—	p.o.	1.0	29.0	29.0
	i.p.	4.2	18.0	3.8				
Diazepam	p.o.	20.0	120.0	5.2	p.o.	1.0	33.0	33.0
	i.p.	10.0	67.0	5.5	—			
Nitrazepam	i.p.	0.81	14.0	19.0				
Phenobarbital	s.c.	30.0	61.0	2.1	p.o.	80.0	80.0	1.2
Methyprylon	s.c.	25.0	41.0	1.8				
Hexobarbital	s.c.	42.0	75.0	1.7				
Emylcamate	i.p.	56.0	78.0	1.2				
Pentobarbital	s.c.	12.0	18.0	1.1				
Chlormezanone	i.p.	62.0	70.0	1.1	p.o.	10.0	20.0	1.5
Meprobamate	i.p.	103.0	105.0	1.0	p.o.	200.0	200.0	—
	p.o.	250.0	300.0	1.2				
Chlorpromazine	p.o.	5.4	8.2	1.5	p.o.	2.0	2.5	1.3
	s.c.	0.21	0.62	3.4				
	i.p.	1.1	2.1	1.8				
Trifluoperazine	s.c.	0.03	0.05	1.9				

(Reproduced from Zbinden and Randall, 1967.)

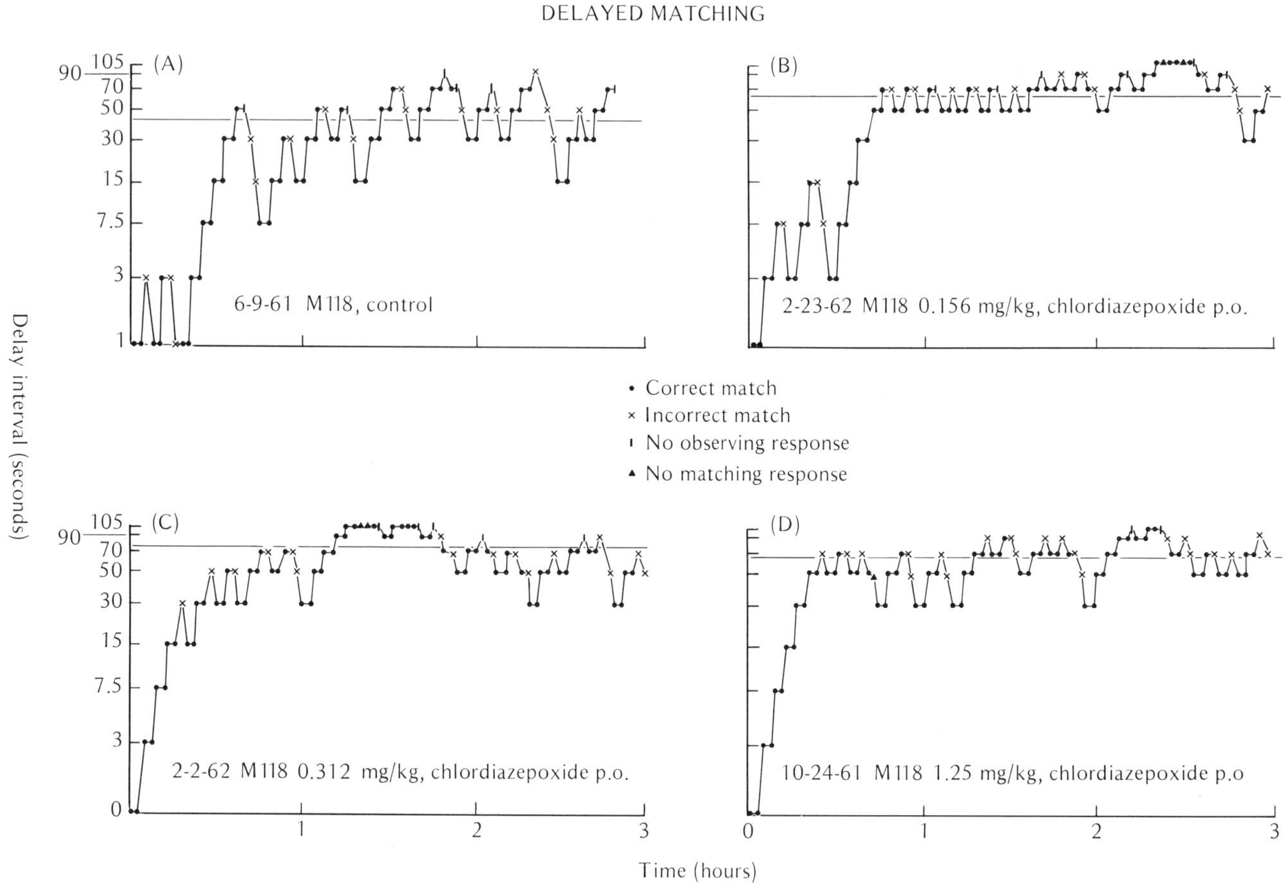

DELAYED MATCHING
(A)
(B)
(C)
(D)
105
90
70
50
30
15
7.5
3
1
0
6-9-61 M118, control
2-23-62 M118 0.156 mg/kg, chlordiazepoxide p.o.
2-2-62 M118 0.312 mg/kg, chlordiazepoxide p.o.
10-24-61 M118 1.25 mg/kg, chlordiazepoxide p.o
• Correct match
× Incorrect match
ı No observing response
▲ No matching response
Delay interval (seconds)
Time (hours)
1
2
3

inforcement, can be shown to affect the two behavioral baselines equally if they are adjusted to control the same rate of ongoing behavior.

Wuttke and Kelleher (1970) suggested that the same baseline phenomenon occurs with the benzodiazepines. In their procedure, one group of pigeons responded under a 5-min interval schedule of food presentation, with every 30th response producing an electric shock (punishment group). Another group responded under the same schedule of food presentation but without electric shock (nonpunishment group). Both groups of birds showed the usual fixed-interval pattern of responding, although the average rate of responding was much lower in the punishment group. The lowest rates at the start of the nonpunished FI, however, were comparable to the highest rates at the end of the punished FI. The benzodiazepines, chlordiazepoxide, diazepam, and nitrazepam, were compared, and all were found to markedly increase responding on the punishment schedule. But increased responding was also seen on the nonpunishment schedule. These rate-increasing effects were analyzed in relation to their respective baselines, and, when this was taken into account, the authors concluded that the effects of the benzodiazepines are to increase low rates of responding, whether they are associated with punishment or reinforcement.

One is reluctant to accept the conclusion that there is not a special relationship between the benzodiazepines and punishment, and more recent results argue against the conclusions described above. First, Wuttke and Kelleher used separate groups of animals for the punishment and nonpunishment schedules. McMillan (1973a), however, trained pigeons on a multiple FI 5-min/FI 5 min reinforcement schedule with red and green key lights. Subsequently, every response during one component of the multiple schedule produced an electric shock which suppressed response rates during that part of the schedule. Chlordiazepoxide, diazepam, and oxazepam all increased the low rates of punished and unpunished responding, but the rate-increasing effect was greater for punished responses. The conclusion is

---

Fig. 9–5 The effect of small doses of chlordiazepoxide on a rhesus monkey in a delayed matching procedure. Each panel shows performance during a 3-hr session. Each point shows the result of a single trial. When the animal made correct responses on two consecutive trials at one delay, the delay presented on the next trial automatically increased one step. Incorrect responses or the lack of an observing response decreased the delay one step. Horizontal lines in each panel are drawn through the average limit of delay. The ordinate (duration of delay interval) is logarithmically scaled. (Reproduced from Zbinden and Randall, 1967.)

that other variables can modify the rate-dependent effects of the benzodiazepines and perhaps these "other variables" relate specifically to drug interactions with punished behavior. This finding has been verified by a number of workers using different schedule parameters to generate rates of responding in the punished and nonpunished components of the multiple schedule. For example, Jeffrey and Barrett (1979) described a schedule on which pigeons peck, alternately, a green-lit key providing food on a fixed-interval schedule with every 30th response shocked, and a blue key where the response at the end of the interval producing food had to be preceded by a pause in responding of at least 10 sec. The overall rates of response output under these two conditions were identical; under both conditions the rate was low, and yet much greater increases of responding were observed in the punishment component.

Miczek (1973) approached this same problem in a rather different way. It has been suggested that a system of cholinergic neurons in the limbohypothalamic circuits may be involved in the suppression of behavior consequent to punishment or nonreinforcement. The ventromedial nucleus of the hypothalamus is thought to be the center of this system, and cholinomimetic and anticholinergic drugs, if injected locally into this nucleus, intensify or abolish such inhibition of behavior. Interestingly, benzodiazepines injected through the same cannula have been shown to act like cholinergic antagonists and reinstate punished responding. Miczek investigated the rate-dependent hypothesis of benzodiazepine action within this framework. He used three different methods of inhibiting responding: (a) immediate punishment of operant responses; (b) nonreinforcement in the presence of an S^Δ; and (c) immediate punishment of a consummatory response. Chlordiazepoxide attentuated the suppression responses induced by immediate punishment but not those associated with nonreinforcement. The conclusion is that "it appears unlikely that the rate-dependency principles can completely account for the observed punishment attenuating effect" of the benzodiazepines.

The benzodiazepines are also reported to exert a specific effect on a form of abnormal behavior induced by adventitious punishment that was originally described by Maier (1949). Rats were given an insoluble problem in a Lashley jumping stand and punished randomly as they performed. Fixated behavior, which took the form of position habits, i.e. jumping persistently to one side, emerged. When a soluble brightness discrimination task was subsequently presented, the rats continued to show the "fixated" position habit, although their jump latencies (longer to the closed panel) indicated that they in fact "knew" when they were jumping to the wrong stimulus. Chlordiazepoxide further reduced the latency to the positive stimulus in a similar study (Feldman, 1964). The experiment was repeated on monkeys trained to press an illuminated key (Feldman and Green, 1966). The spatial position of the lighted key and the reward were randomly programmed, and the animal was punished with tail shock; after 4 days of this procedure, the monkeys showed fixated responses under either stimulus or position control. They were then given a soluble problem, which was the reverse of their fixated response. As in the rat study, chlordiazepoxide lowered response latencies to the positive stimulus, although the monkeys persisted in the fixated response and were unable to learn the discrimination in more than 1000 trials.

On the basis of such evidence, one may conclude that the benzodiazepines are a unique group of antianxiety drugs. Their releasing effect on punished responding is no greater than that obtained with barbiturates. Unlike barbiturates, however, which show in addition a wide range of CNS stimulant and depressant activity, benzodiazepines have a narrower range of behavioral effects, particularly focused on responses to aversive stimuli.

It is important to try to define more precisely the basis of the antianxiety effect of the benzodiazepines. Like amphetamines, they stimulate low rates of responding, but unlike amphetamines, this stimulated behavior includes low rates of punished responding. However, barbiturates and benzodiazepines both share this general response releasing property. The methods of signal detection theory provide a means of distinguishing changes in performance due to loss of response control from loss of sensory control by the environment. It has been shown in two independent studies that chlordiazepoxide at doses which result in a marked released of punished responding are associated with changes in response bias rather than signal detectability (Tye et al., 1977b; Francis and Cooper, 1978). Thus it would appear that anxiolytic drugs do not modify the coding of anxiety-producing stimuli but the responses to those stimuli. It was emphasized when discussing hypnotic drugs, that with the study of a wider range of cognitive tasks and tests of anxiety, the hypnotic minor tranquilizers and the benzodiazepines appear strikingly similar in their behavioral effect. At present we have no neuropharmacological basis to differentiate them and such a comparison would be very useful. Having said this, the overriding fact remains that physical and behavioral dependence on barbiturates is marked whereas it seems to be less so with benzodiazepines. Furthermore, lacking depressant activity, the benzodiazepines do not cause death by overdose. Ultimately, this may prove to be the most significant difference between hypnotic tranquilizers and the benzodiazepines.

THE DEVELOPMENT OF ANIMAL MODELS OF DIRECT RELEVANCE TO HUMAN ANXIETY

Recently, attempts have been made to find tests of anxiety which do not involve the application of electric shocks to animals. Intuitively, procedures such as the Geller-Seifter bear little resemblance to conditions under which people develop anxiety states. Novel stimuli and unfamiliar situation are known to induce anxiety states in animals assessed with psychophysiological measures such as defecation or heart rate and behavioral measures such as reduced exploration. For example, if rats have been trained to respond for food in a Skinner box they will continue to press the lever for food even when a bowl of free food has been placed in the chamber. It is argued that they are anxious about the novel food supply and thus reluctant to take the free food. Chlordiazepoxide greatly enhances the intake of food from the novel food dispenser. A number of studies have claimed that minor tranquilizers have a direct effect on appetite, but it appears that this is not the case and that the increased food intake is a result of the drug's effect on the anxiety experienced in this behavioral situation. In support of this view it has been shown that rats familiar with sweet condensed milk, drink no more under the influence of diazepam, whereas naive animals do.

Of more relevance is a social interaction test described by File and Hyde (1978). Male rats placed in a situation in which neither has established a territory, engage in active social interaction. The most frequent behaviors include sniff, follow, walk over, crawl under, and groom. Aggressive behaviors are less commonly seen. The novelty of the situation can be varied by manipulating the familiarity of the rats with the testing chamber and the level of overhead illumination. Unfamiliar conditions with high illumination produce the lowest interaction scores and familiar dimly lit conditions the highest scores. It is reasoned that the former conditions are more anxiety-provoking. Minor tranquilizers of the depressant class (barbiturates and alcohol in low dosage) increase low levels of social interaction. Chronic treatment with chlordiazepoxide attenuates the reduction in social interaction normally seen in the high light/unfamiliar condition. With acute dosage, chlordiazepoxide produces behavioral sedation which masks the anxiolytic effect. With repeated dosage, however, the sedative effect shows tolerance; the anxiolytic effect is unmasked and remains. These results with acute and chronic benzodiazepine treatment agree with the findings of Margules and Stein (1968) on the Geller-Seifter test. The conditioned emotional response (see Chapter 1, Estes and Skinner, 1941) has traditionally also been used as an animal model of anxiety. The CER is reduced only by acute treatment with benzodiazepines. The behavioral contingencies involved in punishment and CER differ and a number of results suggest that the latter does not provide a reliable test for anxiolytic compounds.

The social interaction test has a number of advantages over the Geller-Seifter procedure. It involves neither deprivation nor application of unnatural aversive stimulus so that controls for possible drug effects on motivation or sensory thresholds are not needed. Of more practical advantage, the social interaction test does not require time-consuming operant conditioning before drug studies can be undertaken. Behavioral pharmacology has a need for simple, biologically relevant behavioral test systems of this kind.

Gray has worked extensively on a discrete trial procedure, termed partial reinforcement effect (PRE) as a behavioral model of anxiety. If rats are trained to run in a straight food-rewarded alley under conditions where only a proportion of trials are rewarded, they extinguish significantly more slowly than rats trained with reinforcement on every trial. To talk anthropomorphically, the uncertainty of reinforcement during training is thought to create an anxiety state which is revealed during the extinction test. PRE is the subject of much theoretical concern and the relationship between nonreward and punishment is currently a focus of interest (Gray, 1977). Neuropharmacological studies show that the dorsal NE bundle innervating hippocampus and cortex plays a central role in the coding of nonreward, which has been shown to be a special form of attentional behavior (Mason and Iversen, 1979). Gray found that performance on the PRE paradigm was correlated with a specific frequency of hippocampal electrical activity (the theta rhythm, 7.7 Hz, driven by the medial septal nuclei) and in experiments he determined the lowest threshold of septal stimulation required to induce 7.7 Hz hippocampal theta rhythm. Barbiturates, ethanol, and benzodiazepines were found to reverse the PRE, and in electrophysiological studies the same doses of these anxiolytic drugs raised the threshold for electrically induced theta rhythm. Fitting together these facts Gray has developed an elegant model of anxiety based on behavioral, electrophysiological, and more recently neuropharmacological findings.

10. Drugs with Antipsychotic or Psychotomimetic Properties

ANTIPSYCHOTIC DRUGS (NEUROLEPTICS)
Classification and neuropharmacological properties

Introduction
The discovery of drugs that are effective in the treatment of psychotic ill-nesses has been perhaps the most important psychopharmacological event of the second half of the 20th century. The dramatic impact that such drugs have had on the treatment of hitherto intractable psychotic illnesses has been responsible in large part for the rapid development of psychopharmacology as an academic discipline in the last 20 years. Before the advent of the antipsychotics, usually known as NEUROLEPTICS, virtually no successful forms of physical treatment of schizophrenia were known, and many mental hospitals had been largely custodial in function. Since the introduction and widespread use of neuroleptic drugs, the in-patient population of such hospitals has declined dramatically.

What are the neuroleptics?
The first widely used drug for the treatment of psychoses was the phenothiazine, CHLORPROMAZINE (Fig. 10–1), and it remains the most important drug in clinical use today. It is estimated that more than 50 million patients around the world have received treatment with this drug since its introduction into clinical practice in the 1950's. The striking success obtained with chlorpromazine led to investigations of several hundred related phenothiazines and other chemical congeners, many of which have proved useful in

SELECTED PHENOTHIAZINE DERIVATIVES

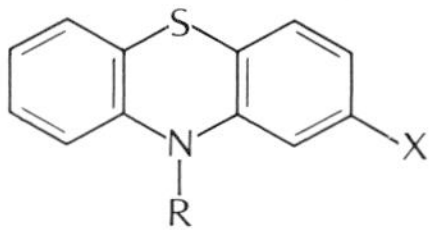

Nonproprietary name	X	R	Antipsychotic dose range* (mg/day)
Promethazine	H	$CH_2CH(CH_3)N(CH_3)_2$	—
Diethazine	H	$(CH_2)_2N(C_2H_5)_2$	—
Promazine	H	$(CH_2)_3N(CH_3)_2$	200-1000
Chlorpromazine	Cl	$(CH_2)_3N(CH_3)_2$	400-1600
Thioridazine	SCH_3	$(CH_2)_2$—(piperidine-N-CH_3) 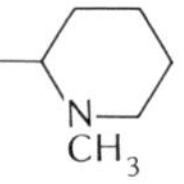	400-1600
Triflupromazine	CF_3	$(CH_2)_3N(CH_3)_2$	75-300
Prochlorperazine	Cl	$(CH_2)_3N$(piperazine)NCH_3 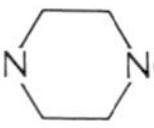	30-200
Trifluoperazine	CF_3	$(CH_2)_3N$(piperazine)NCH_3 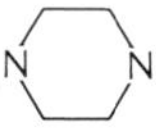	6-30
Perphenazine	Cl	$(CH_2)_3N$(piperazine)$N(CH_2)_2OH$ 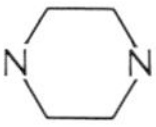	12-64
Fluphenazine	CF_3	$(CH_2)_3N$(piperazine)$N(CH_2)_2OH$ 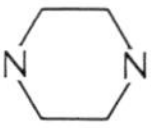	2-20

*For adult hospitalized or severely disturbed patients

Fig. 10–1. The phenothiazine neuroleptic drugs.

clinical practice (Fig. 10–1). Not only phenothiazines, but the related thioxanthenes (e.g. FLUPENTHIXOL) and the chemically unrelated butyrophenones (e.g. HALOPERIDOL) have proved to be neuroleptic (Fig. 10–2). This is not to say that *all* phenothiazines and *all* butyrophenones are neuroleptic; this is far from the case, since quite small structural changes in these compounds can cause a complete loss of neuroleptic activity. For example, all the active members of the phenothiazine series have a chlorine, fluorine, or thio- substituent in the 3-position of the phenothiazine ring; such substituents in any other position on the aromatic ring, for example, the adjacent,

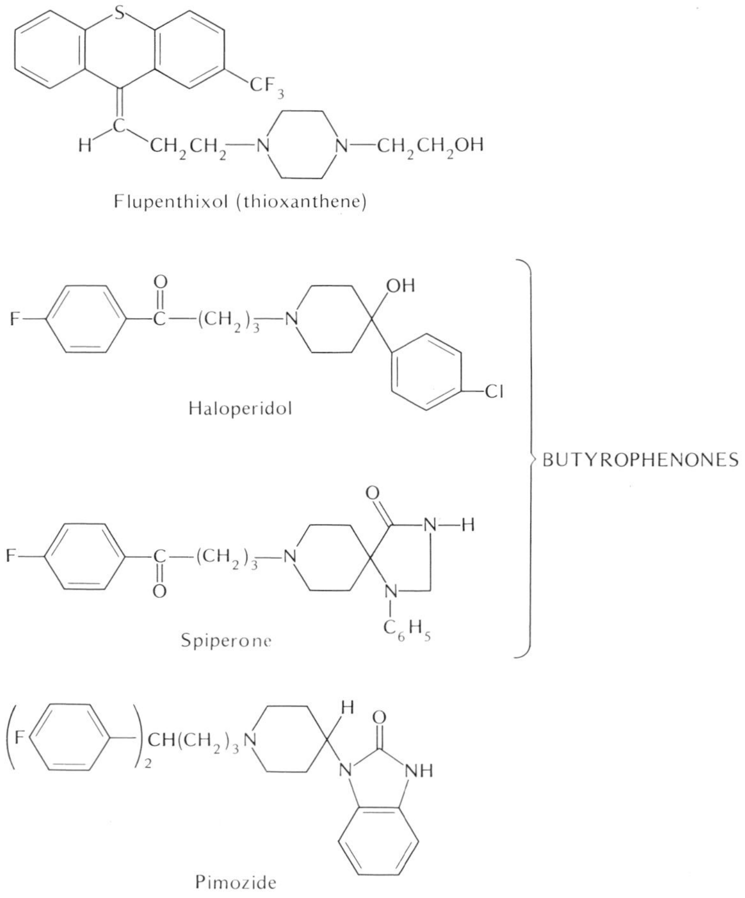

Flupenthixol (thioxanthene)

Haloperidol

BUTYROPHENONES

Spiperone

Pimozide

Fig. 10–2.   Non-phenothiazine neuroleptic drugs.

2-position, are quite ineffective, although these analogues have very similar physical and chemical properties. It is clear, therefore, that the neuroleptic activity of the active compounds in these series is a highly specific molecular property and is not simply related to lipid solubility or other physiochemical properties of the compounds, as is the case for local and general anesthetics, for example.

The neuroleptics are usually administered orally, are well absorbed, and penetrate readily into the CNS. Recently a new method of administering the more potent neuroleptics has been developed; this involves the intra-muscular injection of water-insoluble lipid ester derivatives of the drug in an oil base. Such an injection acts as a "depot" from which the parent drug is gradually released into the bloodstream, thus sustaining therapeutic lev-els of the active drug in the body for periods as long as a month after injec-tion. By using such depot injections, of fluphenazine or flupenthixol, out-patient treatment of schizophrenia has become a practical and rapidly grow-ing possibility.

Are the neuroleptics really antipsychotic?

There is a great deal of confusion about the specificity of action of pheno-thiazines and other neuroleptics in the treatment of schizophrenia and other psychoses. It has been popularly assumed that the drugs do not really alle-viate the symptoms of the psychotic illness, but merely sedate or "tranquil-ize" otherwise recalcitrant patients. Current evidence, however, argues overwhelmingly against this view and suggests that the drugs do have a very specific antipsychotic action not found in other classes of sedative drugs, such as the barbiturates or the anti-anxiety agents (see Snyder, 1974; Davis and Garver, 1978). In a large scale, carefully controlled multi-hospital series of collaborative studies sponsored by the Veterans Administration (VA) and the National Institute of Mental Health (NIMH) in the United States, the effects of phenothiazines and barbiturates were compared in several thou-sand patients (Klein and Davis, 1969). Phenothiazines were more effective in the treatment of schizophrenia than the placebo in a large majority of the studies, whereas phenobarbital was not better than the placebo in any of the studies. Extensive trials of such antianxiety drugs as chlordiazepoxide and diazepam also show these agents to be ineffective in the treatment of schizo-phrenia. The VA-NIMH studies also showed that the phenothiazines were most effective in treating those features of schizophrenia that were classified by Bleuler (1911) as the "fundamental" features of the disease, whereas other symptoms classified as "accessory" or unrelated specifically to the dis-ease responded somewhat less consistently to phenothiazines and symptoms unrelated to schizophrenia per se did not respond at all (Table 10-1). There is thus a large body of evidence to suggest that the neuroleptics exert a unique pharmacological action in schizophrenic patients. This does not nec-essarily mean that these drugs act directly on whatever hypothetical bio-chemical defect may be primarily responsible for the psychotic state, but it does mean that a better understanding of the site of action of the neurolep-tics could prove very valuable in understanding the neural mechanisms un-

Table 10–1. Differential response of schizophrenic symptoms to phenothiazones

Bleuler's classification	Response
Fundamental Symptoms	
Thought disorder	+ + +
Blunted affect	+ + +
Withdrawal	+ + +
Autistic behavior	+ + +
Accessory Symptoms	
Hallucinations	+ +
Paranoid ideation	+
Grandiosity	+
Hostility–Belligerence	0
Nonschizophrenic Symptoms	
Anxiety–Tension–Agitation	0
Guilt–Depression	0

(Adapted from Klein and Davis, 1969.)

derlying this psychosis. Nor is it true that neuroleptics "cure" schizophrenia; there is a high incidence of remission in patients successfully treated with these drugs who then stop taking them. Nevertheless, many schizophrenic patients can sustain a normal life out of hospital by continuous treatment with neuroleptics.

Neuropharmacological actions of neuroleptics in animals

Chlorpromazine and other neuroleptics have been the subject of numerous pharmacological studies. The neuroleptics display a wide range of different activities; chlorpromazine, for example, is a potent α-adrenoceptor antagonist in peripheral tissues, and has anticholinergic, antihistamine, and anti-5-HT activity. In addition, chlorpromazine and some other neuroleptics are quite potent local anesthetics, a property related to the high lipid solubility of these drugs which results in their becoming highly concentrated in the lipid-rich membranes of neurons and other cells. Only one property, however, appears to be shared by all neuroleptic drugs: their ability to antagonize DA receptors in CNS; this is the unifying hypothesis which may explain their unique psychopharmacological properties (see Snyder, 1974; Iversen, 1975; 1978a; Creese et al., 1978). The evidence for this hypothesis is as follows:

1. Biochemical studies show that chlorpromazine and all other neuroleptics

selectively accelerate the rate of release and turnover of DA in animal brain. This is revealed by an increased formation of the DA metabolite homovanillic acid, and an increased rate of conversion of labelled tyrosine to DA following administration of neuroleptic drugs. This increased DA turnover reflects an increased rate of firing of DA neurons as a reflex consequence of blockade of CNS receptors for DA, and direct neurophysiological recording from DA neurons in substantia nigra confirms such a response (Bunney and Aghajanian, 1974).

2. The neuroleptics antagonize the behavioral stimulant actions of amphetamine and apomorphine, drugs which act indirectly or directly to stimulate DA receptors in brain (see Chapter 4). This action of neuroleptics is highly correlated with their clinical effectiveness, and animal tests confirming this effect are widely used by drug companies in predicting new drugs with antischizophrenic potential (Janssen et al., 1965).

3. Biochemical studies of DA receptors in CNS add further support to the hypothesis, since neuroleptic drugs are the most potent inhibitors of the two *in vitro* models: one based on the finding that DA receptors in animal brain are coupled to adenylate cyclase activity (Iversen, 1975), the other based on radioligand binding studies (Creese et al., 1978). Thus, neuroleptics potently inhibit the stimulation of cyclic AMP formation elicited by DA in homogenates of DA-rich areas of brain, and compete for binding of radiolabelled drugs such as ^{3}H-haloperidol and ^{3}H-spiperone to DA receptors in such homogenates. The latter model in particular seems to have high predictive value, since the rank order of potency of neuroleptics in inhibiting ^{3}H-haloperidol binding correlates well with the clinical potencies of neuroleptics in treating schizophrenia (Fig. 10–3). Recent biochemical studies suggest that DA receptors reflected by the adenylate cyclase are of a different category (D1) from those reflected by butyrophenone binding studies (D2) (Kebabian and Calne, 1979) (see Table 2–6). It is not clear what the relative importance of blockade of D1 vs. D2 DA receptors may be in explaining the actions of neuroleptic drugs, since most existing drugs act on both types of DA receptor, albeit with varying potencies. The development of more selective antagonists with preferential actions on D1 or D2 receptors may lead to the emergence of novel neuroleptic agents with different pharmacological profiles from those of existing drugs.

The existing drugs also have a variety of other important neuropharmacological actions. Many are NE antagonists at α-adrenoceptors, although some drugs such as fluphenazine, flupenthixol, and haloperidol are relatively weak in this respect. Other secondary pharmacological actions include

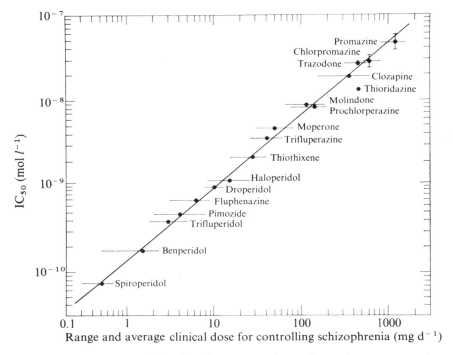

Fig. 10–3   Comparison of the clinical potencies of neuroleptic drugs, measured as average daily dose in treating schizophrenia with potencies of the same drugs in displacing ³H-haloperidol from dopamine receptor sites *in vitro* in calf caudate nucleus membranes (IC50 = drug concentration required to displace 50% of specific ³H-haloperidol binding). (From Seeman et al., 1976.)

antihistamine and anti-HT effects, although the significance or such actions to the overall profile of individual drugs remains unclear.

Behavioral actions of the neuroleptics

In the absence of any appropriate animal model of schizophrenia, the task in behavioral pharmacology is to discover some behavioral parameters that can be used to characterize and differentiate the highly specific antipsychotic drugs from other psychoactive agents. The phenothiazines and related drugs are depressants, but their antipsychotic property is not related to their depressant action. Large doses of barbiturates, despite their potent depressant action, have been found to be quite ineffective in relieving the fundamental symptoms of schizophrenia.

Phenothiazines

Chlorpromazine, the best studied example of this class of neuroleptic drugs, has the general effect of abolishing "behavioral tone" in almost any situation. For example, it reduces spontaneous locomotor activity and other forms of unconditioned behavior in a dose-dependent manner. An effect of chlorpromazine on conditioned behavior was described in an early account of its pharmacology by Courvoisier et al. (1953). A pole-climbing test for the rat was used. After moderate doses of chlorpromazine, rats no longer climbed a pole to avoid shock when a tone sounded; despite this, they still climbed the pole when the shock stimulus was presented. A similar dissociation between impaired avoidance and intact escape behavior after chlorpromazine was also noted by Verhave et al. (1959) in a wheel-turning task.

Chlorpromazine will also reduce behavior maintained by positive reinforcement, as opposed to suppression of responses to aversive stimuli. Food and water intake, sexual behavior, self-stimulation in limbic forebrain areas, and self-administration of such reinforcing drugs as cocaine and amphetamine by the monkey are all reduced by chlorpromazine. It has often been suggested that antipsychotics have a greater effect on behavior maintained by aversive reinforcers than by positive reinforcers, but this does not actually seem to be the case. Morse and Kelleher (1964) maintained squirrel monkeys on FI/FR shock-escape and FI/FR food-reinforcement. The behavioral baselines were indistinguishable and so were the dose-dependent decreases in both behaviors after chlorpromazine. Motivation variables, therefore, seem irrelevant in the characterization of antipsychotic drugs.

The depressant effects of neuroleptics are almost certainly due to blockade of DA receptors in the basal ganglia, which depresses the expression of motor responses. A number of behavioral correlates of DA receptor blockade have come to dominate the screening tests used to detect compounds of potential use as neuroleptics. Many of these tests involve the interaction of amphetamine with DA (e.g. stereotypy, rotational behavior), and have already been described in Chapter 4.

However, the beneficial effects of neuroleptics on the cardinal psychotic symptoms of schizophrenia are not solely due to their ability to block motor output. Behavioral pharmacology has not yet been successful in defining a specific action of neuroleptics which correlates with their antipsychotic effect but does not result from motor retardation.

In the classical behavioral pharmacology literature there are clues which may be worth pursuing in the search for behavioral tests predictive of the non-motor effects of neuroleptics. In addition to their depressant action, the other repeating theme has been that neuroleptics modify the control exerted by stimuli in the environment. A number of the clinically described effects of chlorpromazine—loss of initiative and reactivity, reduction of tension and compulsiveness—can be translated into terms of stimulus control manipulation. One might suppose that social behavior, which is precisely determined by a sequence of external stimuli, would be a sensitive index of antipsychotic activity. Silverman (1965) used such an index in the rat, for which more than forty elements of social behavior can be distinguished and measured. There was no evidence that chlorpromazine reduced all behavior by causing a general motor depression. Nor was there evidence of a general loss of responsiveness to the environment: exploration was unchanged. But the response tendencies induced by certain exteroceptive cues associated with other rats were markedly changed. Mating and aggression were reduced and escape behavior increased. If rats or mice are socially stimulated in crowded living quarters, they are killed more readily by amphetamine. Chlorpromazine antagonizes this effect and the stronger the social stimulation the greater the antagonism. The LD $_{50}$ of amphetamine in isolated mice is increased from 111 to 144 mg/kg, but, in mice housed in groups of three, the LD$_{50}$ for amphetamine rises from 15 to 121 mg/kg after chlorpromazine. Chlorpromazine appears to reduce the responsiveness of individual mice to the stimuli engendered by other mice. There may be a straightforward pharmacological explanation of this interesting effect. Sensory stimuli and amphetamine induce arousal, release of endogenous amines, and increased activity in amine-sensitive neuronal systems. The greater the induced activity, the greater effect the amine-blocking actions of chlorpromazine will be in restoring homeostasis in catecholamine synaptic mechanisms.

Some experiments with conditioned responses have also suggested that chlorpromazine reduces the ability of exteroceptive or interoceptive stimuli to signal that responses are relevant or irrelevant. If pigeons are trained in the presence of a red light to peck for food on an FR 50 schedule and, when the key color changes to blue, the first peck after 15 min is rewarded (FI 15 min), the control performance shows high rates of FR responding followed by the scalloped pattern typical of FI schedules. After 3 mg/kg of chlorpromazine, the difference in the pattern of responding to the two stimuli is reduced. High bursts of responding occurred early in the fixed intervals, for example. The pattern of responding under the influence of the drug was very similar to that observed when the discriminative stimuli were switched off during control sessions.

Some of the experiments of Maffii (1959) using the pole-climbing technique demonstrate that the dampening effect of phenothiazines on stimulus control depends on how important the stimulus is for controlling behavior, a weak discriminative stimulus being abolished more easily than a strong one. Well-trained rats climb the pole even before the conditioned stimulus is presented, and there are thus three discriminative stimuli in the test: (a) general environment of the box, (b) warning signal, and (c) shock. The effective doses of chlorpromazine for eliminating responses to these three stimuli are 1.75, 11.6, and 30.0 mg/kg. The shock is the strongest S^D and the most difficult to disrupt.

Dews and Morse (1961) suggested that antipsychotics "manipulate the relationship between the environment and the animal," and this hypothesis encompasses the results obtained with such drugs on unconditioned behavior, food-reinforced, shock-avoidance, and shock-escape responses.

It seems that the ability of the phenothiazines to modulate the control of external stimuli over behavior may be a better index of their therapeutic value in treating psychotic behavior than their sedative effects, although we do not have information on the effects of recently developed, specific DA-blocking antipsychotics on this test. Emley and Hutchinson (1972) studied the effects of chlorpromazine on Squirrel monkeys exposed to an adventitious shock procedure for inducing aggression (see p. 44). Shocks to the tail every 4 min induce aggression, which manifests itself as hose biting during the shock and somatomotor activity in anticipation of the shock, which results in lever pressing. Chlorpromazine decreases hose biting under these conditions but also increases the anticipatory motor behavior and lever pressing. Major tranquilizers are used in humans to relieve the disruptive emotional excesses induced by irritating environmental events. They could act by depressing such behavior, and the attenuation of hose biting suggests that they do. In addition, they could also enhance attentional or anticipatory behaviors necessary for reward and thereby reduce frustration. These results suggest that they do both, shifting an organism's response tendency from post-event irritability and aggression toward pre-event anticipation, a prerequisite for the acquisition and maintenance of rewarded performance.

Animals such as the pigeon in which behavior is stimulated by neuroleptics are useful in studies of the more subtle behavioral effects of such drugs. For example, their apparent failure to reinstate punished responding in the rat was questioned by Kelleher and Morse (1964) on the assumption that their sedative effect might mask attenuation of suppression. This hypothesis was shown to be incorrect when they tested pigeons on a FR 30/FR 30-punishment multiple schedule and found that, although 30 mg/kg of chlor-

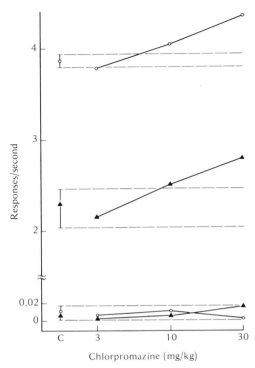

Fig. 10–4   Effects of chlorpromazine on rates of responding under the 30-response, fixed-ratio procedure in which nonpunishment and punishment components alternate. The points at the left of each record are means of control determinations; the solid vertical lines and dashed horizontal lines indicates the ranges of control observations. The ordinate has been broken to expand the scale at the lower values. The two curves above the break show the rates of responding for two pigeons in the nonpunishment component. Circles, pigeon, 234, which had a control rate of 3.9 responses/sec; triangles, pigeon 235, which had a control rate of only 2.3 responses/ sec. The two curves below the break show rates of responding on the punishment components for the same birds. Note that chlorpromazine produced graded increases in rates of responding in nonpunishment components but had no effect on responding in punishment components. (Reproduced from Kelleher and Morse, 1964.)

promazine increased FR 30 responding, there was still no reinstatement of behavior suppressed in the alternate punishment segments (Fig. 10–4). The pigeon has also proved a useful model for studying the effect of phenothiazines on exteroceptive discriminative control. For example, Cook and Kelleher (1962) found that phenothiazines increase responses to a stimulus key that provides information about the availability of reinforcement. Pigeons were trained to peck each of two keys, one food-producing, one stimulus-producing. Positive and negative periods alternated. During these times, both keys were white but pecking the food key during the positive periods produced reinforcement on a 100 VR schedule; during the negative period no reinforcement was produced. Pecking of the stimulus key was programmed so that, during the food period, 20 pecks changed both keys to green and, during the negative period, to red. This behavior to the stimulus key produced information about the availability of food. Under normal conditions, responses are distributed between the two keys. Chlorpromazine increases stimulus key responding and decreases responding for food, so that the discrimination between positive and negative periods was sharpened. Similar results were produced by related phenothiazines (Table 10–2).

The ability to discriminate reinforcing stimuli plays an important part in normal behavior and the limbic DA system has been implicated in such reward mechanisms. Typically neuroleptics depress all behavior patterns associated with obtaining rewards. Wise et al. (1978) used ingenious behavioral methods to try to tease apart effects of the drugs on motor performance and on the ability to respond to the value of stimuli in the environment.

Neuroleptics reduce reinforced responses, but do they have this effect simply because they make responding difficult or because they make the reward less motivating? In a learned lever pressing situation and in a discrete trial runway apparatus, Wise et al. studied the effect on responding of
1. successive extinction sessions (removal of reward)
2. successive treatments with the DA receptor blocking drug pimozide, always in the test situation

Table 10–2. Results with phenothiazine-related compounds

	Increases stimulus key responding	Decreases food-producing responses
Chlorpromazine	Yes	Yes
Prochlorperazine	Yes	Yes
Trifluoperazine	No—decreases	Yes
Promazine	Yes	No effect
Triflupromazine	Yes	Yes

3. successive treatments with pimozide in the home cage and finally in the test situation.

1 and 2 produced a progressive decline in responding but 3 only minimal disruption. The latter result suggests that pimozide blocks conditioned behavior not because the animal's motor capacity is impaired but because the normal association between the test situation and reward has been repeatedly blocked. Under condition 3 DA receptor blockade had been present but not in the context of the rewarded test situation, and hence the reward had not lost its ability to maintain responding.

Before continuing to discuss the specific features of some of the more recently developed DA antagonist drugs, some general statement can be made about the action of neuroleptics. Recent work reinforces the view that these drugs do not act solely by depressing motor performance, although they certainly have such an action. A number of findings suggest that they also modify the control exerted over behavior by discriminative stimuli, possibly most important, by reinforcing stimuli. An interaction with DA receptors would appear to be involved in all these effects, although it is premature to assume an exclusive interaction with DA. However, the exciting possibility is raised that different classes of DA receptors in different forebrain sites may account for these dissociable effects of neuroleptics on motor output and the coding of meaningful stimuli.

Butyrophenones

These antipsychotic drugs were introduced in the mid 1960's and have not been investigated as extensively as the phenothiazines. However, the behavioral properties of these drugs appear very similar to those of the phenothiazines. The butyrophenones are generally more specifically active as DA antagonists than chlorpromazine, and this may explain their potency in blocking such drug effects as amphetamine-induced stereotypy, which are thought to involve DA receptors primarily. Hanson et al. (1966) compared the relative potency of a series of depressant drugs on Sidman avoidance in the Squirrel monkey. Haloperidol was found to be 6.74 times as potent as chlorpromazine. It is interesting that the butyrophenones stimulate spontaneous motor behavior at very low doses, whereas the action of the phenothiazines is purely depressant. It is possible that dissociation of these two groups of antipsychotics will not be evident from behavioral studies but that it may be more readily accomplished in terms of their neuropharmacological action.

Behavioral profiles of different classes of neuroleptics

It is not easy to characterize the effects of neuroleptic drugs on normal behavior. They are basically depressant, but there is good reason to believe
that this behavioral effect may be secondary to some more subtle modulation of behavioral control. This is more than an academic problem for drug
companies in search of more effective and specific antipsychotic drugs. A
specific battery of animal tests for predicting antipsychotic drugs would be
of immense practical importance, and various screening procedures, of
course, already exist. Antipsychotic drugs strongly antagonize amphetamine-induced stereotypy, and this fact has provided a useful screening test
for evaluating new drugs. Janssen et al. (1965) described in detail the use of
behavioral tests in animals to predict neuroleptic activity. The tests themselves are simple: (a) Drug-induced *catalepsy* and ptosis; (b) antagonism of
amphetamine-induced stereotypy; (c) drug effect on shock avoidance in
jumping box; (d) antagonism of apomorphine-induced stereotypy; (e) drug
alterations of food intake; (f) open-field activity (rearing or ambulation); (g)
drug effects on mortality caused by E and NE injections; (h) antagonism of
tryptamine-induced limb convulsions; and (i) resistance to rotational trauma.
Forty antipsychotic drugs, principally of the phenothiazine and butyrophenone classes, were tested, and an ED_{50} (i.e. the dose of drug producing one-
half the maximal response or a specified response in 50% of animals) was
obtained for each test. These values were used to plot "activity spectra," and
it was found that the two classes of drug produced clearly distinguishable
spectra as illustrated in the mean patterns for all phenothiazines and all
butyrophenones (Fig. 10–5).

Neuropharmacological animal model systems have also proved useful for
quantifying neuroleptic actions. One unifying hypothesis of the behavioral
effects produced by neuroleptic drugs is that they act by blocking DA receptors in the CNS. A recent useful biochemical model for assessing such antagonist actions has come from the finding that neuroleptic drugs block the
stimulating effects of DA on cyclic AMP production in homogenates of rat
brain striatum or rat mesolimbic nuclei. It has been shown for a series of
neuroleptics that they differ over a 500-fold range in their ability to inhibit
the striatal dopamine-sensitive adenylate cyclase.

Clozapine and thioridazine: atypical neuroleptics

Clozapine and thioridazine are interesting neuroleptic drugs with moderate
DA receptor blocking potencies combined with relatively high potencies as

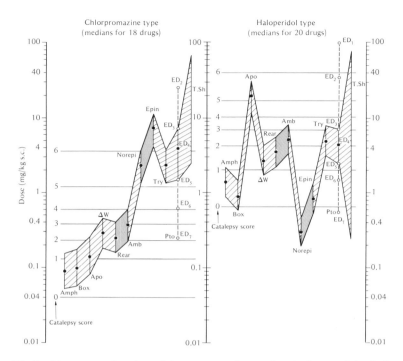

Fig. 10–5   Mean neuroleptic activity spectra of neuroleptic drugs of the haloperi-
dol-type (*right*) and the chlorpromazine-type (*left*)

Amph: ED_{50} amphetamine test   Amb: ED_{50} ambulation, open-field test
Box: ED_{50} jumping box test   Norepi: ED_{50} norepinephrine test
Apo: ED_{50} apomorphine test   Epin: ED_{50} epinephrine test
ΔW: ED_{50} ΔW-test, food intake   Try: ED_{50} tryptamine test
Rear: ED_{50} rearing, open-field
                  test

The confidence limits ($P = 0.05$) of each ED_{50} are represented by a vertical line:

Pto: ED_x-values, palpebral ptosis test: the lowest open circle represents ED_7 the
    next circle ED_6 then ED_5 then (black circle) ED_4 then ED_3 ED_2 and ED_1

T.Sh.: the vertical line represents the estimated active dose range (lowest active to
    highest active dose), rotational traumatic shock test.

Catalepsy score: ED_x (ED_0 to ED_6), catalepsy test. The position of each ED_x is represented by a horizontal line crossing the entire spectrum.

(Reproduced from Janssen et al., 1965).

antimuscarinic drugs. Unlike most neuroleptics they do *not* block ampheta-mine-induced stereotypy or rotational behavior, nor do they induce cata-lepsy except at very high doses. It has been proposed that their ability to block both DA and ACh receptors cancels out their effects in structures where DA and ACh are in reciprocal balance. This is the case in the stria-tum, the crucial structure for the expression of amphetamine-induced ster-eotypy, and accounts for their failure to block this behavior. Such a DA/ACh interaction is thought to be functionally less important in limbic areas. Ac-cordingly clozapine and thioridazine are able to block amphetamine-in-duced arousal mediated by the limbic DA system. However, the interesting point about these drugs is that they are clinically effective antipsychotics despite their failure to block striatal DA functions. More important is the fact that, unlike most neuroleptic drugs, they have little tendency to pro-duce Parkinson's disease-like extrapyramidal side effects in man, presum-ably because their built-in anticholinergic properties do not lead to any im-balance in the DA/ACh interactions in striatum. Efforts continue to determine whether these drugs have other unique properties. Clozapine and thioridazine, like typical neuroleptics, are active on avoidance tasks (Stille et al., 1971). On the other hand, clozapine has been reported to in-crease responding on a DRL schedule for juice reward, whereas chlor-promazine and thioridazine depress responding over a wide dose range (Canon, 1979).

Tardive dyskinesia

Prolonged treatment of schizophrenic patients with neuroleptics results in the emergence of a number of bizarre and uncontrollable movements in a substantial percentage of patients (estimates vary from 25–75%). These ab-normal movements most commonly affect the oral-buccal musculature, but may extend to the neck and hands. The term TARDIVE DYSKINESIA (TD) was introduced in the 1960's to describe this syndrome. The condition is to be distinguished from the parkinsonian-like state frequently seen in the initial stages of treatment with neuroleptics but which disappears with continuing treatment, to be followed later in some patients by TD. It is thought that blockade of DA transmission accounts for the initial parkinsonism and that sustained blockade of transmission results ultimately in some form of DA receptor supersensitivity, and thus paradoxically TD may represent the signs of dopaminergic overactivity in striatum, giving rise to the increased output of abnormal motor behavior. TD can be treated by increasing the dose of the neuroleptic; the rationale being that this is necessary to dampen the supersensitive DA receptors. Abnormal DA function unbalances the DA/ACh interaction in striatum, and consequently cholinergic medication has also been used in the treatment of TD. There is a pressing need for more satisfactory pharmacological management of this condition and it is hoped that a better understanding of the neuropharmacological connections of the basal ganglia may lead to the development of new drugs.

Efforts have been made to develop an animal model for TD. Monkeys treated for many months with high doses of haloperidol develop abnormal movements, strikingly similar to those seen in patients. Neuroleptics are now often given to schizophrenic patients in the form of intramuscular depot injections, designed for slow, sustained release of the drug. Rats exposed to an equivalent depot injection treatment with the phenothiazine fluphena-zine, develop abnormal movements of the mouth, jaw muscles, and front paws (Iversen et al., 1980). Clow et al. (1979) have described a method for chronically treating rats with the phenothiazine, trifluoperazine, adminis-tered in the drinking water. These animals eventually also give evidence of abnormal movements, and the method is a promising one for biochemical studies of long-term adaptive changes in DA mechanisms during chronic exposure to neuroleptics. The results indicate that the predicted increases in DA receptor numbers and sensitivity do occur on this drug regime.

HALLUCINOGENIC DRUGS AND CANNABIS
Classification and neuropharmacological properties

This is a remarkably diverse collection of drugs, and it is not easy to define the term "hallucinogenic." Perhaps the term "phantasticant" would give a more encompassing description of these agents, which share a common ac-tion in man in leading to a change in consciousness involving a change in reality, often associated with hallucinations. As Ray (1972) puts it, "The phantasticants . . . replace the present world with an alternative—one that is equally real but different. Both the drug-induced and the nondrug world can be attended to at the same time, and there is memory for the drug-induced reality after the drug effect diminishes." We have chosen to include marijuana and the tetrahydrocannabinols in this section, although these drugs do not fit clearly into the group.

Considering the popular attention the hallucinogens have received and the considerable social impact their widespread use has had, we remain remarkably ignorant of the scientific basis for the action of any of these drugs.

d-Lysergic acid diethylamide (LSD) and indolamine hallucinogens

The striking hallucinogenic properties of LSD have been known since 1938 when the Swiss chemist Hoffman synthesized this substance from naturally occurring lysergic acid, an alkaloid extracted from the ergot fungus that affects rye and other grains. In man, the d-isomer of LSD remains the most potent hallucinogenic substance known—100 to 500 μg alter sensory perception and the sense of reality greatly, with prominent visual hallucinations. The mode of action of LSD is still unknown, but it is likely that it acts on 5-HT transmitter mechanisms in the brain. The LSD molecule contains an indole nucleus, as does 5-HT (see Fig. 10–6). Gaddum and his colleagues found that LSD was a potent antagonist of the action of 5-HT on intestinal smooth muscle, and it was originally thought that the CNS activity of LSD might be related to an antagonist effect on 5-HT receptors in the CNS. The major argument against such a proposal stems from the finding that a related substance, the bromo derivative (Fig. 10–6) of LSD, is effective as a 5-HT antagonist in peripheral test systems, but is not hallucinogenic. Bromo-LSD penetrates the blood–brain barrier, so its lack of CNS action cannot be attributed to nonpenetration into the brain. Neurophysiological studies have shown that LSD may actually mimic the effects of 5-HT at certain synapses in the brain. Aghajanian et al. (1970) found that LSD, like 5-HT, stimulates the firing of certain brainstem neurons that receive an input from the 5-HT-containing cells in the raphe nuclei. On the other hand, also like 5-HT, LSD inhibits the rate of firing of the raphe 5-HT neurons themselves. These effects could be elicited by the administration of very small doses of LSD (10 μg/kg) systemically, or by direct iontophoretic application of exceedingly small amounts of LSD onto the neurons in the brainstem. Biochemical evidence also supports the view that LSD acts as an agonist, since it slows the rate of turnover of 5-HT in rat brain, a change consistent with the "receptor feedback" concept described in Chapter 2, by which agonist drugs are expected to slow turnover and antagonists to accelerate turnover of the CNS transmitters with whose receptors they interact.

Radioligand binding studies with ^{3}H-d-LSD have revealed the presence of high-affinity binding sites in various regions of brain (Bennett and Snyder, 1975). These sites show properties consistent with an interaction of LSD with 5-HT receptors, since 5-HT and 5-HT antagonists potently inhibit LSD

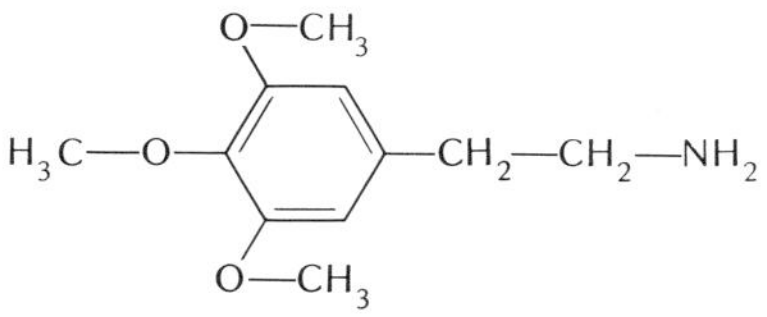

Fig. 10–6   Hallucinogenic drugs.

The structures shown include:

Mescaline

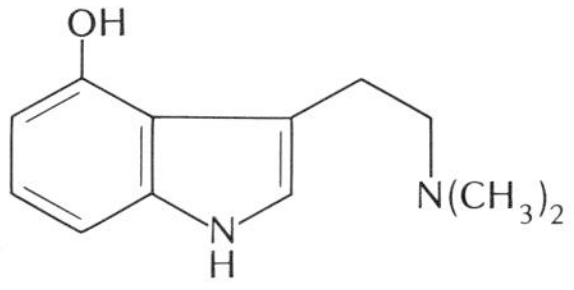

Psilocyin

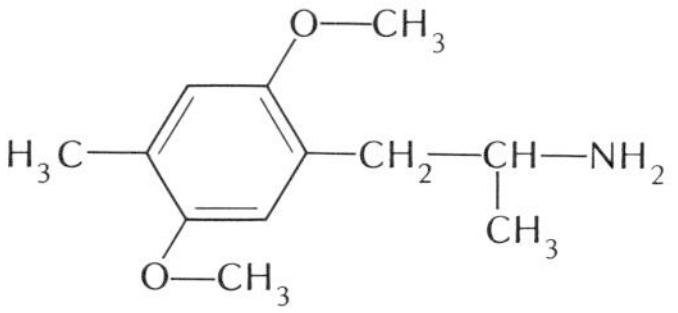

DOM (STP)
(2-amino-1-[2′,5′-dimethoxy-4′-methyl]-
phenylpropane)

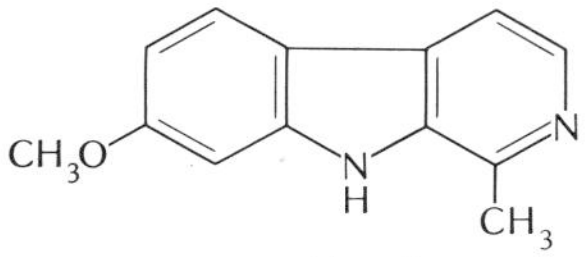

Harmine

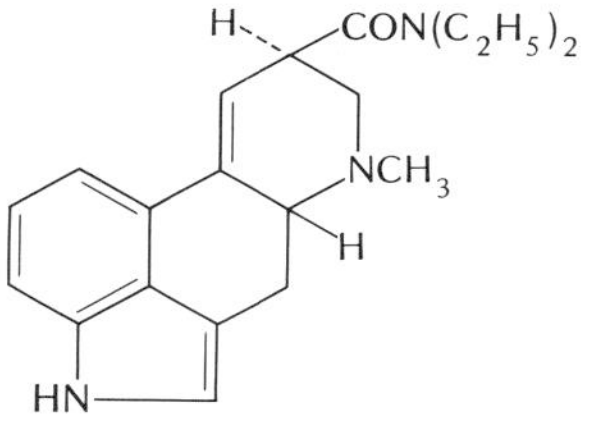

**d-Lysergic acid
diethylamide (LSD)**

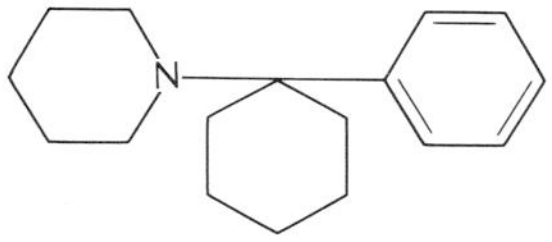

**Phencyclidine
(Sernyl)**

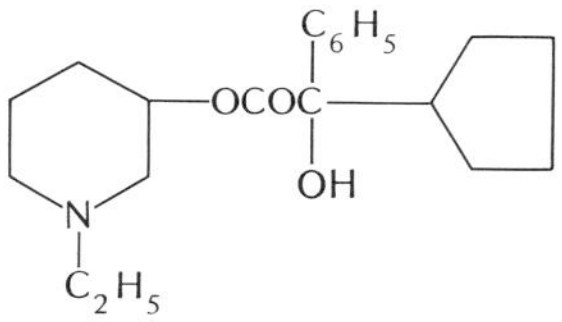

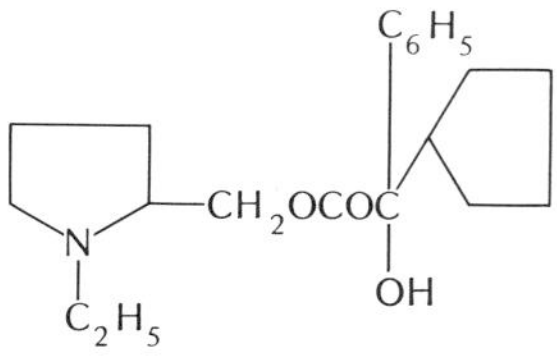

Piperidyl glycolate esters
(Ditran is a mixture of these
two compounds)

binding. Recently Peroutka and Snyder (1979) suggested that LSD may bind with high affinity to both categories of 5-HT receptors (5-HT$_1$ and 5-HT$_2$) whereas conventional 5-HT antagonist drugs bind preferentially to only the 5-HT$_2$ category. In addition, LSD has been shown to have moderate affinity for DA receptors in CNS, where it has the properties of a partial agonist, eliciting dopamimetic effects at low doses and DA antagonist properties at higher doses. These effects, however, require doses of LSD that are much higher than those needed to cause the hallucinogenic actions, and are thus unlikely to be of primary importance.

Apart from LSD, there are a number of other indolamine hallucinogens, including N-dimethyltryptamine (about 250 times less potent than LSD in man) and psilocyin. The latter is derived as the active material from psilocybin, the phosphorylated precursor present in the sacred mushrooms of Central America, which are about one-hundred times less potent than LSD. Another alkaloid, harmine, and related substances also have hallucinogenic properties (Fig. 10–6).

Tolerance to LSD develops rapidly in man, and repeated daily doses become completely ineffective after 3 to 4 days. A phenomenon known as cross-tolerance develops between LSD, psilocyin, and mescaline—meaning that after tolerance has developed to one of these drugs the others are also tolerated. The existence of cross-tolerance between several different hallucinogenic drugs is strong pharmacological evidence that they share some common mechanism of action.

Mescaline and other methoxylated phenylethylamines

The hallucinogenic properties of mescaline are well known, although the compound is, in fact, one of the least potent of the hallucinogens, requiring a dose of some 350 mg in man—or more than one thousand times the amount for LSD.

Mescaline was derived initially from the dried cactus or "peyote" used by the Aztecs and later by North American Indians in religious rites. Mescaline and many other related hallucinogenic derivatives of phenylethylamine have since been synthesized. Many of these synthetic compounds are related to amphetamine, which itself can cause hallucinations when consumed in large doses by addicts, although the amphetamine-induced hallucinations are predominantly tactile and auditory, rather than visual (see Chapter 4). Some of these compounds are listed in Table 10–3. The substances DOET and DOM are particularly interesting. These compounds are far more po-

Table 10–3. Mescaline and related methoxylated phenylethylamines

Compound	Hallucinogenic potency in man*
Mescaline (3,4,5-trimethoxyphenylethylamine)	1
3,4,5-TMA (trimethoxyamphetamine)	2.2
2,4,6-TMA	13
2,4,5-TMA	17
2,3,6-TMA	10
2,3,5-TMA	4
2,5-DMA (dimethoxyamphetamine)	8
2,4-DMA	5
DOM (2,5-dimethoxy-4-methyl amphetamine)	50–100
DOET (2,5-dimethoxy-4-ethyl amphetamine)	100
2,4-5-MMDA (2-methoxy, 4–5-methylene dioxyamphetamine)	12
2,3-4-MMDA	10
2,3-4-MMDA	3

(Data from Snyder et al., 1970.)
*Potency is defined in mescaline units to indicate how many times more potent than mescaline the above compounds are in man; the average hallucinogenic dose of mescaline is 350 mg.

tent than mescaline, and although they seem to produce the "insight" or increased self-awareness characteristic of the LSD syndrome, they are far less effective than other hallucinogenic drugs in causing visual hallucinations. Mescaline and other hallucinogenic phenylethylamine derivatives bear an obvious structural resemblance to the catecholamine transmitters, but there is no pharmacological evidence that their CNS actions are related to an effect on adrenergic mechanisms. Since cross-tolerance develops between mescaline and LSD, a common mode of action, perhaps on the indolamine systems, seems more likely.

Other hallucinogens
Many substances that are unrelated to the indolamines or phenethylamines have been found to be hallucinogenic. Such an action is commonly seen with the more potent CNS anticholinergic drugs that block muscarinic ACh receptors: these include a series of piperidyl glycolate esters such as DI-TRAN, SCOPOLAMINE (Fig. 2–13), and QUINUCLIDINYL BENZILATE (QNB), although not all anticholinergic drugs are hallucinogenic. The drug PHEN-CYCLIDINE (Fig. 10–6) was developed for use as an anesthetic, but also produces disorganization of thought and loss of contact with reality. The

mechanism of action is unknown, although it has come to prominence as a major drug of abuse in the United States in recent years.

Marijuana and the synthetic tetrahydrocannabinols

The dried leaves and flowers of the hemp plant, *Cannabis sativa*, are known as marijuana. The more potent hashish is a resin derived from *Cannabis* flowers, which contain a high concentration of the psychoactive ingredients. These ingredients have been chemically identified, and the principal active material is Δ^9-tetrahydrocannabinol (Fig. 10–7). Very little is known of the mode of action of this and related *Cannabis* derivatives on the CNS. Δ^9-Tetrahydrocannabinol apparently is metabolized and excreted only slowly in man, with as much as one-half of an injected dose of the radioactively labelled drug remaining in the body two days after administration. There is also some evidence that chronic drug use may induce liver hydroxylating enzymes that can convert tetrahydrocannabinol to a psychopharmacologically active hydroxylated derivative.

Behavioral pharmacology

Animal behavior studies of the hallucinogens are exceptionally difficult to interpret because of the intensely subjective nature of the effects of these

Fig. 10–7 *Cannabis sativa* derivatives.

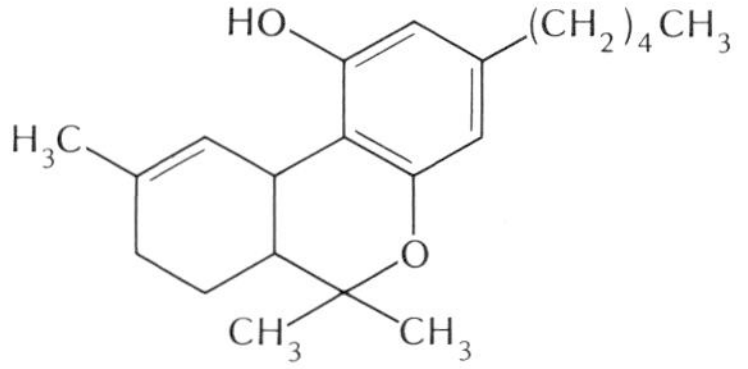

Δ^9-Trans-tetrahydrocannabinol

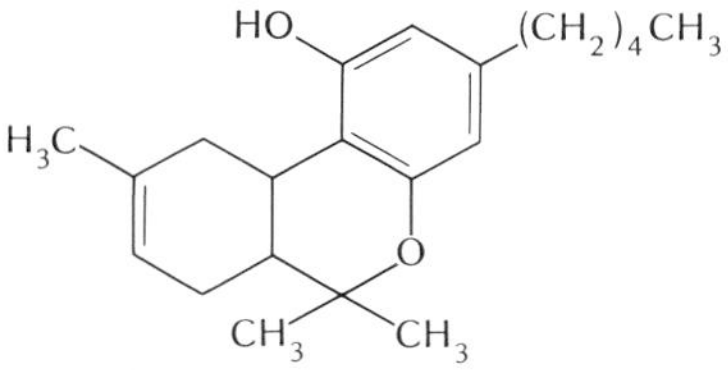

Δ^8-Trans-tetrahydrocannabinol

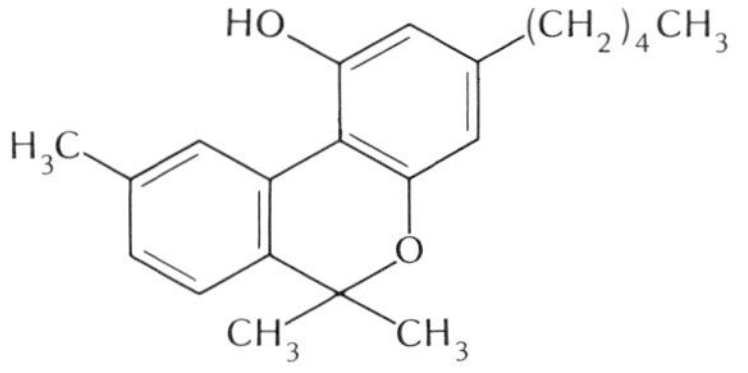

Cannabinol

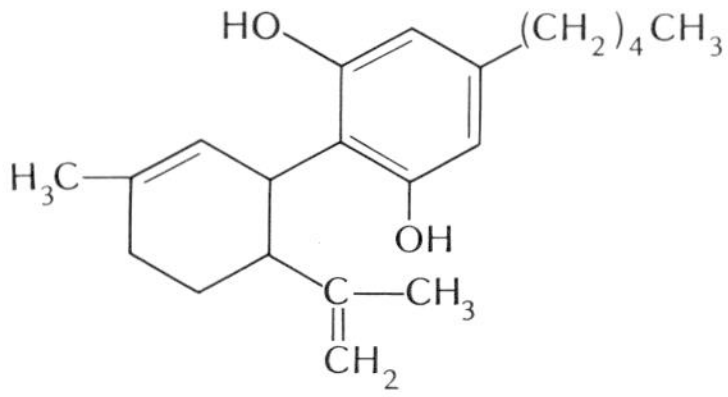

Cannabidiol

substances. Although animals may indeed be subject to the visual and auditory hallucinations and bizarre perceptual changes caused by such drugs in man, this is clearly not objectively measurable. The best we can do is to attempt to determine whether such drugs induce a characteristic pattern of changes in behavior that can be observed and measured—although this must always be a poor shadow of the information that can be derived from studies in man.

Mescaline and related drugs

The symptoms of acute intoxication may be divided into two phases: the first is characterized by mild autonomic disturbances; the second includes the effects upon the CNS, which are generally depressive in nature. Mc-Millan (1973a) reports that mescaline depresses behavior controlled by reinforcement or punishment. In the second phase, dogs and cats are rendered docile and tame. Rats are described as catatonic, yet paradoxically show hyperactivity to noises. Much higher doses appear to dampen the responses to painful stimuli. In mice, compulsive scratching has been observed, and this is antagonized by chlorpromazine.

The changed response to stimuli may also underline the aberrant conditioned avoidance behavior observed in several species after mescaline administration. Rats were trained to make an avoidance response to an auditory signal to avoid electric shock. After 100 mg/kg of mescaline, they reacted to the auditory signal as if it were an electric shock, squealing and jumping. Dogs showed similar behavior to tones signaling shock to the paw.

Smythies et al. (1967) reported a biphasic change in conditioned avoidance response (CAR) latencies after mescaline. Initially, 25 mg/kg causes loss of CAR with increased response latencies, but this is followed by a decrease in reaction time below control values. Substitution of either the 4- or 5-methoxy group in mescaline with an OH group abolishes the biphasic effect on CAR and produces a drug with little psychotomimetic activity in either animals or man. By contrast, modification of the molecule by introduction of a methyl group in the alpha position of the side chain yields compounds structurally related to amphetamine with potent psychotomimetic effects in both animals and man.

DOM (2,5-dimethoxy-4-methylamphetamine) is a drug that produces intense excitement and elation. Small doses produce what may well be hallucinatory behavior in cats: staring gaze, sudden jumping in the cage, and attempts to catch imaginary objects. The EEG activity after these doses is very similar to that produced by such sympathomimetic amines as amphetamine. With higher doses, motor convulsions, which cannot be antagonized by chlorpromazine, occur.

Lysergic acid diethylamide, LSD

As in the case of mescaline, the symptoms of LSD intoxication can be divided into two categories, one relating to the autonomic nervous system and the other, mood change, to the CNS. The latter include hallucinations, intellectual disturbances, and changes of mood which may vary from euphoria to anxiety and depression, which may perhaps depend on the individual's personality.

The principal subjective symptoms are perceptual, and images of extraordinary complexity and plasticity are seen. Because of this the drug is termed hallucinogenic, even though the appearance of real hallucinations, i.e. formed images independent of external stimuli, are not common at usual doses. Auditory as well as visual effects are common, and intellectual processes are impaired. In subhuman primates, LSD appears to produce hallucinatory behavior. In baboons $10-40$ μg/kg produces hyperexcitability; there is mild ataxia and grasping of nonexistent objects in the air. At slightly higher doses, spatial orientation (climbing, swinging, and jumping) is impaired, but these doses do not inactivate the animals.

The sensory disturbances have prompted neurophysiological studies of the effects of the drug on the afferent sensory pathways. In the cat (Evarts, 1957), spontaneous activity in the lateral geniculate body was severely depressed by 30 μg/kg of LSD injected intra-arterially; this observation has been verified by other workers. Horn and McKay (1973) asked more specific questions about how LSD changes the sensory receptive fields of lateral geniculate nucleus neurons. At this level in the visual system, neurons show characteristic concentric circular receptive fields in which the center either gives an "on" or "off" response to a spotlight, and the surround the complementary responses. All doses of LSD depressed spontaneous neuronal activity. At doses of less than 100 μg, the responses of the center and surround of the receptive fields to photic stimulation were not strongly correlated, suggesting that the drug influences the sensory transformation properties of the lateral geniculate nucleus. The authors pointed out that since the properties of cortical visual neurons are jointly determined by the spontaneous activity and sensory transformation in more peripheral parts of the visual system, the effects of LSD on the lateral geniculate nucleus could at least partly account for the disturbed perceptual experience associated with LSD intake in animals and man (Hoffer and Osmond, 1967).

Observational studies with cats demonstrate that LSD, and drugs structurally or functionally related to LSD, causes highly characteristic unconditioned responses, not seen with other classes of psychoactive drugs (Jacobs et al., 1976). Certain behaviors such as staring, grooming, and head and body shakes have a relatively high frequency of occurrence in control animals and are increased by LSD. Other behaviors, particularly limb flicks, abortive grooming, and investigatory or play behavior occur with a very low frequency normally and are greatly enhanced by LSD. Limb flicks, a response used normally to remove a foreign substance from the paw, were increased from a mean of 0.2/hr to 45.8/hr by a dose of LSD of 50 μg/kg. These effects are not due to the peripheral action of LSD because the congener of LSD, D-2-bromo-LSD, which has only peripheral actions, has no such behavioral effects. Depletion of brain 5-HT results in an action similar to that of LSD, suggesting a functional interaction between this drug and serotonergic substrates of the CNS. This effect of LSD is long lasting and shows rapid tolerance, both features of the psychedelic response to LSD in humans.

Trulson and Jacobs (1979) provided further evidence for a relationship between 5-HT neuronal activity and LSD-induced abnormalities in behavior. Recording from the dorsal raphe in the behaving cat, they found reductions in the activity of 5-HT neurons during the behavioral responses to LSD (10–50 μg/kg) and to 5-methoxy-N,N-dimethyltryptamine. However, the behavioral response outlasted the electrophysiological response, and on repeated administration LSD continued to elicit the neurophysiological response when the behavioral response to the drug had shown tolerance. These observations support the notion of an interaction between LSD and 5-HT neurons, but suggest that other neuropharmacological effects are also involved in the overall response to LSD.

A number of studies have reported that LSD induces changes in conditioned discriminative behavior; visual tasks have been most extensively studied. Brown and Bass (1967) reported a psychophysical method for training monkeys to make scaling judgments along a size dimension. The letter E was prepared in a constant size and in 3, 5, 10, 15, 20, and 25% size decrements from that constant. Eight monkeys were trained to choose the smaller E from an array of two constants and one comparison stimuli. Failure to select the proper value within 30 sec or an incorrect choice resulted in a 5-sec shock, which could be escaped from by a correct response. LSD in doses as low as 0.1 mg/kg increased reaction time in this task.

Fuster (1959) also found that LSD increased reaction time and decreased accuracy in monkeys responding to tachistoscopically presented objects.

Doses of 2 to 8 μg/kg disrupted performance on a cone/pyramid discrimination test presented for 20-msec exposures. Fuster attributed this failure to the demanding level of attention required in the tachistoscopic task, but success depends as much on the accuracy of visual discrimination and quickness of response as on attentiveness. In more recent experiments with monkeys, in which ample time was allowed for attention and response, LSD in doses of 10 to 40 μg/kg disrupted a difficult size discrimination, although an easy one was unaffected. It has been suggested that, in difficult discriminations, even when there is plenty of time to respond, animals shift their attention from relevant to irrelevant dimensions and that LSD facilitates such attentional shifts.

It is not known if changes of these kinds reflect sensory or psychological effects of the drug or both. Bridger (1971) evaluated the existing literature with this distinction in mind. He pointed out that in animals LSD (and mescaline) can produce either excitatory or inhibitory effects depending on dose and type of behavior. The inhibitory (but not the excitatory) effects show tolerance as do the psychedelic effects in humans, and it is thus suggested that the excitatory effects in animals mimic most closely the psychotomimetic actions in man. Smythies and Sykes (1964) showed that LSD (as well as mescaline) produces inhibition of well established two-way shuttlebox conditioned avoidance behavior in rats. The inhibition is immediately followed by an excitatory phase, with short avoidance latencies. The inhibition shows rapid tolerance after repeated injections of mescaline. If a more stressful situation is used such as initial acquisition of shock avoidance, then LSD and mescaline produce only excitatory effects (Evarts, 1958; Domino et al., 1965; Bridger, 1971). Stress appears to transform the biphasic response to hallucinogens into a purely excitatory one, which does not show tolerance, and this may well model the psychotomimetic effects of the drugs in man.

Key (1961) is one of the few experimenters to study the effect of LSD on a range of sensory and discriminative tasks. A shock avoidance task was used in cats trained to cross a 9-in. barrier to avoid a 0.5 mA shock. Three conditions were studied:

1. Sensory generalization. After being trained to cross on presentation of a 600-Hz pure tone, the response to tones between 200 and 2000 Hz were tested in extinction.

2. Discrimination I. The cat was trained to cross on presentation of a 600-Hz tone. Then a 400-Hz tone was introduced, and the cat was trained not to cross at that signal.

3. Discrimination II. With two other tones, the cat was again trained to cross to one and not to cross to the other in order to avoid shock. But, in this task, trials on both tones were given from the start of training.

It was found that 15 μg/kg of LSD slowed extinction in the stimulus generalization test, i.e. more responses were made to the conditioned and the generalization stimuli, but the shape of the generalization curve remained the same. Thus, although the animal apparently still discriminated between the stimuli, the significance threshold of auditory signals changed. With discrimination method I, 15 μg/kg of LSD resulted in crossings to both tones, whereas the discrimination trained by Method II remained unaffected. It is suggested that the negative tone in Method I was never very significant to the animal because it was introduced after the conditioned response had been established. With the general increase in stimulus significance induced by LSD, responses to this negative stimulus were shown. By contrast, under Method II, the negative tone was already highly significant to the cat because responses to it had been extinguished. As in other studies, LSD did not affect discriminations based on two highly significant cues in well-trained animals.

There are a number of other experiments reporting varying results with LSD; it is reasonable to assume that variations in the animals and the training procedures account for the wide range of results obtained. In such discrimination experiments, several workers have noted the considerable invididual variation of the primate response to LSD. This has also been noted in experiments on cognitive tasks (Black et al., 1969). Several laboratories have investigated the effect of LSD on delay tasks of various kinds. Evarts (1957) reported that doses as large as 950 μg did not impair delayed response cued by the direct method, i.e. the monkey watches the experimenter hide a peanut reinforcement in one of two spatial locations and then, after a delay, is allowed to retrieve the peanut. If, however, indirect cueing is used, i.e., a discriminative stimulus, such as a form, is presented to indicate where the reinforcement is to be found, then LSD has a much more disruptive effect. In fact, the most severe disruption has been found when indirect delayed response is tested automatically, rather than by a human tester, in the Wisconsin General Test apparatus (WGTA). Black has suggested that a direct-cued DR involves a short-term associative process between reinforcement and position, whereas an indirect-cued DR involves long-term associative processes. LSD apparently affects the latter and not the former (Fig. 10–8). Similarly, delayed alternation tested in the automatic WGTA with a 2-sec delay was found to be affected by LSD (Jarvik and

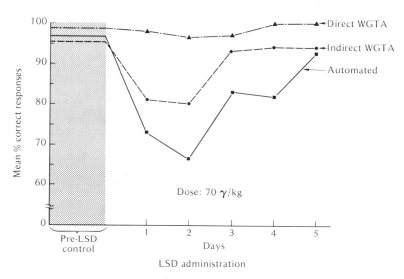

Fig. 10-8   Performance curves on three versions of the delayed response task in a group of four monkeys. At an intermediate dose of LSD, 70 μg/kg, note the clear differential effect, with impairment occurring in the performance of the indirect and automated tasks and the virtual absence of effect on direct task scores. (Reproduced from Black et al., 1969.)

Chorover, 1960). At some doses, both the accuracy and number of alternation responses were depressed, but at lower doses accuracy, but not response rate, was affected. By contrast, amphetamine and chlorpromazine were found to depress rate but not accuracy. It was suggested that delay tasks are very sensitive to LSD because the drug changes sensitivity to internal and external distracting stimuli. Several workers have noted the rapid development of tolerance to LSD, which is true also in man. It has also been repeatedly noted that the disruptive effects of LSD on discriminative and cognitive tasks persist several weeks after drug administration.

Bridger (1971) has suggested that hallucinogens produce these affects by enhancing the association between unconditioned (UCS) and conditioned (CS) stimuli thus making it difficult for the animal to distinguish between them. Under mescaline animals have been observed to respond to a conditioned stimulus as though it were the unconditioned aversive stimulus used in the paradigm.

Electrophysiological evidence has been cited in support of this idea. When condtioning has been established, differential patterns of activity occur in cortex in response to the CS and UCS but limbic areas are relatively inactive, although they are active in the initial stage of avoidance training. It is suggested that LSD and mescaline disrupt the normal balance of activity between cortical and subcortical sites and thus impede the perception of the UCS and CS. Stress exacerbates the response to hallucinogens, probably because the limbic areas are further excited.

Cannabis

In man, *Cannabis* produces a feeling of well being, improved ideation, and a facilitation of motor activity. After large doses, sense of time and space are eventually lost, and torpor ensues. Animals show a similar combination of depressant and excitatory effects. There is an increase in spontaneous activity, which is hindered by a motor deficit. The animals run around swaying and falling on their sides. These contradictory effects of *Cannabis* are emphasized by the observation that it potentiates both the depressant action of barbiturates and the excitatory action of amphetamine. In early behavioral studies with *Cannabis*, the tendency of the natural compound to decompose when exposed to air made it difficult to evaluate the dose required to produce psychological changes in animals. The synthesis of crystalline Δ^9-THC, the major active component of *Cannabis*, and Δ^8-THC, a minor active component, have been important for the development of animal studies.

The pure compounds Δ^9-THC and Δ^8-THC produce behavior similar to that seen after hallucinogenic drugs are administered in a range of species, and they also disrupt complex behavior involving memory or discrimination. In this respect, *Cannabis* resembles LSD, and, like LSD, it has pronounced effects on the theta wave EEG.

Scheckel et al. (1968) studied the two active cannabinoids in either squirrel or rhesus monkeys trained with operant methods on (a) continuous shock avoidance, (b) titration of shock threshold; and (c) delayed matching of color. On the continuous shock avoidance task, low doses of 4 or 8 mg/kg of Δ^9-THC depressed the avoidance response rate by more than 50%. The monkeys appeared depressed. With higher doses (16–64 mg/kg), the monkeys were highly stimulated, and avoidance responding was often at twice the control rates. The animals were excited and behaved as though they were having visual hallucinations. With 2, 4 and 8 mg/kg Δ^8-THC, stimulation was observed without the depression seen at lower doses. On the Weiss and Laties shock titration procedure, 4–8 mg/kg of either compound gave evidence of increased shock tolerance, but it is doubtful if this represents a genuine analgesic effect—the response to shock merely varies more. Delayed matching of color suffered most, being severely disrupted for 4 days by a single dose of 4 mg/kg of Δ^9-THC. In addition to their general depressant or stimulant properties associated with hallucinations, Δ^8- and Δ^9-THC appear to affect high-order cognitive performance most profoundly.

McMillan et al. (1970) reported that the key pecking behavior of pigeons performing on a multiple FI/FR schedule was severely depressed by 1.8 mg/kg of Δ^9-THC. The depressant effect is not specific to reinforced behavior, for McMillan (1973a) has shown that on both elements of a multiple FI/ FI punishment schedule Δ^9- and Δ^8-THC depress responding. Tolerance to the drug developed rapidly, however, and, after the 5th daily dose, response rates had returned to within the range of the control undrugged rate. The dose of drug was then gradually increased, and, by day 25, a dose of 36 mg/ kg rarely depressed responding; indeed, in some sessions, rates of responding were increased. When the drug was stopped, no withdrawal symptoms were observed.

The rapid development of tolerance and the eventual rate-increasing effect of the drug resemble the effects of morphine in pigeons, although unlike cannabis the narcotics produce strong withdrawal symptoms.

References

BOOKS AND MONOGRAPHS

Barchas, J.D., P.A. Berger, R.D. Ciaranello, and G.R. Elliott, eds. (1977). *Psychopharmacology: From Theory to Practice*. New York: Oxford University Press.

Clark, W.G. and J. del Guidice, eds. (1978). *Principles of Psychopharmacology*, 2nd ed. New York: Academic Press.

Cooper, J., F.E. Bloom, and R. Roth (1978). *The Biochemical Basis of Neuropharmacology*, 3rd ed. New York: Oxford University Press.

Iversen, L.L., S.D. Iversen, and S.H. Snyder, eds. (1975–78). *Handbook of Psychopharmacology*, vol. 1–14. New York: Plenum Press.

Lipton, M.A., A. Di Mascio, and K.F. Killam, eds. (1978). *Psychopharmacology: a Generation of Progress*. New York: Raven Press.

Thompson, T. and P.E. Dews, eds. (1977). *Advances in Behavioral Pharmacology*, vol. 1. New York: Academic Press.

ARTICLES

Aghajanian, G.E. (1975). In *Handbook of Psychopharmacology*, vol. 3 (L. Iversen, S. Iversen, and S. Snyder, eds.). New York: Plenum Press.

Aghajanian, G.K., W.E. Foote, and M.H. Sheard (1970). Action of psychotogenic drugs on single midbrain raphe neurones. *J. Pharmac. Exp. Ther.* 171:178–87.

Ahlskog, J.E. (1974). Food intake and amphetamine anorexia after selective forebrain norepinephrine loss. *Brain Res.* 82:211–240.

Akil, H., D.J. Mayer, and J.C. Liebeskind (1976). Antagonism of stimulation-produced analgesia by naloxone, a narcotic antagonist. *Science* 191:961–962.

Akiskal, H.S. and W.T. McKinney (1975). Overview of recent research in depression. *Arch. Gen. Psychiat.* 32:285–305.

Angrist, B.M. and S. Gershon (1970). The phenomenology of experimentally induced amphetamine psychosis—preliminary observations. *Biol. Psychiat.* 2:95–107.

Angrist, B.M., G. Sathananthan, and S. Gershon (1973). Behavioural effects of L-DOPA in schizophrenic patients. *Psychopharmacology* 31:1–12.

Appel, J.B. and L.A. Dykstra (1977). Drugs, discrimination and signal detection theory. In *Advances in Behavioral Pharmacology*, vol. 1 (T. Thompson and P.B. Dews, eds.). New York: Academic Press, pp. 139–166.

Azmitia, E.C. (1978). The serotonin-producing neurons of the midbrain median and dorsal raphe nuclei. In *Handbook of Psychopharmacology*, vol. 9, (L.L. Iversen, S.D. Iversen, and S.H. Snyder, eds.). New York: Plenum Press, pp. 233–314.

Azrin, N.H. (1956). Some effects of two intermittent schedules of immediate and non-immediate punishment. *J. Psychol.* 42:3–21.

Azrin, N.H. (1958). Some effects of noise on human behavior. *J. Exp. Anal. Behav.* 1:183–200.

Azrin, N.H. and D.F. Hake (1969). Positive conditioned suppression using positive reinforcers as the unconditioned stimuli. *J. Exp. Anal. Behav.* 12:167–173.

Azrin, N.H. and W.C. Holtz (1966). Punishment. In *Operant Behavior: Areas of Research and Application* (W.K. Honig, ed.). New York: Appleton pp. 300–447.

Azrin, N.H., W.C. Holtz, and D.F. Hake (1963). Fixed-ratio punishment. *J. Exp. Anal. Behav.* 6:141–48.

Azrin, N.H., R.R. Hutchinson, and D.F. Hake (1966). Extinction-induced aggression. *J. Exp. Anal. Behav.* 9:191–204.

Azrin, N.H., R.R. Hutchinson, and R. McLaughlin (1965). The opportunity for aggression as an operant reinforcer during aversive stimulation. *J. Exp. Anal. Behav.* 8:171–80.

Baltzer, V. and L. Weiskrantz (1970). Negative and positive behavioral contrast in the same animals. *Nature* 228:581–82.

Baltzer, V., Huber, H., and Weiskrantz, L., Effects of various drugs on behavioral contrast using a double-crossover procedure. *Behav. Neural Biol.* 27:330–341 (1979).

Barfield, R.J. and B.D. Bachs (1968). Sexual behavior: Stimulation by painful electric shock to the skin in male rats. *Science* 161:393–95.

Barondes, S.H. and H.D. Cohen (1968). Memory impairment after subcutaneous injection of aceloxycyloheximide. *Science* 160:556–557.

Barrett, J.E. (1977a). Effects of *d*-amphetamine on responding simultaneously maintained and punished by presentation of electric shock. *Psychopharmacology* 54:119–124.

Barrett, J.E. (1977b). Behavioral history as a determinant of the effects of *d*-amphetamine on punished behavior. *Science* 198:67–69.

Beecher, H.K. (1959). *Measurement of Subjective Responses*, New York: Oxford University Press.

Belluzi, J.D., N. Grant, V. Garsky, D. Sarantakis, E.D. Wise, and L. Stein (1976). Analgesia induced in vivo by central administration of enkephalin in rat. *Nature* 260:625–626.

Bender, L. (1947). Childhood schizophrenia. *Amer. J. Orthopsychiat.* 17:40–56.

Bennett, J.P. Jr. and S.H. Snyder (1975). Stereospecific binding of *d*-lysergic acid diethylamide (LSD) to brain membranes: relationship to serotonin receptors. *Brain Research* **94**:523–544.

Berger, B.D. and L. Stein (1969). An analysis of the learning deficits produced by scopolamine. *Psychopharmacologia (Berl.)* **14**:271–83.

Berlyne, D.E. (1955). The arousal and satiation of perceptual curiosity in the rat. *J. Comp. Physiol. Psychol.* **48**:238–46.

Berthelson, S. and W.A. Pettinger (1977). A functional basis for classification of α-adrenergic receptors. *Life Sciences* **21**:595–598.

Black, P., S.N. Cianci, P. Spyropoulos, and J.D. Maser (1969). Behavioral effects of LSD in subhuman primates. *Drugs and the Brain*. (P. Black, ed.). Baltimore: Johns Hopkins Press, pp. 291–99.

Blackman, D. (1974). *Operant Conditioning. An Experimental Analysis of Behaviour*. London: Methuen.

Bleuler, E. (1911). *Dementia Praecox or the Group of Schizophrenias*. New York: International Unviersity Press. (English trans. by J. Zinkin, 1950.)

Blough, D.S. (1957). Some effects of drugs on visual discrimination in the pigeon. *Ann. N.Y. Acad. Sci.* **66**:733–39.

Blough, D.S. (1966). *Operant Behavior: Areas of Research and Application* (W.K. Honig, ed.) New York: Appleton, pp. 345–379.

Booth, D.A., C.W.T. Pilcher, G.D. D'Mello, and I.P. Stolerman (1977). Comparative potencies of amphetamine, fenfluramine and related compounds in taste aversion. Experiments in rats. *Br. J. Pharmac.* **61**:669–677.

Bradley, P.D. (1968). Synaptic transmission in the central nervous system and its relevance for drug action. *Int. Rev. Neurobiol.* **11**:1–56.

Bradley, P.B. and J. Elkes (1957). The effects of some drugs on the electrical activity of the brain. *Brain* **80**:77–117.

Brady, J.V. (1958). Ulcers in "executive" monkeys. *Scient. Amer.* **199**:95–100.

Bridger, W.H. (1971). Psychotomimetic drugs, animal behavior, and human psychopathology.

Bridger, W.H. and I.J. Mandel (1971) Excitatory and inhibitory effects of mescaline on shuttle avoidance in the rat. *Biological Psychiatry* **3**:379–385.

Bridges, K.M.B. (1932). Emotional development in early infancy. *Child Develop.* **3**:324–41.

Broadhurst, P. (1961). Abnormal animal behavior. In *Handbook of Abnormal Psychology*. (H. J. Eysenck, ed.). New York: Basic Books, pp. 726–63.

Bronson, G.W. (1968). The development of fear in man and other animals. *Child Develop.* **39**:409–31.

Brown, H. and W.C. Bass (1967). Effect of drugs on visually controlled avoidance behavior in rhesus monkeys: A psychophysical analysis. *Psychopharmacologia (Berl.)* **11**:142–53.

Bunney, B. and G. Aghajanian (1974). In *Frontiers in Catecholamine Research*. (E. Usdin and S. Snyder, eds.). Oxford: Pergamon.

Bunney, W.E. and J.M. Davis (1965). Norepinephrine in depressive reactions. *Arch. Gen. Psychiat.* **13**:483–94.

Bunney, B.S., G.K. Aghajanian, and R.H. Roth (1973). *Nature* (New Biology) **245**:123–25.

Burridge, S.L. and J.E. Blundell (1979). Amphetamine anorexia: antagonism by typical but not atypical neuroleptics. *Neuropharmacology* 18:453–457.

Butcher, L.L. (1978). Recent advances in histochemical techniques for the study of central cholinergic mechanisms. In *Cholinergic Mechanisms and Psychopharmacology*, (D.J. Jenden, ed.) New York: Plenum Press, pp. 93–124.

Cairncross, K.D., A. Wren, C. Forster, B. Cox, and H. Schnieden (1979). The effect of psychoactive drugs on plasma cortico sterone levels and behavior in the ulbectomised rat. *Pharmacol. Biochem. Behav.*, 10:355–359.

Canon, J.G. (1979). A comparison of clozapine, and thioridazine upon DRL performance in the squirrel monkey. *Psychopharmacology*, 64:55–60.

Cappell, H. and A.E. Le Blanc (1971). Conditioned aversion to saccharin by a single administration of mescaline and *d*-amphetamine. *Psychopharmacologia (Berl.)* 22:352–356.

Carey, R.J. (1976). Effects of selective forebrain depletions of norepinephrine and serotonin on the activity and food intake effects of amphetamine and fenfluramine. *Pharmac. Biochem. Behav.* 5:519–523.

Carey, R.J. (1978). A comparison of the food intake suppression produced by giving amphetamine as an aversion treatment versus as an anorexic treatment. *Psychopharmacology* 56:45–48.

Carey, R.J. and E.B. Goodall (1976). Amphetamine-induced taste aversion: a comparison of *d*-versus *d*-amphetamine. *Pharmacol. Biochem. Behav.*, 2:325–330.

Carlsson, S.G. (1972). Effects of apomorphine on exploration. *Phys. & Behav.* 9:127–29.

Carlton, P.L. (1963). Cholinergic mechanism in the control of behavior by the brain. *Psychol. Rev.* 70:19–39.

Chance, M.R.A. and A.P. Silverman (1964). The structure of social behaviour and drug action. In *Animal Behaviour and Drug Action*. Ciba Foundation Symposium. London: J and A Churchill Ltd., pp. 65–79.

Chance, W.T., G.M. Krynack, and J.A. Rosecrans (1978). Effects of medial raphé and raphé magnus lesions on the analgesic activity of morphine and methadone. *Psychopharmacology* 56:133–137.

Cherek, D.R., T. Thompson, and G.T. Heistad (1973). Responding maintained by the opportunity to attack during an interval food reinforcement schedule. *J. Exp. Anal. Behav.* 19:113–24.

Clark, B.J. (1976). Pharmacology of β-adrenergic blocking drugs. In β-*Adrenoceptor Blocking Agents*, (P.R. Saxena and R.P. Forsyth, eds.) Amsterdam: North Holland, pp. 45–60.

Clark, F.C. and B.J. Steele (1966). Effects of *d*-amphetamine on performance under a multiple schedule in the rat. *Psychopharmacologia* (Berl.) 9:157–69.

Clavier, R.M. and A. Routtenberg (1976). Brainstem self-stimulation attenuated by lesions of medial forebrain bundle but not by lesions of locus coeruleus or the cardel ventral norepinephrine bundle. *Brain Res.* 101:251–271.

Clow, A., P. Jenner, A. Theodorov, and C.D. Marsden (1979). Striatal dopamine receptors become supersensitive while rats are given trifluoperazine for six months. *Nature* 278:59–61.

Colpaert, F.C. and J.A. Rosecrans, eds. (1978). *Stimulus Properties of Drugs: Ten Years of Progress*. Amsterdam: North Holland.

Colpaert, F.C., C.J.E. Niemegeers, and P.A.J. Janssen (1978). Discriminative stimulus properties of cocaine and d-amphetamine, and antagonism by haloperidol: a comparative study. *Neuropharmacology* **12**:937–942.

Conti, J.C., E. Strope, R.N. Adams, and C.A. Marsden (1978). Voltammetry in brain tissue: chronic recording of stimulated dopamine and 5-hydroxy-tryptamine release. *Life Sciences* **23**:2705–2716.

Cook, L., A. Davidson, D.J. Davis, and R.T. Kelleher (1960). Epinephrine, norepinephrine, and acetylcholine as conditioned stimuli for avoidance behavior. *Science* **131**:990–91.

Cook, L. and R.T. Kelleher (1962). Drug effects on the behavior of animals. *N.Y. Acad. Sci.* **96**:315–35.

Cook. L. and R.T. Kelleher (1963). Effects of drugs on behavior. *Ann. Rev. Pharm.* **3**:205–22.

Cooper, B.R., J.M. Cott, and G.R. Breese (1976). Effects of catecholamine-depleting drugs and amphetamine on self-stimulation of brain following various 6-hydroxydopamine treatments. *Psychopharmacologia (Berl.)* **37**:235–248.

Corfield-Sumner, P.K. and I.P. Stolerman (1978). Behavioral Tolerance. In *Contemporary Research in Behavioural Pharmacology.* (D.E. Blackman and D.J. Sangel, eds.). New York: Plenum Press, pp. 391–442.

Costall, B., D.H. Fortune, and R.J. Naylor (1978). The induction of catalepsy and hyperactivity by morphine administered directly into the nucleus accumbens of rats. *Eur. J. Pharmacol.* **49**:49–64.

Courvoisier, S., J. Fournel, R. Ducrot, M. Kolsky, and P. Koetschet (1953). Propriétés pharmacodynamiques du chlorhydrate de Chloro-3 (Dieméthylamino-3-propyl)-10 phénothiazines (4.560 R. P.) *Arch. Intern. Pharmacodynamie* **92**:305–61.

Creese, I. and S.D. Iversen (1975). The pharmacological and anatomical substrates of the amphetamine response in the rat. *Brain Research* **83**:419–436.

Creese, I., O.R. Burt, and S.H. Snyder (1978). Biochemical actions of neuroleptic drugs: focus on the dopamine receptor. In *Handbook of Psychopharmacology*, vol. 10 (L.L. Iversen, S.D. Iversen, and S.H. Snyder, eds.). New York: Plenum Press, pp. 37–89.

Crespi, L.P. (1944). Amount of reinforcement and level of performance. *Psychol. Rev.* **51**:341–57.

Dahlström, A. and K. Fuxe (1964). A method for the demonstration of monoamine containing nerve fibres in the central nervous system. *Acta. Physiol. Scand.* **60**:293–95.

Davenport, R.K. and E.W. Menzel (1963). Stereotyped behavior of the infant chimpanzee. *Arch. Gen. Psychiat.* **8**:99–104.

Davis, J.M. (1974). In *Frontiers in Catecholamine Research.* (E. Usdin and S.H. Snyder, eds.). Oxford: Pergamon.

Davis, J.M. and D.L. Garver (1978). Neuroleptics: clinical use in psychiatry. In *Handbook of Psychopharmacology*, vol. 10 (L.L. Iversen, S.D. Iversen, and S.H. Snyder, eds.) New York: Plenum Press, pp. 126–164.

Deutsch, J.A. (1971). The cholinergic synapse and the site of memory. *Science* **174**:788–94.

de Wied, D. (1974). Pituitary-adrenal system hormones and behavior. In *The Neurosciences, Third Study Program.* (F.O. Schmitt and F.G. Worden, eds.). Cambridge (Mass.): MIT Press, pp. 653–66.

de Wied, D. (1978). Behavioural effects of neuropeptides related to β-LPH. *Centrally Acting Peptides*, (J. Hughes, ed.) New York: Macmillan Press Ltd. pp. 241–251.

de Wied, D. and W.H. Gispen (1977). Behavioral effects of peptides. In *Peptides in Neurobiology* (Harold Gainer, ed.) New York: Plenum Press, pp. 397–448.

Dews, P.B. (1955a). Studies on behavior. I. Differential sensitivity to pentobarbital of pecking performance in pigeons depending on the schedule of reward. *J. Pharmac. Exp. Ther.* **113**:393–401.

Dews, P.B. (1955b). Studies on behavior. II. The effects of pentobarbital, methamphetamine and scopolamine on performance in pigeons involving discriminations. *J. Pharmac. Exp. Ther.* **115**:380–89.

Dews, P.B. (1958). Studies on behaviour. IV. Stimulant actions of methamphetamine. *J. Pharmac. Exp. Ther.* **122**:137–47.

Dews, P.B. (1964). A behavioural effect of amobarbital. *N-S Arch. Exp. Path. u. Pharmak.* **248**:296–307.

Dews, P.B. (1978). Origins and future of behavioural pharmacology. *Science* **22**:1115–1122.

Dews, P.B. and W.H. Morse (1961). Behavioural pharmacology. *Ann. Rev. Pharm.* **1**:145–74.

Dill, R.E. and E. Costa (1977). Behavioural dissociation of the enkephalinergic systems of nucleus accumbens and nucleus caudatus. *Neuropharmacology* **16**:323–326.

Dinsmoor, J.A. (1952). A discrimination based on punishment. *Quart. J. Exp. Psychol.* **4**:27–45.

Domino, E.F., A.J. Karoly, and E.L. Walker (1958). Differential effects of some CNS depressants on a quantitative shock avoidance response in the dog. *J. Pharmac. Exp. Ther.* **122**:20 A.

Domino, E.F., D.F. Caldwell, and R. Henke (1965). Effects of psychoactive agents on acquisition of conditioned pole jumping in rats. *Psychopharmacologia (Berl.)* **8**:285–89.

Drawbaugh, R. and H. Lal (1974). Reversal by narcotic antagonist of a narcotic action elicited by a conditioned stimulus. *Nature* **247**:65–67.

Dunn, A.J. (1976). The chemistry of learning and the formation of memory. In *Molecular and Functional Neurobiology* (W.H. Gispen, ed.). Amsterdam: Elsevier, pp. 348–387.

Dunn, A.J. (1980), The neurochemistry of learning and memory: an evaluation of recent data. *Ann. Rev. Psychol.* (in press).

Dunn, A.J., E.J. Green, and R.L. Isaacson (1979). Intracerebral adrenocorticotropic hormone mediates novelty—induces grooming in the rat. *Science* **203**:281–283.

Ellinwood, E.H. (1971). Effect of chronic methamphetamine intoxication in rhesus monkeys. *Biol. Psychiatr.* **3**:25–32.

Ellinwood, E.H., A Sudilovsky, and L. Nelson (1972) Behavioral analysis of chronic amphetamine intoxication. *Biol. Psychol.* **4**:215–30.

Ellison, G., M.S. Eison, and H.S. Huberman (1978). Stages of intoxication: delayed appearance of abnormal social behaviors in rat colonies. *Psychopharmacology* **56**:293–299.

Emley, G.S. and R.R. Hutchinson (1972). Basis of behavioral influence of chlorpromazine. *Life Sciences* **11**:43–47.

Emson, P. (1979). Peptides as neurotransmitter candidates in the mammalian CNS. *Progress in Neurobiology* 13:61–116.

Emson, P.C. and O. Lindvall (1979). Distribution of putative neurotransmitters in the neocortex. *Neuroscience* 4:1–30.

Estes, W.K. and B.F. Skinner (1941). Some quantitative properties of anxiety. *J. Exp. Psychol*. 29:390–400.

Evarts, E.V. (1957). A review of the neurophysiological effects of lysergic acid diethylamide (LSD) and other psychomimetic agents. *Ann. N.Y. Acad. Sci*. 66:479–95.

Evarts, E.V. (1958). Neurophysiological correlates of pharmacologically-induced behavioral disturbances. *Proc. Ann. Res. Nerv. Ment. Dis*. 36:347–80.

Falk, J.L. (1972). The nature and determinants of adjunctive behavior. In *Schedule effects: Drugs, Drinking and Aggression*. (R.M. Gilbert and J.D. Keehn, eds.). Toronto: University of Toronto Press.

Feldman, R.S. (1964). Further studies on assay and testing of fixation-preventing psychotropic drugs. *Psychopharmacologia (Berl.)* 6:130–42.

Feldman, R.S. and K.F. Green (1966). Effects of chlordiazepoxide on fixated behavior in squirrel monkeys. *J. Psychopharm*. 1:37–45.

Ferster, C.B. (1966). Animal behavior and mental illness. *Psychol. Rec*. 16:345–56.

File, S.E. (1979). Effects of $ACTH_{4-10}$ in the social interaction test of anxiety. *Brain Res*. 171:157–160.

File, S.E. and J.R.G. Hyde (1978). Can social interaction be used to measure anxiety? *Brit. J. Pharmacol*. 62:19–24.

File, S.E. and A.G. Wardill (1975). Validity of head-dipping as a measure of exploration in a modified hole board. *Psychopharmacologia* 44:53–59.

Findley, J.D. (1966). Programmed environments for the experimental analysis of human behavior. In *Operant behavior: Areas of Research and Application*. (W.K. Honig, ed.). New York: Appleton, pp. 827–43.

Fitzsimons, J.T. (1975). The renin-angiotensin system and drinking behaviour. *Prog. Brain Res*. 42:215–233.

Fitzsimons, J.T. (1976). The physiological basis of thirst. *Kidney Int*. 10:3–11.

Flood, J.F., E.L. Bennett, A.E. Orme, M.R. Rosenzweig, and M.E. Jarvik (1978). Memory: modification of anisomycin-induced amnesia by stimulants and depressants. *Science* 199:324–326.

Fonnum, F. and J. Storm-Mathisen (1978). Localization of GABA-ergic neurons in the CNS. In *Handbook of Psychopharmacology*, vol. 9 (L.L. Iversen, S.D. Iversen, and S.H. Snyder, eds.) New York: Plenum Press, pp. 357–401.

Francis, R.L. and S.J. Cooper (1979). Chlordiazepoxide-induced disruption of discrimination behavior: a signal detection analysis. *Psychopharmacology* 63:307–310.

Fuster, J.M. (1959). Lysergic acid and its effects on visual discrimination in monkeys. *J. Nerv. Ment. Dis*. 129:252–56.

Garattini, S., E. Borroni, T. Mennini, and R. Samanin. (1978). Differences and similarities between anorectic agents. In *Central Mechanisms of Anorectic drugs* (S. Garattini and R. Samanin, eds.). New York: Raven Press, pp. 127–143.

Garcia, J. and F.R. Ervin (1968). Gustatory-visceral and telereceptor-cutaneous conditioning: adaptation in internal and external milieus. *Behav. Biol*. 1:389–415.

Garcia, J. and R.A. Koelling (1966). Relation of cue to consequence in avoidance learning. *Psychon. Sci.* 4:123–24.

Geller, I. (1962). Use of approach avoidance behavior (conflict) for evaluating depressant drugs. In *Sixth Hannemann Symposium on Psychosomatic Medium*. (Nadine, ed.). Chap. 33.

Geller, I. and J. Seifter (1960). The effects of meprobromate, barbiturates, *d*-amphetamine and promazine on experimentally induced conflict in the rat. *Psychopharmacologia* 1:482–92.

Geller, I., E. Backman, and J. Seifter (1963). Effects of reserpine and morphine on behaviour suppressed by punishment. *Life Sciences* 4:226–31.

Gelelr, I., J.T. Kulak, and J. Seifter (1962). The effects of chlordiazepoxide and chlorpromazine on a punishment discrimination. *Psychopharmacologia (Berl.)* 25:112–16.

Gessa, G.L., E. Paglietti, and B. Pellegrino Quarantotti (1979). Induction of copulatory behavior in sexually inactive rats by naloxone. *Science* 204:203–205.

Glaser, D.C. (1910). The formation of habits at high speed. *J. Comp. Neur.* 20:165–84.

Goldberg, S.R. and C.R. Schuster (1967). Conditioned suppression by a stimulus associated with nalorphine in morphine-dependent monkeys. *J. Exp. Anal. Behav.* 10:235–42.

Goldstein, A. and P. Sheehan (1969). Tolerance to opioid narcotics. 1. Tolerance to the "running fit" caused by levorphanol in the mouse. *J. Pharmac. Exp. Ther.* 169:175–84.

Goldstein, A., L. Aranow, and S.M. Kalman (1974). In *Principles of Drug Action*, 2nd ed. New York: Harper & Row.

Gracely, R.H., R. Dubner, and P.A. McGrath (1979). Narcotic analgesia: fentanyl reduces the intensity but not the unpleasantness of painful tooth pulp sensations. *Science* 203:1261–1263.

Gray, J.A. (1977). Drug effects on fear and frustration: possible limbic site of action of minor tranquilizers. *Handbook of Psychopharmacology*, vol. 8. (L.L. Iversen, S.D. Iversen and S.H. Snyder, eds.) New York: Plenum Press, pp. 433–529.

Grevert, P. and A. Goldstein (1978). Endorphins: naloxone fails to alter experimental pain or mood in humans. *Science* 199:1093–1095.

Hanson, H.M., J.J. Witoslawski, E.H. Campbell, and A.G. Itkin (1966). Estimation of relative antiavoidance activity of depressant drugs in squirrel monkeys. *Arch. Intern. Pharmacodynamie* 161:7–16.

Harlow, H.F. and M.K. Harlow (1965). The affectional systems. In *Behaviour of Non-human Primates*, vol. 2 (A.M. Schrier, H.F. Harlow, and F. Stollnitz, eds.). New York: Academic Press.

Hearst, E. (1964). Drug effects on stimulus generalization gradients in monkeys. *Psychopharmacologia (Berl.)*. 6:57–70.

Hearst, E., M.B. Koresko, and R. Poppen (1964). Stimulus generalization and the response-reinforcement contingency. *J. Exp. Anal. Behav.* 7:369–80.

Heise, G.A. and E. Boff (1962). Continuous avoidance as a base-line for measuring behavioral effects of drugs. *Psychopharmacologia* 3:264–82.

Heise, G.A. (1975). Discrete trial analysis of drug action. *Fed. Proc.* 34:1898–1903.

Herman, B.H. and J. Panksepp (1978). Effects of morphine and naloxone on separation distress and approach attachment: evidence for opiate mediation of social affect. *Pharm. Biochem. Beh.* 9:213–220.

Hilgard, E.R. and G.H. Bower (1966). *Theories of Learning* 3rd ed. New York: Appleton.

Hill, R.T. (1970). Facilitation of conditioned reinforcement as a mechanism of psychomotor stimulation. In *Amphetamines and Related Compounds*. Proceedings of the Mario Negri Institute for Pharmacological Research, Milan, Italy. (E. Costa and S. Garattini, eds.). New York: Raven Press, pp. 781–95.

Hoebel, B.G. (1978). The psychopharmacology of feeding. In *Handbook of Psychopharmacology*, vol. 8 (L.L. Iversen, S.D. Iversen and S.H. Snyder, eds.). New York: Plenum Press, pp. 55–129.

Hoffer, A. and H. Osmond (1967). *The Hallucinogens*. New York/London: Academic Press.

Hökfelt, T. and A. Ljungdahl (1972). *Histochemie* 29:325–39.

Hökfelt, T., R. Elde, O. Johansson, A. Ljungdahl, M. Schultzberg, K. Fuxe, M. Goldstein, G. Nilsson, B. Pernow, L. Terenius, D. Ganten, S.L. Jeffcoate, J. Rehfeld, and S. Said (1978). Distribution of peptide-containing neurons. In *Psychopharmacology: A Generation of Progress* (M.A. Lipton, A. DiMascio and K.F. Killam, eds.). New York: Raven Press.

Holtz, W.C. and N.H. Azrin (1961). Discriminative properties of punishment. J. Exp. Anal. Behav. 4:225–32.

Horn, G. and J.M. McKay (1973). Effects of lysergic acid diethylamide on the spontaneous activity and visual receptive fields of cells in the lateral geniculate nucleus of the cat. *Exp. Brain Res.* 17:271–84.

Hosobuchi, Y., J.E. Adams, and R. Linchitz (1977). Pain reliefs by electrical stimulation of the central gray matter in humans and its reversal by naloxone. *Science* 197:183–186.

Hrdina, P.D., von Kulmiz, and R. Stretch (1979). Pharmacological modification of experimental depression in infant macaque. *Psychopharmacology* 64:89–93.

Huberman, H., M.S. Eison, K. Bryan, and G. Ellison (1977). A slow-release silicone pellet for chronic amphetamine administration. *Eur. J. Pharmacol.* 45:237–242.

Hughes, J., ed. (1978). *Centrally Acting Peptides*. London: Macmillan.

Hulme, M., A. Sahgal, and S.D. Iversen (1979). Effects of sodium amylobarbitone on memory processes in the pigeon. *Psychopharmacology* 62:71–78.

Hunt, H.F. and J.V. Brady (1955). Some effects of punishment and intercurrent "anxiety" on a simple operant. *J. Comp. Physiol. Psychol.* 48:305–10.

Hunter, B., S.F. Zornetzer, M.E. Jarvik, and J.L. McGaugh (1977). Modulation of learning and memory: effects of drugs influencing neurotransmitters. In *Handbook of Psychopharmacology*, vol. 8 (L.L. Iversen, S.D. Iversen and S.H. Snyder, eds.) New York: Plenum Press, pp. 531–577.

Hutchinson, R.R., N.H. Azrin, and G.M. Hunt (1968a). Attack produced by intermittent reinforcement of a concurrent operant response. *J. Exp. Anal. Behav.* 11:489–95.

Hutchinson, R.R., N.H. Azrin, and J.W. Renfrew (1968b). Effects of shock intensity and duration on the frequency of biting attack by squirrel monkeys. *J. Exp. Anal. Behav.* 11:83–88.

Hutt, C. and S.J. Hutt (1965). Effects of environmental complexity on stereotyped behaviour of children. *Ann. Behav.* 13:1–4.

Iversen, L.L. (1975). Dopamine receptors in the brain. *Science* 188:1084–1089.

Iversen, L.L. (1978a). Biochemical and pharmacological studies: the dopamine hypothesis. In *Schizophrenia: towards a New Synthesis* (J.K. Wing, ed.). London: Academic Press, pp. 89–116.

Iversen, L.L. and A.V.P. Mackay (1979). Pharmacodynamics of antidepressants and antimanic drugs. In *Psychopharmacology of Affective Disorders*, (E.S. Paykel and A. Coppen, eds.). Oxford: Oxford University Press, pp. 60–90.

Iversen, S.D. Brain dopamine and behavior (1977). In *Handbook of Psychopharmacology*, vol. 8 (L.L. Iversen, S.D. Iversen and S.H. Snyder, eds.). New York: Plenum Press, pp. 333–384.

Iversen, S.D. (1978b). Animal models of relevance to biological psychiatry. *Handbook of Biological Psychiatry*, vol. 1 (H. M. van Praag, M. H. Lader, O. J. Rafaelsen, and E. J. Sachar, eds,). New York: Marcel Dekker, pp. 303–335.

Iversen, S.D. and L.L. Iversen (1975). Central neurotransmitters and the regulation of behaviour. In *Handbook of Psychobiology* (M.S. Gazzaniga and C. Blakemore, eds.). New York: Academic Press, pp. 153–200.

Iversen, S.D., R. Hughes, and R. Howells (1980). The behavioural consequences of long-term treatment with neuroleptic drugs. In *The Long-Term Effects of Neuroleptics* New York: Raven Press (in press).

Jacobs, B.L., M.E. Trulson, and W.C. Stern (1976). An animal model for studying the actions of L.S.D. and related hallucinogens. *Science* 194:741–743.

Janowsky, D.S., M.K. El-Yousel, J.M. Davis, and H.J. Sekerke (1973). Provocation of schizophrenic symptoms by intravenous methlyphenidate. *Arch. Gen. Psychiat.* 28:185–91.

Janssen, P.A.J., C.J.E. Niemegeers, and K.H.L. Schellekens (1965). Is it possible to predict the clinical effects of neuroleptic drugs (major tranquillizers) from animal data? Part I. "Neuroleptic activity spectra" for rats *Arzneim-Forsch.* 15:104–17.

Jarvik, M.E. (1964). The influence of drugs upon memory. In *Animal Behavior and Drug Action.* (H. Steinberg, ed.). London: Churchill, pp. 44–60.

Jarvik, M.E. and S. Chorover (1960). Impairment by lysergic acid diethylamide of accuracy in performance of a delayed alternation test in monkeys. *Psychopharmacologia (Berl.)* 1:221–30.

Jeffrey, D.R. and J.E. Barrett (1979). Effects of chlordiazepoxide on comparable rates of punished and unpunished responding. *Psychopharmacology* 64:9–11.

Jessell, T.M. and L.L. Iversen (1977). Opiate analgesics inhibit substance P release from rat trigeminal nucleus. *Nature* 268:433–434.

Joyce, E.M. and S.D. Iversen (1979). The effect of morphine applied locally to mesencephalic dopamine cell bodies on spontaneous motor activity in the rat. *Neurosii. Letters* 14:207–212.

Kandel, E.R. (1978). A cell-biological approach to learning. Grass Lecture Monograph I, Society for Neuroscience, Bethesda, Maryland.

Kanof, P.D. and P. Greengard (1978). Brain histamine receptors as targets for antidepressant drugs. *Nature* 272:329–331.

Katzman, R., R.D. Terry, and K.L. Bick, eds. (1978). *Alzheimer's Disease: Senile Dementia and Related Disorders* New York: Raven Press.

Kebabian, J.W. and D.B. Calne (1979). Multiple receptors for dopamine *Nature* **277**:93–96.

Kelleher, R.T. and W.H. Morse (1964). Escape behavior and punished behavior. *Fed. Proc.* **23**:808–17.

Kelleher, R.T. and W.H. Morse (1968). Determinants of the specificity of behavioral effects of drugs. *Ergebn. der Physiol.* **60**:1–56.

Kelley, A.E., L. Stinus, and S.D. Iversen (1980). Interactions between d-ala-met-enkephalin, A10 dopaminergic neurones, and spontaneous behaviour in the rat. *Behav. Brain Res.* 1 (in press).

Kelly, J.S. and L.P. Renaud (1973). *Brit. J. Pharmac.* **48**:369–86.

Kelly, P.H., P.W. Seviour, and S.D. Iversen (1975). Amphetamine,and apomorphine responses in the rat following 6-OHDA lesions of the nucleus accumbens septi and corpus striatum. *Brain Research* **94**:507–522.

Kesner, R.P., D.J. Priano, and J.R. De Witt (1976). Time-dependent disruption of morphine tolerance by electroconvulsive shock and frontal cortical stimulation. *Science* **194**: 1079–1081.

Kety, S.S. (1972). The possible role of the adrenergic systems of the cortex in learning. *Res. Publ. Ass. Nerv. Ment. Dis.* **50**:376–389.

Key, B.J. (1961). The effect of drugs on discrimination and sensory generalization of auditory stimuli in cats. *Psychopharmacologia (Berl.)* **2**:352–63.

Kimble, G.A. (1961). *Hilgard and Marquis Conditioning and Learning*. New York: Appleton, Chaps. 3, 4.

Klein, D.F. and J.M. Davis (1969). *Diagnosis and Drug Treatment of Psychiatric Disorder*. Baltimore: Williams & Wilkins, pp. 52–138.

Klugh, H.E. and R.A. Patton (1959). Escape behavior of monkeys from low intensity tone. *Psychol. Rep.* **5**:573–78.

Koob, G.F., P.J. Fray, and S.D. Iversen (1976). Tail-pinch stimulation: sufficient motivation for learning. *Science* **194**:637–639.

Koob, G.F., P.J. Fray, and S.D. Iversen (1978). Self-stimulation at the lateral hypothalamus and locus coeruleus after specific unilateral lesions of the dopamine system. *Brain Res.* **146**:123–140.

Kovács, G.L., B. Bohus, and D.H.G. Versteeg (1979). Facilitation of memory consolidation by vasopressin: mediation by terminals of the dorsal noradrenergic bundle. *Brain Res.* **172**:73–85.

Krieger, D.T. and A.S. Liotta (1979). Pituitary hormones in brain: where, how and why? *Science* **205**:366–372.

Kuhar, M.J. and L.C. Murrin (1978). Sodium dependent high affinity choline uptake. *J. Neurochem.* **30**:15–22.

Kumar, R. (1969). Exploration and latent learning: differential effects of dexamphetamine on components of exploratory behavior in rats. *Psychopharmacologia Berl.)* **16**:54–72.

Lal, H., ed. (1977). Discriminative stimulus properties of drugs. New York: Plenum Press.

Larochelle, L., P. Bedard, L. J. Poirier, and T.L. Sourkes (1971). Correlative neuroanatomical and neuropharmacological study of tremor and catatonia in the monkey. *Neuropharm.* **10**:273–88.

Lehmann, J. and H.C. Fibiger (1979). Acetylcholinesterase and the cholinergic neurone. *Life Sciences* **25**:1939–1947.

Levine, S. (1962). The effects of infantile experience on adult behavior. In *Experimental Foundations of Clinical Psychology.* (A.J. Bachrach, ed.). New York: Basic Books.

Liddell, H.S. (1954). Conditioning and Emotions. *Scient. Amer.*

Liebeskind, J.C. and L.A. Paul (1977). Psychological and physiological mechanisms of pain. *Ann. Rev. Psychol.* **28**:41–60.

Liebowitz, S.F. and C. Rossakis (1979). Pharmacological characterization of perifornical hypothalamic dopamine receptors mediating feeding inhibition in the rat. *Brain Res.* **172**:115–130.

Lindvall, O. and A. Björklund (1974). The organization of the ascending catecholamine neuron systems in the rat brain as revealed by the glyoxylic acid fluorescence method. *Acta Physiol. Scand. Suppl.* **412**:1–48.

Lindvall, O. and A. Björklund (1978). Organization of catecholamine neurons in the rat central nervous system. In *Handbook of Psychopharmacology*, vol. 9. (L.L. Iversen, S.D. Iversen and S.H. Snyder, eds.) New York: Plenum Press, pp. 139–232.

Livett, B. (1973). *Brit. Med. Bull.* **39**(2).

Lyon, M. and A. Randrup (1972). The dose-response effect of amphetamine upon avoidance behavior in the rat seen as a function of increasing stereotypy. *Psychopharmacologia (Berl.)* **23**:334–47.

Lyon, M. and T.W. Robbins (1977). The action of central nervous system stimulant drugs. A general theory concerning amphetamine effects. *Current Developments in Psychopharmacology*, vol. 2 (W. Essman and L. Valzelli, eds.). New York: Spectrum pp. 89–163.

McCaman, R.E., D.G. McKenna, and J.K. Ono (1977). A pressure system for intracellular and extracellular ejection of picoliter volumes. *Brain Research* **136**:141–147.

McCleary, R.A. (1966). Response-modulating functions of the limbic system: initiation and suppression. *Progress in Physiological Psychology*, vol. 1. New York: Academic Press, pp. 209–272.

McKearney, J.W. (1968a). Maintenance of responding under a fixed interval schedule of electric shock presentation. *Science* **160**:1249–51.

McKearney, J.W. (1968b). The relative effects of *d*-amphetamine, imipramine and harmaline on tetrabenazine suppression of schedule-controlled behavior in the rat. *J. Pharmac. Exp. Ther.* **159**:429–40

McKearney, J.W. (1970). Rate-dependent effects of drugs: modification by discriminative stimuli of the effects of amobarbital on schedule-controlled behavior. *J. Exp. Anal. Behav.* **14**:167–175.

McKearney, J.W. and J.E. Barrett (1975). Punished behavior: increases in responding after d-amphetamine. *Psychopharmacology* **41**:23–26.

McKearney, J.W. and J.E. Barrett (1978). Schedule-controlled behavior and the effects of drugs. In *Contemporary Research in Behavioural Pharmacology.* (D.E. Blackman and D.J. Salger, eds.). New York: Plenum, pp. 1–68.

McMillan, D.E. (1973a). Drugs and punished responding. I. Rate-dependent effects under multiple schedules. *J. Exp. Anal. Behav.* 19:133–45.

McMillan, D.E. (1973b). Drugs and punished responding. III. Punishment intensity as a determinant of drug effect. *Psychopharmacologia (Berl.)* 30:61–74.

McMillan, D.E. and W.H. Morse (1967). Some effects of morphine and morphine antagonists on schedule-controlled behavior. *J. Pharmac. Exp. Ther.* 157:175–84.

McMillan, D.E., L.S. Harris, J.M. Frankenhein, and J.S. Kennedy (1970). 1-δ⁹-Trans-tetrahydrocannabinol in pigeons: tolerance to the behavioral effects. *Science* 169:501–503.

Mackintosh, N.J. (1974). *The Psychology of Animal learning*. London: Academic Press.

Mackintosh, N.J. (1978). Conditioning, *Psychology Survey*, No. 1 (B.M. Foss, ed.) 43–57.

Maffi, C. (1959). The secondary conditioned response of rats and the effects of some psychopharmacological agents. *J. Pharm. Pharmac.* 11:129–30.

Maier, N.R.F. (1949). *Frustration: The Study of Behavior without a Goal*. New York: McGraw Hill.

Makanjuola, R.O.A., G. Hill, R.C. Dow, G. Campbell, and G.W. Ashcroft (1977). The effects of psychotropic drugs on exploratory and stereotyped behaviour of rats studied on a hole-board. *Psychopharmacology* 55:67–74.

Malmo, R.B. (1959). Activation: a neuropsychological dimension. *Psychol. Rev.* 66:367–86.

Marchbanks, R. (1975). In *Handbook of Psychopharmacology*, vol. I (L. Iversen, S. Iversen, and S. Snyder, eds.) New York: Plenum.

Margules, D.L. and L. Stein (1968). Increase of "anti-anxiety" activity and tolerance of behavioural suppression during chronic administration of oxazepam. *Psychopharmacologia* 13:74–80.

Martin, J.T. (1978). Imprinting behaviour: pituitary-adrenocortical modulation of the approach response. *Science* 200:565–566.

Mason, S.I. and S.D. Iversen (1979). Theories of the dorsal bundle extinction effect. *Brain Res. Reviews* 180:107–137.

Masserman, J.H. (1943). *Behavior and Neurosis*. Chicago: University of Chicago Press.

Masserman, J.H. and C. Pechtel (1956). An experimental investigation of factors influencing drug action. *Psychiat. Res. Rep.* 95–113.

Mayer, D.J., T.L. Wolfle, H. Akil, B. Carder, and J.C. Liebeskind (1971). Analgesia from electrical stimulation in the brainstem of the rat. *Science* 174:1351–1354.

Melzack, R. and P.D. Wall (1965). Pain mechanisms: a new theory. *Science* 150:971–979.

Meyerson, B.J. and M. Eliasson (1978). Pharmacological and hormonal control of reproductive behavior. *Handbook of Psychopharmacology*, vol. 8 (L.L. Iversen, S.D. Iversen, and S.H. Snyder, eds.). New York: Plenum Press, pp. 159–232.

Miczek, K.A. (1973). Effects of scopolamine, amphetamine and chlordiazepoxide on punishment. *Psychopharmacologia (Berl.)* 28:373–89.

Miller, N.E. and A. Carmona (1967). Modification of a visceral response, salivation in thirsty dogs, by instrumental training with water reward. *J. Comp. Physiol.*

Psychol. **63**:1–6.

Miller, N.E. and L. DiCara (1967). Instrumental learning of heart rate changes in curarized rats: shaping, and specificity to discriminate stimulus. *J. Comp. Physiol. Psych.* **63**:12–19.

Milner, P. (1970). *Physiological Psychology.* New York: Holt, Rinehart and Winston.

Milner, P. (1971). *Physiological Psychology,* Intn'l ed. New York: Holt, Rinehart & Winston.

Möhler, H. and T. Okada (1977). Benzodiazepine receptors: demonstration in the central nervous system. *Science* **198**:849–851.

Mondadori, C. and P.G. Waser (1979). Facilitation of memory processing by posttrial morphine: possible involvement of reinforcement mechanisms? *Psychopharmacology* **63**:297–300.

Moore, K.E. (1963). Toxicity and catecholamine releasing actions of dextro and levo amphetamine in isolated and aggregated mice. *J. Pharmacol. Exp. Ther.* **142**:6–00.

Moore, K.E. (1978). Amphetamines: biochemical and behavioral actions in animals. In *Handbook of Psychopharmacology,* vol. 11 (L.L. Iversen, S.D. Iversen, and S.H. Snyder, eds.), New York: Plenum Press, pp. 41–98.

Moore, R.Y. and F.E. Bloom (1978). Central catecholamine neuron systems: anatomy and physiology of the dopamine systems. *Ann. Rev. Neurosci.* **1**:129–169.

Moore, R.Y. and F.E. Bloom (1979). Central catecholamine neuron systems: anatomy and physiology of the norepinephrine and epinephrine systems. *Ann. Rev. Neurosci.* **2**:113–168.

Morse, W.H. (1964). Effects of amobarbital and chlorpromazine on punished behavior in the pigeon. *Psychopharmacologia (Berl.)* **6**:286–94.

Morse, W.H., J.W. McKearney, and R.T. Kelleher (1977). Control of behavior by noxious stimuli. In *Handbook of Psychopharmacology,* vol. 7, (L.L. Iversen, S.D. Iversen and S.H. Snyder, eds.). New York: Plenum Press, pp. 151–181.

Moss, R.L. (1978). Effects of hypothalamic peptides on sex behavior in animal and man. In *Psychopharmacology: a Generation of Progress* (M.A. Lipton, A. DiMascio and K.F. Killam, eds.). New York: Raven Press, pp. 431–440.

Mowrer, O.H. (1939). A stimulus-response analysis of anxiety and its role as a reinforcing agent. *Psychol. Rev.* **46**:553–65.

Myer, J.S. (1966). Punishment of instinctive behavior: suppression of mouse-killing by rats. *Psychon. Sci.* **4**:385–86.

Myer, J.S. (1968). Associative and temporal determinants of facilitation and inhibition of attack by pain. *J. Comp. Physiol. Psychol.* **66**:17–21.

Myer, J.S. and D. Ricci (1968). Delay of punishment for the goldfish. *J. Comp. Physiol. Psychol.* **66**:417–21.

Myers, R.D. (1975). Blood-brain barrier: techniques for the intracerebral administration of drugs. In *Handbook of Psychopharmacology,* (L.O. Iversen, S.D. Iversen and S.H. Snyder, eds) vol. 2, New York: Plenum Press, pp. 1–28.

Nakajima, S. (1975). Amnesic effect of cycloheximide in the mouse mediated by adrenocortical hormones. *J. Comp. Physiol. Psychol.* **83**:378–385.

Nicoll, R.A. (1978). Sedative-hypnotics: animal pharmacology. In *Handbook of Psychopharmacology,* vol. 12 (L.L. Iversen, S.D. Iversen and S.H. Snyder, eds.), New York: Plenum Press, pp. 187–234.

Nieouillon, A., A. Cheramy, V. Leviel, and J. Glowinski (1979). Effects of the unilateral nigral application of dopaminergic drugs on the in vivo release of dopamine in the two cardate nuclei of the cat. *Eur. J. Pharmacol.* **53**:289–296.

O'Brien, C.P. (1976). Experimental analysis of conditioning factors in human narcotic addiction. *Pharm. Rev.* **27**:533–543.

O'Kelly, L.I. and L.C. Steckle (1939). A note on long-enduring emotional responses in the rat. *J. Psychol.* **8**:125–31.

Ögren, S.O. and K. Fuxe (1977). On the role of brain noradrenaline and the pituitary-adrenal axis in avoidance learning. I: studies with corticosterone. *Neurosci. Lett.* **5**:191–196.

Oldendorf, W.H. (1971). Brain uptake of radiolabelled amino acids, amines and hexoses after arterial injection. *Am. J. Physiol.* **221**:1629–1639.

Oldendorf, W.H. (1975). Permeability of the blood brain barrier. In *The Nervous System*, vol. 1 (D.B. Tower, ed.). New York: Raven Press, pp. 279–289.

Oliverio, A. (1968). Effects of scopolamine on avoidance conditioning and habituation of mice. *Psychopharmacologia (Berl.)* **12**:214–26.

Overton, D.A. (1966). State-dependent learning produced by depressant and atropine-like drugs. *Psychopharmacologia (Berl.)* **10**:6–31.

Panksepp, J., B. Herman, R. Conner, P. Bishop and J.P. Scott (1978). The biology of social attachments: opiates alleviate separation distress. *Biol. Psychiatry* **13**:607–618.

Pappas, G.D. and S.T.G. Waxman (1972). In *Structure and Function of Synapses* (G.D. Pappas and D.P. Purpura, eds.). New York: Raven Press. p. 11.

Peroutka, S.J. and S.H. Snyder (1979). Multiple serotonin receptors: differential binding of ^{3}H-5-hydroxytryptamine, ^{3}H-lysergic acid diethylamide and ^{3}H-spiroperidol. *Mol. Pharmac.* **16**:687–699.

Perry, E.K., B.E. Tomlinson, G. Blessed, K. Bergmann, P.H. Gibson, and R.H. Perry (1978). Correlation of cholinergic abnormalities with senile plaques and mental test scores in senile dementia. *Brit. Med. J.* **2**:1457–1459.

Peters, A. (1970). In *Contemporary Research Methods in Neuroanatomy.* (W.J.H. Nauta and S.O.E. Ebbesson, eds.). New York: Springer-Verlag, p. 65.

Phillips, A.G. and H.C. Fibiger (1978). The role of dopamine in maintaining intracranial self-stimulation in the central tegmentum, nucleus accumbens, and medial prefrontal cortex. *Canad. J. Psychol.* **32**:58–66.

Pilcher, C.W.T. and I.P. Stolerman (1976). Recent approaches to assessing opiate dependence in rats. In *Opiates and Endogenous Opioid Peptides.* (eds.) Elsevier/ North Holland Biomedical Press, Amsterdam, pp. 327–334.

Pollard, G.T. and J.L. Howard (1979). The Geller-Seifter conflict paradigm with incremental shock. *Psychopharmacology* **62**:117–121.

Porsolt, R.D., G. Anton, N. Blavet, and M. Jalfre (1978). Behavioural despair in rats: a new model sensitive to antidepressant treatments. *Eur. J. Pharmac.* **47**:379–391.

Poschel, B.P.H. and F.W. Ninteman (1963). Norepinephrine: a possible excitatory neurohormone of the reward system. *Life Sciences* **3**:782–88.

Randrup, A. and I. Munkvad (1970). Biochemical, anatomical and psychological investigations of stereotyped behavior induced by amphetamines. In *Amphetamines and Related Compounds*. (E. Costa and S. Garratini, eds.). New York: Raven Press, pp. 695–713.

Ray, D.S. (1972). *Drugs, Society and Human Behavior*. St. Louis: Mosby.

Rech, R.H. (1965). Amphetamine effects on poor performance of rats in a shuttlebox. *Psychopharmacologie (Berl.)* 9:110–17.

Rech, R.H. and K.E. Moore (1971). *An Introduction to Psychopharmacology*. New York: Raven Press, p. 99.

Reicher, M.A. and E.W. Holman (1977). Location preference and flavor aversion reinforced by amphetamine in rats. *Anim. Learn. Behav.* 5:343–346.

Revusky, S.H. (1968). Aversion to sucrose produced by contingent x-irradiation: temporal and dosage parameters. *J. Comp. Physiol. Psychol.* 65:17–22.

Reynolds, G.S. (1968). *A Primer of Operant Conditioning*. Glenview (Ill.): Scott Foresman.

Rigter, H. (1978). Attenuation of amnesia in rats by systemically administered enkephalins. *Science* 200:83–85.

Robbins, T.W. (1977). A critique of the methods available for the measurement of spontaneous motor activity. In *Handbook of Psychopharmacology*, vol. 7 (L.L. Iversen, S.D. Iversen, and S.H. Snyder, eds.). New York: Plenum Press, pp. 37–82.

Robbins, T.W. (1978). The acquisition of responding with conditioned reinforcement: effects of pipradol, methylphenidate, *d*-amphetamine, and nomifensine. *Psychopharmacology* 58:79–87.

Robbins, T. and S.D. Iversen (1973). A dissociation of the effects of *d*-amphetamine on locomotor activity and exploration in rats. *Psychopharmacologia (Berl.)* 28:155–64.

Roberts, D.C.S., M.E. Corcoran, and H.C. Fibiger (1977). On the role of ascending catecholaminergic systems in intravenous self-administration of cocaine. *Pharmac. Biochem. Behav.* 6:615–620.

Roberts, E., T.N. Chase, and D.B. Tower eds. (1976). *GABA in Nervous System Function*, New York: Raven Press.

Roche, K.E. and A.I. Leshner (1979). ACTH and vasopressin treatments immediately after a defeat increase future submissiveness in male mice *Science* 204:1343–1344.

Rodgers, R.J. (1977). Attenuation of morphine analgesia in rats by intra-amygdaloid injection of dopamine. *Brain Res.* 130:156–162.

Rolls, E.T., B.J. Rolls, P.H. Kelly, S.G. Shaw, K.J. Wood, and R. Dale (1976). The relative attenuation of self-stimulation, eating and drinking produced by dopamine-receptor blockade. *Psychopharmacologia (Berl.)*, 38:219–230.

Rossier, J., E.D. French, G. Rivier, N. Ling, R. Guillemin, and F.E. Bloom (1977). Foot-shock induced stress increases β-endorphin levels in blood but not brain. *Nature* 270:618–620.

Routtenberg, G.A. and R. Santos-Anderson (1977). The role of prefrontal cortex in intracranial self-stimulation. A case history of anatomical localization of motivational substrates. In *Handbook of Psychopharmacology*, vol. 8 (L.L. Iversen, S.D.

Iversen, and S.H. Snyder, eds.). New York: Plenum Press, pp. 1–24.

Rushton, R and H. Steinberg (1964). Modification of behavioural effects of drugs by past experience. In *Animal Behaviour and Drug Action*. (H. Steinberg, ed.). London: Churchill, pp. 207–18.

Rutledge, C.O. and R.T. Kelleher (1965). Interactions between the effects of methamphetamine and pentobarbital on operant behavior in the pigeon. *Psychopharmacologia (Berl.)* 7:400–408.

Rylander, G. (1969). Clinical and medico-criminological aspects of addictions to central stimulating drugs. In *Abuse of central stimulants* (Sjoquist and M. Tottie, eds.). New York: Raven Press, pp. 251–273.

Sachar, E.J. and M. Baron (1979). The biology of affective disorders. *Ann. Rev. Neurosci.* 2:205–218.

Schachter, S. and J.E. Singer (1962). Cognitive, social and physiological determinants of emotional state. *Psychol. Rev.* 69:379–99.

Scheckel, C.L. (1965). Self-adjustment of the interval in delayed matching: Limit of delay for the rhesus monkey. *J. Comp. Physiol. Psychol.* 59:415–18.

Scheckel, C.L., Boff, E., Dahlen, P. and Smart, T. (1968). Behavioral effects in monkeys of racemates of two biologically active marijuana constituents. *Science* 160:1467–69.

Schildkraut, J. (1978). Current status of the catecholamine hypothesis of affective disorders. In *Psychopharmacology: a Generation of Progress* (M.A. Lipton, A. Di Mascio and K.F. Killam, eds.). New York: Raven Press, pp. 1223–1234.

Schiørring, E. (1971). Amphetamine-induced selective stimulation of certain items with concurrent inhibition of others in an open-field test with rats. *Behaviour* 39:1–17.

Schiørring, E. and A. Hecht (1979). Behavioural effects of low, acute doses of morphine in nontolerant groups of rats in an open-field test. *Psychopharmacology* 64:67–71.

Schopler, E. (1965). Early infantile autism and receptor processes. *Arch. Gen. Psychiat.* 13:327–35.

Schou, M. (1963). Normothymotics, "mood-normalizers." Are lithium and imipramine drugs specific for affective disorders. *Brit. J. Psychiat.* 109:803–809.

Schuster, C.R. and J.H. Woods (1968). The conditioned reinforcing effects of stimuli associated with morphine reinforcement. *Int. J. Addictions* 3:223–30.

Seeman, P., T. Lee, M. Chau-Wong, and K. Wong (1976). Antipsychotic drug doses and neuroleptic/dopamine receptors. *Nature* 261:717–718.

Segal, M. (1976). Interactions of ACTH and norepinephrine on the activity of rat hippocampal cells. *Neuropharmacology* 15:329–333.

Segal, M. and F.E. Bloom (1976). The action of norepinephine in the rat hippocampus. IV. The effects of locus coeruleus stimulation on evoked hippocampal unit activity. *Brain Res.* 107:513–525.

Seligman, M.E.P. (1975). *Helplessness*. San Francisco: W.H. Freeman.

Setler, P.E. (1978). The neuroanatomy and neuropharmacology of drinking. In *Handbook of Psychopharmacology*, vol. 8 (L.L. Iversen, S.D. Iversen and S.H. Snyder, eds.). New York: Plenum Press, pp. 131–158.

Shapiro, M.M. (1961). Salivary conditioning in dogs during fixed-interval reinforcement contingent upon lever pressing. *J. Exp. Anal. Behav.* 4:361–64.

Shute, C.C.D. and P.R. Lewis (1967). The ascending cholinergic reticular systems: Neocortical, olfactory and subcortical projections. *Brain* 90:487–520.

Sidman, M. (1956). Drug-behavior interaction. *Ann N.Y. Acad. Sci.* 65:282–302.

Sidman, M. (1960). Normal sources of pathological behavior. *Science* 132:61–68.

Siegel, R.K. (1978). Cocaine hallucinations. *Am J. Psychiat.* 135:309–314.

Siegel, S. (1976). Morphine analgesic tolerance: its situation specificity supports a Pavlovian conditioning model. *Science* 193:323–325.

Skrede, K.K. and R.H. Westgaard (1971). The transverse hippocompal slice: a well-defined cortical structure maintained *in vitro*. *Brain Res.* 35:584–588.

Smotherman, W.P. and S. Levine (1978). ACTH and $ACTH_{4-10}$ modification of neophobia and taste aversion responses in the rat. *J. Comp. Physiol. Psychol.* 92:22–33.

Smythies, J.R., R.J. Bradley, V.S. Johnston, and F. Leonard (1967). The behavioural effects of some derivatives of mescaline and *N,N*-dimethyltryptamine in the rat. *Life Sciences* 6:1887–93.

Smythies J.R. and E.A. Sykes (1964). The effect of mescaline upon the conditioned avoidance response in the rat. *Psychopharmacologia* 6:163–172.

Snyder, S.H. (1972). Catecholamines in the brain as mediators of amphetamine psychosis. *Arch. Gen. Psychiat.* 27:169–179.

Snyder, S.H. (1974). Catecholamines as mediators of drug effects in schizophrenia. In *Neurosciences: Third Study Program*. (F.O. Schmitt and F. Worden, eds.). Cambridge (Mass.): MIT Press, pp. 721–32.

Snyder, S.H. and J.P. Bennett, Jr. (1976). Neurotransmitter receptors in the brain: biochemical identification. *Ann. Rev. Physiol.* 38 153–175.

Snyder, S.H. and S. Childers (1979). Opiate receptors and endorphins. *Ann. Rev. Neurosci.* 2.

Snyder, S.H., E. Richelson, H. Weingaffner, and L.A. Faillace (1970). Psychotropic methoxyamphetamines: structure and activity in man. In *Amphetamines and Related Compounds*. (E. Costa and S. Garrattini, eds.). New York: Raven Press, pp. 905–28.

Solomon, R.L. (1964). Punishment. *Amer. Psychol.* 19:239–53.

Stein, L. (1968). Chemistry of reward and punishment. In *Psychopharmacology: A Review of Program, 1957–1967*. (D.H. Efron, ed.). Washington, D.C.: U.S. Government Printing Office.

Stein, L. and O.S. Ray (1960). Brain stimulation reward "thresholds" self-determined in rat. *Psychopharmacologia* 1:251–256.

Stein, L. and C.D. Wise (1969). Release of norepinephrine from hypothalamus and amygdala by rewarding medial forebrain bundle stimulation and amphetamine. *J. Comp. Physiol. Psychol.* 67:189–98.

Stein, L., C.D. Wise, and J.D. Belluzzi (1977). Neuropharmacology of reward of punishment. In *Handbook of Psychopharmacology*, vol. 8 (L.L. Iversen, S.D. Iversen, and S.H. Snyder, eds.). New York: Plenum Press, pp. 25–54.

Stein, L., C.D. Wise, and B.D. Berger (1973). Anti-anxiety action of benzodiazepines: decrease in activity of serotonin neurons in the punishment system. In *The Benzodiazepines*. New York: Raven Press, pp. 299–326.

Stille, G., H. Lavenev and E. Eichenberger, (1971). The pharmacology of 8-chloro-11(4-methyl-1-piperazinyl)-5H-dibenzo[b,e][1,4] diazepine (clozapine) *Farmaco. Ed. Sci.* **26**:603–625.

Storm-Mathisen, J. (1979). Localization of putative transmitters in the hippocampal formation. In *Functions of the Septo-hippocampal System*, CIBA Foundation Symposium 58 (New Series). Amsterdam: Elsevier/Excerpta Medica.

Storm-Mathisen, J. and L.L. Iversen (1979). Glutamic acid and excitatory nerve endings: selective uptake of ^{3}H-glutamic acid revealed by light and electron microscopic autoradiography. *Neuroscience* **4**:1237–1253.

Stretch, R. and G.J. Gerber (1973). Drug-induced reinstatement of amphetamine self-administration behaviour in monkeys. *Canad. J. Psychol.* **27**:168–79.

Summerfield, A. (1964). Drugs and human behaviour. *Brit. Med. Bull.* **20**:70–74.

Tabakoff, B., J. Yanai, and R.F. Ritzmann (1978). Brain noradrenergic systems as a prerequisite for developing tolerance to barbiturates. *Science* **200**:449–451.

Taylor, K.M. and S.H. Snyder (1971). Differential effects of D- and L-amphetamine on behavior and on catecholamine disposition in dopamine and noradrenaline containing neurons of rat brain. *Brain Res.* **28**:295–309.

Terrace, H.S. (1963). Errorless discrimination learning in the pigeon: effects of chlorpromazine and imipramine. *Science* **140**:318–19.

Trulson, M.E. and B.L. Jacobs (1979). Dissociations between the effects of LSD on behaviour and raphé unit activity in freely moving cats. *Science* **205**:515–518.

Tye, N.C. and S.D. Iversen (1975). Some behavioural signs of morphine withdrawal blocked by conditional stimuli. *Nature* **255**:416–418.

Tye, N.C., B.J. Everitt, and S.D. Iversen (1977a). 5-hydroxytryptamine and punishment. *Nature* **268**:741–743.

Tye, N.C., A. Sahgal, and S.D. Iversen (1977b). Benzodiazepines and discrimination behaviour: dissociation of response and sensory factors. *Psychopharmacology* **52**:191–194.

Ullman, A.D. (1951). The experimental production and analysis of a "compulsive eating symptom" in rats. *J. Comp. Physiol. Psychol.* **44**:575–81.

Ulrich, R.E., R.R. Hutchinson, and N.H. Azrin (1965). Pain-elicited aggression. *Psychol. Rev.* **15**:111–26.

Ungerstedt, U. (1971). On the anatomy, pharmacology and function of the nigrostriatal dopamine system. *Acta. Physiol. Scand. Suppl.* 367.

Ungerstedt, U., L.L. Butcher, S.G. Butcher, N-E Anden, and K. Fuxe (1969). Direct chemical stimulation of dopaminergic mechanisms in the neostriatum of the rat. *Brain Res.* **14**:461–71.

Vaillant, G.E. (1964). A comparison of cholorpromazine and imipramine on behaviour of the pigeon. *J. Pharmac. Exp. Ther.* **146**: 377–84.

Van Praag, H.M. (1978). Amine hypotheses of affective disorders. In *Handbook of Psychopharmacology*, vol. 13 (L.L. Iversen, S.D. Iversen, and S.H. Snyder, eds.). New York: Plenum Press, pp. 187–297.

van Ree, J.M., B. Bohus, D.H.G. Versteeg, and D. de Wied (1978). Neurohypophyseal principles and memory processes. *Biochem. Pharmac.* **27**:1793–1800.

Verhave, T., J.E. Owen, and E.B. Robbins (1959). The effect of morphine sulphate on avoidance and escape behavior. *J. Pharmac. Exp. Ther.* **125**:248–257.

Wade, M. (1947). The effect of sedatives upon delayed response in monkeys following removal of the prefontal lobes. *J. Neurophysiol.* **10**:57–61.

Warburton, D.M. (1972). The cholinergic control of internal inhibition. In *Inhibition and Learning* (R. Boakes and M.S. Halliday, eds.). London: Academic Press, pp. 431–60.

Watson, S.J., H. Akil, P.A. Berger, and J.D. Barchas (1979). Some observations on the opiate peptides and schizophrenia. *Arch. Gen. Psychiatry* **36**:35–41.

Weiskrantz, L. (1968). Emotion. *Analysis of Behavioral Change* (L. Weiskrantz, ed.). New York: Harper and Row, pp. 50–90.

Weiskrantz, L., C.G. Gross, and V. Baltzer (1965). The beneficial effects of meprobramate on delayed response in the frontal monkey. *Quart. J. Exp. Psychol.* **17**:118–24.

Weiss, B. and A. Heller (1969). Methodological problems in evaluating the role of cholinergic mechanisms in behavior. *Fed. Proc.* **28**:135–46.

Weiss, B. and V.G. Laties (1958). Fractional escape and avoidance on a titration schedule. *Science* **128**:1575–76.

Weiss, B. and V.G. Laties (1961). Behavioral thermoregulation. *Science* **133**:1338–44.

Weiss, B. and V.G. Laties (1964a). Drug effects on the temporal patterning of behavior. *Fed. Proc.* **23**:801–807.

Weiss, B. and V.G. Laties (1964b). Analgesic effects on monkeys of morphine nalorphine and a benzomorphan narcotic antagonist. *J. Pharmac. Exp. Ther.* **143**:169–73.

Weiss, J.M., E.E. Krieckhaus, and R. Conte (1968). Effects of fear conditioning on subsequent avoidance behaviour and movement. *J. Comp. Physiol. Psychol.* **65**:413–21.

Wikler, A. (1965). Conditioning factors in opiate addiction and relapse. In *Narcotics*. (D.M. Wilner & G.G. Kassebaum, eds.). New York: McGraw-Hill, pp. 85–100.

Wikler, A. and F.T. Pescor (1963). Classical conditioning of a morphine abstinence phenomenon, reinforcement of *opioid*-drinking behaviour and relapse in morphine-addicted rats. *Psychopharmacologia (Berl.)* **10**:325–84.

Wing, J.K., ed. (1978). *Schizophrenia: Towards a New Synthesis*, London: Academic Press.

Wise, R.A., R.A. Yokel, and H. de Wit (1976). Both positive reinforcement and conditioned aversion from amphetamine and from apomorphine in rats. *Science* **191**:1273–1275.

Wise, R.A., J. Spindler, H. De Wit, and G.J. Grber (1978). Neuroleptic-induced anhedonia in rats: pimozide blocks reward quality of food. *Science* **201**:262–264.

Woods, J.H. and R.E. Tessel (1974). Fenfluramine: amphetamine congener that fails to maintain drug-taking behavior in the rhesus monkey. *Science* **185**:1067–1069.

Wuttke, W. and R.T. Kelleher (1970). Effects of some benzodiazepines on punished and unpunished behavior in the pigeon. (1970) *J. Pharmac. Exp. Ther.* **172**:397–405.

Yaksh, T.L. and T.A. Rudy (1976). Analgesia mediated by a direct spinal action of narcotics. *Science* **192**:1357–1358.

Yaksh, T.L. and T.A. Rudy (1978). Narcotic analgesia: CNS sites and mechanisms of action as revealed by intracerebral injection techniques. *Pain* **4**:299–359.

Yaksh, T.L., J.C. Yeung, and T.A. Rudy (1977). Medial thalamic lesions in the rat: effects on the nociceptive threshold and morphine antinociception. *Neuropharmacology* **16**:107–114.

Yamamura, H.I., S.J. Enna, and M.J. Kuhar (1978). *Neurotransmitter Receptor*

Binding New York: Raven Press.

York, J.L. and E.W. Maynert (1978). Alterations in morphine analgesia produced by chronic deficits of brain catecholamines or serotonin: role of analgesimetric procedure. *Psychopharmacology* **56**:119–125.

Zarevics, P. and P.E. Setler (1979). Simultaneous rate-independent and rate-dependent assessment of intracranial self-stimulation: evidence for the direct involvement of dopamine in brain reinforcement mechanisms. *Brain Res*. **169**:499–512.

Zbinden, G. and Randall, L.O. (1967). Pharmacology of Benzodiazepines: laboratory and clinical correlations. *Adv. Pharm*. **5**:213–91.

Zimmerberg, B., A.J. Strumof and S.D. Glick (1978). Cerebral asymmetry and left-right discrimination. *Brain Res*. **140**:194–195.

Zornetzer, S.F. (1978). Neurotransmitter modulation and memory: a new neuropharmacological phrenology. In *Psychopharmacology: a generation of progress*, (M.A. Lipton, A. DiMascio, and K.F. Killam, eds.). New York: Raven Press, pp. 637–649.

Index